Decision Making Through Problem Based Learning in Hematology

Arun Gupta

Decision Making Through Problem Based Learning in Hematology

A Step-by-Step Approach in patients with Anemia

Springer

Arun Gupta
Department of Hematology
Mubarak Al Kabeer Hospital
Hawally, Kuwait

ISBN 978-981-99-8935-5 ISBN 978-981-99-8933-1 (eBook)
https://doi.org/10.1007/978-981-99-8933-1

This Springer imprint is published by the registered company Springer Nature Singapore Pte Ltd.
The registered company address is: 152 Beach Road, #21-01/04 Gateway East, Singapore 189721, Singapore

Paper in this product is recyclable.

Foreword 1

It is a great pleasure to write a brief foreword for this excellent hematology book written by Dr. Arun Gupta. Hematology was being practiced by both physicians and pathologists differently in different parts of the world until its recognition as a separate medical specialty. Long back, Dr. Arun Gupta started his professional career in hematology as a hematopathologist. Thus, his knowledge and expertise in laboratory hematology are immensely sound. Presently, practicing as a consultant and teacher in clinical hematology, his expertise in the correlation of patients' clinical presentation with precisely chosen laboratory investigations is of unique advantage. Now is the era of bedside teaching, interactive group discussions, and literature search for accurate information and its translation into diagnostic and management practices in patient care. His book is most appropriately titled "Decision Making Through Problem Based Learning (PBL) in Hematology—a Step-by-Step Approach." This book is what it really states. His description of 25 cases with step-by-step resolution of the patient's problems in a unique sequential manner is exemplary.

About the book itself: Apart from the wonderful layout of the patients' clinical presentation followed by step-by-step description of relevant laboratory investigations leading to firm diagnostic information, I consider two more features that attract appreciation and special mention. These include (a) the wonderful photographs, particularly of the microscopic pictures along with intelligent graphic illustrations, and (b) inclusion of some cases of not-so-common types of anemia such as cold agglutinin disease, paroxysmal cold hemoglobinuria, and anemia related to copper deficiency.

To happily mention, last but not least is that I feel immensely happy and privileged that Dr. Arun Gupta has been one of my favorite students and then after, a highly dedicated and committed colleague. Fortunate is the teacher whose student excels him like a father whose son beats him in reaching higher professional standing.

Professor and Consultant in Hematology, Kuwait (Retired) — Ramesh Arya

Foreword 2

Hematology, the study of blood and blood-related disorders, demands not only a deep understanding of the science but also the ability to apply that knowledge in real-world scenarios.

This book introduces a dynamic approach. It transcends traditional didactics, emphasizing hands-on problem-solving. It offers a comprehensive and innovative guide to navigating the complex world of hematology, with a specific focus on anemia patients. Problem-based learning (PBL) empowers learners to actively engage with and solve actual clinical challenges.

This invaluable resource reflects the transformative power of problem-based learning. Whether you are a seasoned healthcare professional seeking to enhance your skills or a student embarking on a journey in hematology, it equips you with the tools necessary to make sound decisions, ultimately leading to improved patient outcomes.

Welcome to a new approach to hematology education and practice.

Professor Kuwait University, Safat, Kuwait

Rajaa Marouf

Foreword 3

Dr. Arun Gupta has written a unique textbook of anemias that will have a useful role for medical students and even for postgraduate students in the early phase of their training. The case-based approach to anemias is an innovative and effective way of teaching medical students the fundamentals of the pathophysiology and pathology of anemias. The approach and framing of the questions are logical and follow a stepwise rational approach. Dr. Gupta's description and delivery are unique and provide a valuable resource for students on anemias. Case scenarios on anemias are well written and adopt a problem-oriented approach and provide the framework on which students can build.

K. Krishnan

Emeritus Professor of Medicine,
East TN State University,
Johnson City, TN, USA

Foreword 4

I am delighted to introduce this book, "Decision Making Through Problem Based Learning in Hematology: A Step-by-Step Approach in Patients with Anemia," by Dr. Arun Gupta. This book is a valuable resource for those who want to learn more about the diagnosis and management of anemia, a common and often complex hematological condition. The book covers various aspects of anemia, from its pathophysiology and symptoms to its evidence-based management. The book adopts a problem-based learning approach, which encourages the reader to apply their knowledge and skills to real-life scenarios and cases. The book also provides key points and summaries for each chapter, as well as a unique question–answer format that facilitates comprehension and retention. The book is suitable for students, teachers, clinicians, and researchers who are interested in hematology and anemia. It is also a useful reference for exam preparation and clinical practice. I congratulate Dr. Gupta for his excellent work and contribution to the field of hematology. I hope that you will enjoy reading this book and find it informative and helpful.

Faisal A. Alsayegh

Consultant Hematologist Associate Professor,
College of Medicine, Kuwait University,
Hawally, Kuwait

Foreword 5

ले जनरल नरेन्द्र कोतवाल, एस एम, वी एस एम
निदेशक एवं कमांडेंट
Lt Gen Narendra Kotwal, SM, VSM
Director & Commandant
Tele : 020 - 26363301 (O)
020 - 26360515 (R)
Mob. : 9910996639
Email : narendrakotwal@gmail.com

सशस्त्र सेना चिकित्सा महाविद्यालय
पुणे - ४११०४०
भारत
Armed Forces Medical College
Pune - 411 040
India

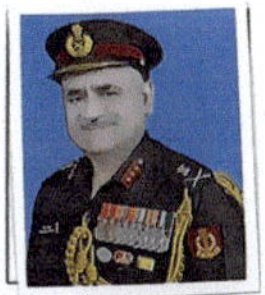

FOREWORD

1. Hematology is a link between numerous subspecialities of medicine. Since ages, this has been an inseparable and indispensable branch of medical science. Almost everyone suffers from anemia once in their lifetime, be it a young or old.

2. The new system of medical training makes it mandatory for trainees to learn interpretation of laboratory data as soon as they enter second year of their training. At that time a book which provides information in simplified way is of much help to students. The postgraduates who specialize in hematology need in depth understanding of diseases and since anemia is the most common of all hematological diseases, this book will be of immense help to both postgraduates as well as physicians interested in managing patients of anemia.

3. I am very happy that Dr Arun Gupta who is my colleague and friend from our days together as undergraduate students has come up with such wonderful piece of work. Dr Arun Gupta pursued his postgraduate qualification from PGIMER Chandigarh, India and has acquired distinction of being certified as Diplomate National Board from National Board Pathology, India. He has acquired proficiency in hematology while working as member of faculty in Medical College Srinagar, India and as a Consultant Haematologist in middle east.

4. With his experience of over 25 years of working as a Consultant and teacher in hematology, he has acquired immense experience in both laboratory and clinical hematology and his experience, which is reflected in this book, will be of utmost benefit to readers. This book titled 'Problem based learning in Hematology-a step-by-step approach in patients with Anemia' covers wide range of topics on anemia from common types to rare ones, written in easy to recall question-answer format with excellent images and supportive graphic illustrations. I am sure this book will become a single compiled source of information for all readers as it has been written with incredible depth and breadth of knowledge, as well as with clarity and eloquence of expression.

5. I congratulate Dr Arun Gupta for bringing up such brilliant and original contribution to the field of Hematology and wish him good luck for all future endeavors.

(Narendra Kotwal)
Lt Gen
Director & Commandant
Lt Gen Narendra Kotwal

Place: Pune

Date: 30 Sep 2023

AFMC,
Pune, India

Foreword 6

It is indeed a privilege to write a foreword for a book being authored by a colleague who has been a close associate right from the undergraduate days to the postgraduate journey together.

Dr. Arun Gupta, an alumni of Postgraduate Institute of Medical Education and Research (PGIMER), Chandigarh, India, has been an acclaimed clinical hematologist and hematopathologist for the past more than 20 years working in different capacities in Kuwait.

A very avid postgraduate and undergraduate teacher, he has been a keen researcher as well and has to his credit many international publications of high impact.

This book mainly lays stress on different types of anemias, their pathophysiology, and laboratory workup. The focus laid down in the problem-based learning (PBL) in each type of anemia is noteworthy. It is going to be of immense help not only for pathology residents but for clinical residents as well.

Dr. Arun Gupta has put in lots of hard work in making things look so simplified, especially the elaborate account of 25 cases of anemia with a stepwise approach for their evaluation and diagnosis.

The quality of photomicrographs has been excellent and so is their graphic description.

I wish Dr. Arun Gupta a huge success for his editorial venture.

Professor Pathology Medical College,
Jammu, India

Subhash Bhardwaj

Preface

This is an era of evolving teaching methods for medical students. The scenario is drifting away from traditional classroom teaching. Now, medical students are exposed to patients in clinics and wards as early as in the second year of their training, and a problem-based learning (PBL) has been advocated to impart more analytical power to students. PBL fosters critical thinking, clinical reasoning, and teamwork skills. PBL also helps to integrate basic science and clinical knowledge in a meaningful way. Unfortunately, students at that stage of training do not have the acumen to do concise literature search, have few or no comprehensive sources of information, and need guidance to access the wealth of knowledge available for programmed hematology training. This is time consuming and frustrating for many.

This book is written with an aim to bridge the gap in acquiring information, which can be transformed into clinical practice in a simple straightforward manner. It is based on problem-based learning in patients with anemia and will provide all relevant information at one platform. In this book, you will find 25 case scenarios that cover various aspects of anemia, followed by step-by-step investigations and their interpretation, trigger questions, key concepts, and references. Each case emphasizes a systematic approach for the analysis of laboratory information to exclude possible differential diagnoses and how to correlate results of tests done with final diagnosis.

The evaluation of each case is discussed in a question–answer format, as is expected in exams. Presentation is in the form of tables, diagrams, microscopic images including morphology, flow cytometry results, and molecular defects. An important aspect of the book is the explanation of each answer based on evidence from literature.

A brief description of the disease on its pathophysiology, clinical symptoms, and signs and most recent information is included in each chapter in a question–answer format followed by helpful points for quick reference for practicing clinicians and students in wards, clinics, and emergencies.

This book will be most useful for undergraduate medical students during hematopathology training and introductory phase in clinical medicine and hematology, postgraduate residents in hematology and medicine, and undergraduate and postgraduate allied health students who want to enhance their knowledge and skills in diagnosing anemia using PBL. This will also be quite resourceful for practicing hematologists and teachers in medical and paramedical institutions and will benefit immensely in translating diagnostic proficiency into management practice in patient care.

I have written this book with my experience of more than 25 years of teaching undergraduate and postgraduate medical students in hematology and practice in clinical and laboratory hematology. I hope that this book will help you improve your analytical skills and enhance confidence in diagnosing anemia in your patients. I welcome your feedback and suggestions for improvement. Please contact me at drarun1962@yahoo.com with your comments.

Hawally, Kuwait Arun Gupta

Acknowledgments

I would like to express my deepest gratitude to the following people who have supported me throughout the journey of writing this book:

First and foremost, I want to thank my wife, Dr. Geeta, who has always encouraged me to pursue my passion for writing. I could not have done this without her love and support.

I have to give credit to my children, Sheena and Anshul, who helped me a lot in shaping the book structure and initial formatting. They were quite excited about the book and challenged me to think deeper.

I am indebted to Dr. Ramesh Arya, Dr. Rajaa Marouf, and late Professor KC Das, whose immense experience as a teacher and colleague taught me in depth hematology, which inspired me to translate my knowledge into writing this book.

I wish to thank all doctors working with me, Dr. Eman Kamal, Dr. Rasha Joudah, Dr. Mona Mahmoud, and Dr. Sarah Sayed, who provided assistance in procuring the best set of slides for photography at every step.

I am grateful to all friends, colleagues, and well-wishers who spared their precious time to write a note of Foreword for this book.

Last but not least, I am thankful to the editors and publishers who have worked hard in a very professional way to give perfect look to this book and provided invaluable feedback and suggestions that made a considerable improvement in this piece of work.

Hawally, Kuwait Arun Gupta

Contents

Chapter 1
Iron Deficiency Anemia

A 38-year-old lady reports to the hematology clinic with complaints of tiredness, dizziness, easy fatigability, and mild dyspnea on exertion of 1-month duration. She also gave history of menorrhagia during the preceding 3 months. Recently, she had been diagnosed to have type-2 diabetes mellitus and mild hypertension, for which she is receiving antidiabetic and antihypertensive medications. Physical examination showed pallor. There is no jaundice or palpable organomegaly. Table 1.1 shows result of CBC done at presentation:

Table 1.1 CBC

CBC parameter	Patient's result	Reference range
WBC	5.9	3.7–10 × 10^9/L
RBC	3.39	4.5–5.4 × 10^{12}/L
HB	85	130–170 g/L
Hct	0.27	0.36–0.46 L/L
MCV	73	83–101 fL
MCH	22	27–32 pg
MCHC	302	315–345 g/L
RDW	19	11.6–14.6%
PLT	500	130–430 × 10^9/L
MPV	8	7–11 fL
Poly #	3.5	1.7–6 × 10^9/L
Lymp#	1.9	1–3 × 10^9/L
Mono#	0.3	0.2–1.0 × 10^9/L
EO#	0.2	0.02–0.5 × 10^9/L
BASO#	0	0.02–0.1 × 10^9/L
RETIC%	0.6	0.5–1.5%

A. Gupta, *Decision Making Through Problem Based Learning in Hematology*, https://doi.org/10.1007/978-981-99-8933-1_1

1.1 Questions

Q1. Interpret the CBC result given above and suggest investigations for further evaluation in such case.

Answer: The CBC result shows low values for red cell count, hemoglobin, hematocrit, MCV, MCH, MCHC, and reticulocyte count. Values for red cell distribution width (RDW) and platelet count are high. These findings suggest microcytic hypochromic anemia with reticulocytopenia.

Most common causes of microcytic hypochromic anemia include [1]:

1. Iron deficiency anemia (IDA)
2. Thalassemia
3. Sideroblastic anemia
4. Anemia of chronic disorders (ACD)
5. Lead poisoning

The next best line of investigations should include examination of peripheral blood film, estimation of serum levels of iron, ferritin, transferrin and transferrin saturation, and CRP. Baseline investigations for functions of liver, kidney, thyroid, pancreas, and bone are also required to exclude chronic pathology.

Q2. Given are images from peripheral blood film (Figs. 1.1, 1.2, 1.3, 1.4), serum levels of iron, ferritin, transferrin and transferrin saturation, and CRP (Table 1.2). Baseline investigations for functions of liver, kidney, thyroid, pancreas, and bone are also presented (Table 1.3). Interpret these results and suggest provisional diagnosis?

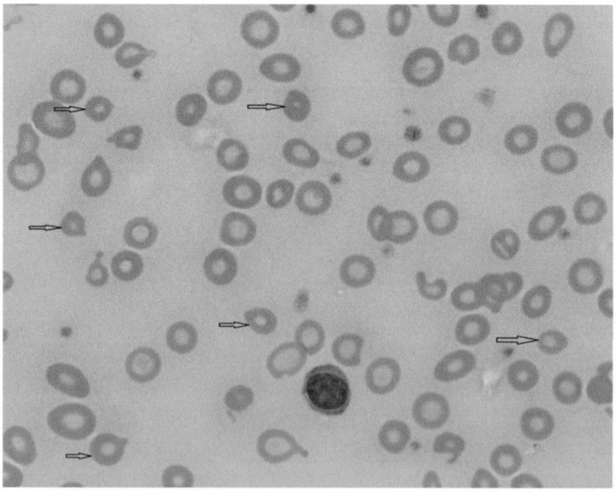

Fig. 1.1 PBF. Microcytes. Leishman stain ×100

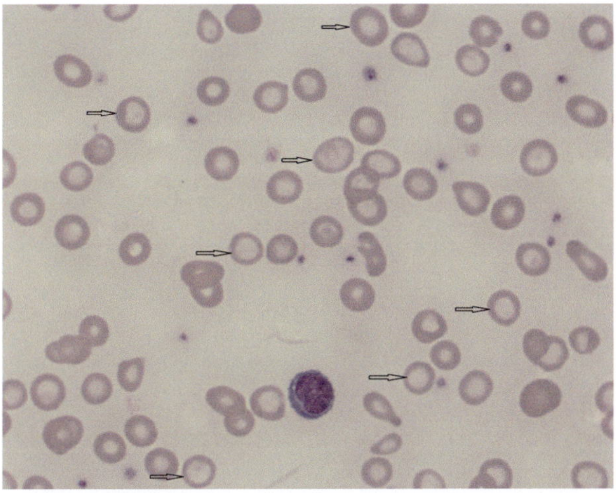

Fig. 1.2 PBF. Hypochromic cells. Leishman stain ×100

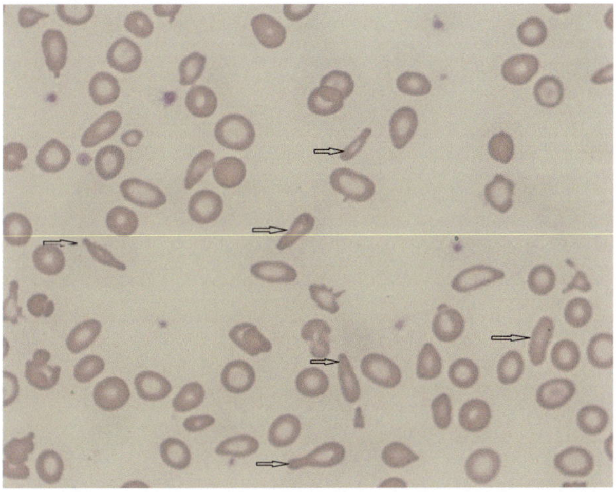

Fig. 1.3 PBF. Poikilocytes. Leishman stain ×100

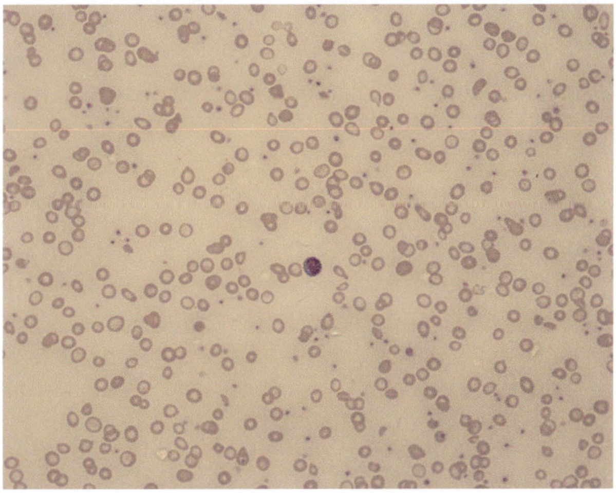

Fig. 1.4 PBF. Low density of red cells. Leishman stain ×40

Table 1.2 Serum iron profile, CRP and ESR

Test	Patient's result	Ref range
S. Iron	2.0	11–31 µmol/L
Transferrin	2.3	2.1–3.6 g/L
Trans. Sat% (TSAT)	3.0	20–40%
Ferritin	11.5	24–336 ng/mL
ESR	30	0–20 mm/h
CRP	2	0–10 mg/L

Table 1.3 Biochemical tests

Test	Patient's result	Ref range
Glu	6.0	3.9–6.1 mmol/L
Urea	2.9	2.5–6.6 mmol/L
Creat	90	60–120 µmol/L
Na^+	139	136–146 mmol/L
Ca^+	2.3	2.2–2.6 mmol/L
Mg^+	1.0	0.08–1.1 mmol/L
T. Prot	68	63–80 mmol/L
Alb	41	35–47 mmol/L
Choles	2.5	1.5–5.2 mmol/L
TG	0.9	0.4–1.7 mmol/L
Urates	370	150–400 mmol/L
T Bil	12	3–20 µmol/L
D. Bil	5	0–5 µmol/L
Alk Ph	41	26–88 IU/L
ALT	29	10–60 IU/L
AST	32	10–42 IU/L
GGT	20	7–64 IU/L
LDH	120	90–180 IU/L
Hapto	0.5	0.2–2.0 g/L
T4	10.6	7.8–16 pmol/L
TSH	3.99	0.27–4.2 ulU/ml

Answer: The blood films show reduced density of red cells. Smears show anisocytosis* with many microcytic** red cells. Few poikilocytes*** are also seen. There is mild to moderate hypochromia.**** Results of iron studies show low serum iron, transferrin saturation, and ferritin. Results of biochemical tests show values within normal range. Anemia due to infections/ inflammation is excluded as CRP is normal. Mild increase in ESR is due to anemia. Based on these results, provisional diagnosis of anemia secondary to iron deficiency is suggested.

However, other pathologies which can be associated with IDA need to be investigated under appropriate clinical setting. Further tests may be required to exclude dual deficiency (B12 + folic acid), hemoglobinopathies like thalassemia (hemoglobin electrophoresis), and estimation of serum levels of lead. A bone marrow examination will be required to evaluate possibility of sideroblastic anemia and assess iron stores and for further evaluation in case patient does not respond to iron therapy.

**Anisocytosis: Variation in size of red cells.*

***Microcytes: Red cells smaller than 6 micron. Rough visual estimation is done by comparing size of red cells with size of nucleus of a resting lymphocyte.*

****Poikilocytosis: Variation in shape of red cells. These may include slightly oval/elongated, pencil shaped, elliptical shaped, and cells resembling tear drops.*

*****Hypochromia: Red cells that have greater central area of pallor (reduced hemoglobinization) It can be mild, moderate, or severe. Normal pallor is 30–33% of total diameter of cell.*

Q3. Given are results of serum B12, folic acid, red cell folate, serum lead levels (Table 1.4), result of HPLC (Fig. 1.5), and images from bone marrow aspirate (Figs. 1.6 and 1.7). Interpret these results and suggest final diagnosis.

Table 1.4 Serum B12, folate, and lead levels

Test	Patient's result	Reference range
S. B12	565	150–700 pmol/L
S. Folate	31.7	10–42 nmol/L
RBC folate	2554	1187–2854 nmol/L
Lead	0	0–10 mcg/L

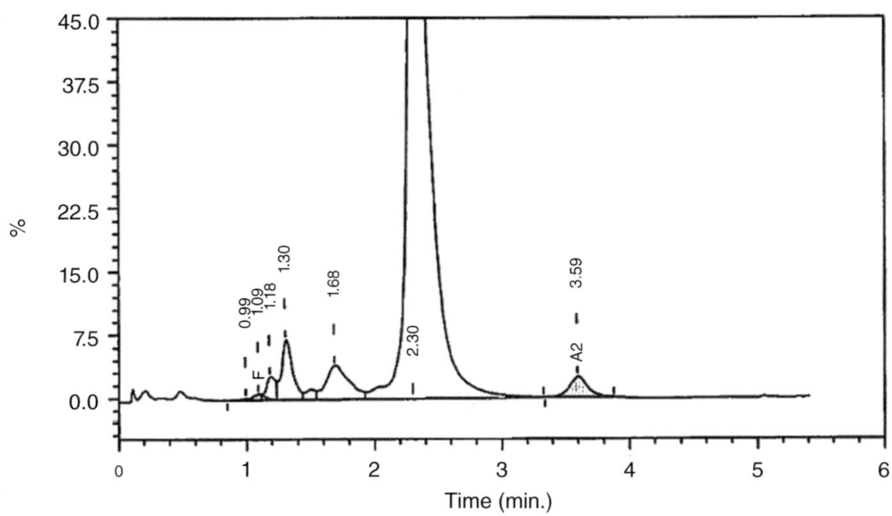

Fig. 1.5 Respresentative HPLC. Hb A: 96.5%, HbA2: 2.5%

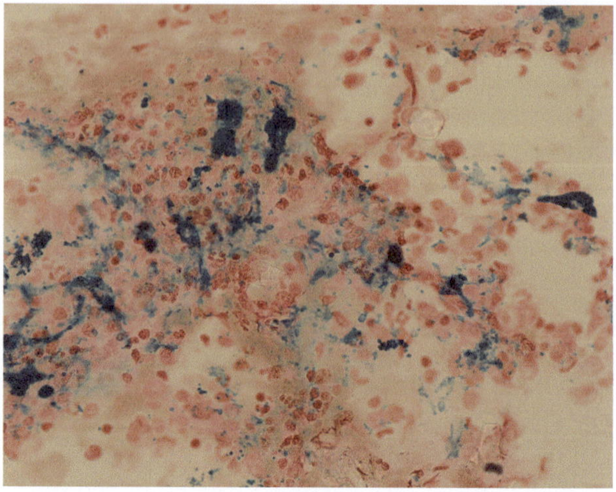

Fig. 1.6 BM aspirate (control). Normal iron stores. Prussian blue stain ×40

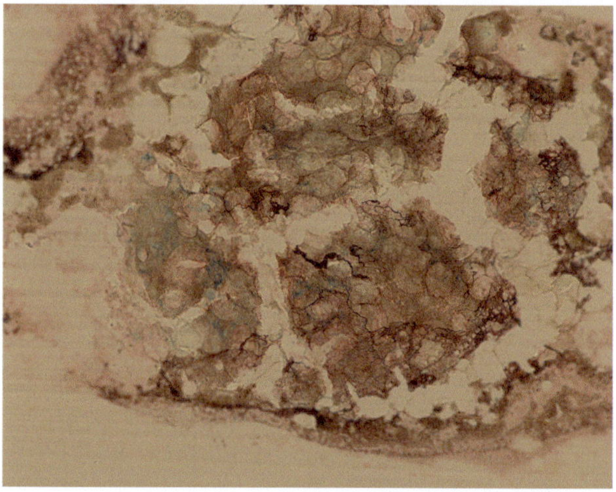

Fig. 1.7 BM aspirate (Patient) Markedly reduced iron stores. Prussian blue stain ×40

Answer: The results of serum B12, folic acid, RBC folate, and lead are within normal reference range, thus excluding the posssibilies of dual deficiency anemia and anemia due to lead toxicity. The HPLC shows normal percentage of HbA and Hb A2, thus eliminating thalassemia as an etiology.The bone marrow iron stores as shown by Prussian blue stain are markedly reduced, thus substantiating iron deficiency as a cause of anemia in this case. As no sideroblasts are seen, the possibility of sideroblastic anemia is also ruled out.

Thus microcytic hypochromic anemia along with reduced serum iron, transferrin saturation, and iron stores (ferritin and hemosiderin) confirms diagnosis of iron deficiency anemia in this case.

Once diagnosis of IDA is established, next investigations are done to evaluate the cause of iron deficiency.

Q4. What are the major causes of IDA and what specialized tests may be required to establish iron deficiency as a cause of anemia?

Answer: Some of the common causes of IDA are [2, 3]:

1. Blood loss. In males, it is from the gastrointestinal system (ulcers in the stomach/ duodenum, prolonged ingestion of medications like aspirin, hemorrhoids, polyps, occult malignancies, etc.). In females, the most common cause is menorrhagia.
2. Worm infestation as hookworm.
3. Bleeding from the kidney or into the lungs can also produce iron deficiency.
4. Other causes include reduced intake as in malnutrition, conditions that interfere with the absorption of iron as achlorhydria, long-term use of antacids, excessive intake of tea/ coffee, H. pylori-associated gastritis, gastrectomy, and intestinal conditions which result in poor absorption such as following gastric bypass surgery, celiac disease, Whipple's disease, and Crohn's disease.
5. Iron deficiency can occur in pregnancy and during growth in the adolescent period.
6. Diseases such as thalassemia, sideroblastic anemia, and chronic inflammations/infections result in ineffective utilization of iron.
7. Rare causes include regular dialysis and repeated phlebotomies.

   So if the cause of iron deficiency is not clear from history, a battery of investigations will be required. These include

1. Stool examination for ova/cysts and occult blood
2. Upper and lower gastrointestinal endoscopy and biopsy (H. pylori)
3. Urine examination for hematuria
4. Serological tests for celiac disease, autoimmune atrophic gastritis, and H. pylori
5. Rarely radiological investigations for intra-abdominal and pelvic pathologies

Q5. A summary of additional tests done to evaluate bleeding and celiac disease in this patient is presented (Table 1.5). Interpret the results and suggest cause of IDA in this patient.

Table 1.5 Results of additional tests

Test	Result
Stool examination for ova/cysts and occult blood	Negative
Upper and lower GI endoscopy	Normal
Urine routine examination	Normal
Serological tests for celiac disease, autoimmune diseases, and H. pylori	Normal
Ultrasound abdomen and pelvis	Uterine fibroids

Answer: The test results show uterine fibroids by pelvic ultrasound. All other tests are normal. This patient has history of menorrhagia. So a final diagnosis of IDA secondary to menorrhagia due to uterine fibroids is confirmed.

Q6. Some specialized tests are also performed in evaluation of microcytic hypochromic anemia. What is the role of red cell ferritin, serum transferrin receptors (STRf), red cell zinc protoporphyrin/heme ratio, and free erythrocyte porphyrin (FEP) in differentiating various causes of microcytic hypochromic anemia?

Answer: When hemoglobin synthesis is impaired, red cell ferritin increases, e.g., thalassemia [1] or sideroblastic anemia. This excess of iron will appear as siderotic granules. These are known as Pappenheimer bodies. They stain purplish blue with Leishman and blue with Prussian blue [5].

In IDA, the number of serum transferrin receptors (STfR) increases. In fact, any condition in which there is hyperplasia of erythroid precursors such as iron deficiency anemia and thalassemia will show an increased number of STfR**.** These can be identified with anti-CD71 antibodies. Serum transferrin receptors are normal in anemia due to chronic inflammation. It is of immense value in distinguishing iron deficiency from anemia of chronic disease [2, 3, 8].

In IDA, zinc substitutes for iron in protoporphyrin IX, and the concentration of zinc protoporphyrin relative to heme increases. So Zn-protoporphyrin/heme ratio increases. This test is more sensitive than ferritin level and is not altered in chronic inflammation/ infections [7, 9].

Free erythrocyte protoporphyrin (FEP) is raised in iron deficiency anemia but not in thalassemia. Other conditions in which it is raised include lead poisoning, chronic infection, and rarely in dyserythropoietic and sideroblastic anemias [10–12].

Q7. What is the role of hepcidin, ferroportin-1, and hephaestin in pathophysiology of IDA?

Answer: In IDA, hepcidin levels are decreased. Normally hepcidin reduces release of iron from intestinal epithelial cells to plasma and also inhibits release of iron from macrophages. It probably acts by binding to ferroportin and enhances its destruction. In anemia due to inflammation, hepcidin production is increased many folds, and this results in sequestration of iron into macrophages and inhibition of release of iron from intestinal epithelial cells into circulation [13, 14].

Ferroportin1 helps in transport of iron across the cell membrane. Hephaestin is present in villous cells of small intestine. It is involved in conversion of Fe^{2+} to Fe^{3+} [15, 16].

Q8. What are the pathophysiological effects of IDA?

Answer: Iron is an essential component of hemoglobin and myoglobin. It has important role in many enzymatic reactions involving peroxidase, mitochondrial dehydrogenase, monoamine oxidase, etc. In IDA, heme production is decreased, there is ineffective erythropoiesis, and the red cell rigidity and auto hemolysis are increased. There is overall decreased red cell survival [17].

1.2 Correlation of Results of Investigations with Symptoms and Signs in Iron Deficiency Anemia

Q9. What are the common symptoms of IDA and how do these correlate with diagnosis in this patient?

Answer: Common symptoms in IDA are easy fatiguability, weakness, pale skin, dizziness, cravings for clay, brittle nails, hair loss, poor appetite, frequent infections, etc. [18, 19].

Long standing deficiency produces cheilitis, atrophic glossitis, Plummer-Vinson pharyngeal webs [20, 21].

This patient has tiredness, dizziness, easy fatigability, and mild dyspnea on exertion. These symptoms are due to decreased oxygen carrying capacity of hemoglobin. When oxygen supply is reduced, the muscles depend on anaerobic respiration also. So capacity to perform normal day-to-day activity decreases. The body tries to acquire more oxygen through respiratory effort, and patient becomes dyspnea on exertion.

Q10. How do the CBC parameters correlate with diagnosis of IDA in this patient and how do they help in differentiating IDA from thalassemia?

Answer: In IDA, low hemoglobin correlates with low values for red cell count, MCV, MCH, and MCHC. The RDW is high. Platelets may be normal or increased (reactive increase). Our patient has all these findings which correlate well with the diagnosis. In thalassemia, red cell number is disproportionately high in relation to decreased hemoglobin. MCV and MCH are low but MCHC and RDW are usually normal. Platelet count remains within normal range [22].

Q11. How is mild, moderate, and severe hypochromia assessed on blood film?

Answer: There are no clear guidelines for such assessment. However, a rough visual estimation is done by looking at the hemoglobinized (colored) part of the red cell. In normal red cells, the central pallor is not more than one-third (30–33%) of the total diameter of the cell. In mild deficiency, the pale part is little more than one-third. In severe hypochromia, only a thin rim of hemoglobinized part is seen. A moderate hypochromia is considered if pale area is seen covering red cell between mild and severe hypochromia [23].

Q12. This patient has high red cell distribution width (RDW). What is the significance of RDW in IDA?

Answer: Red cell distribution width reflects variation in size of red cells in blood. More the variation, higher the value for RDW. In IDA, as there is variation in size and shape of red cells, the RDW is higher than normal. This helps in differentiating it from thalassemia minor and anemia of chronic disease, where RDW is usually normal.

Q13. How are reticulocyte count and reticulocyte hemoglobin helpful in diagnosis and management of IDA?

Answer: In mild iron deficiency, reticulocyte count is usually normal or on lower side, but in severe deficiency, it may be lower than normal. Also it is helpful in assessing the response of bone marrow when a patient of IDA is treated with iron. The reticulocyte count should start increasing within 5 to 10 days of beginning of iron therapy, and the hemoglobin should increase by about 2 g/dL within 3 to 4 weeks. Anemia is considered refractory if the response is not satisfactory [24]. A new additional parameter, reticulocyte hemoglobin content, has come up which is helpful in identifying iron deficient erythropoiesis. It is especially helpful when the traditional biochemical parameters are noninformative [25, 26]. Reticulocyte hemoglobin content is not influenced by other factors such as inflammation, infection and malignancy etc. It indicates the amount of iron available to the newly formed red cells in bone marrow.

Q14. This patient has a high platelet count. What is the cause of thrombocytosis in IDA?

Answer: Platelets are derived from megakaryocytes. Iron deficiency increases the megakaryopoietic differentiation. A possibility of cytokine-mediated increase in megakaryopoiesis has been proposed [27].

Q15. How are CRP, ESR, and biochemical tests helpful in evaluation of microcytic hypochromic anemia and differentiating it from ACD?

Answer: CRP is produced in liver. Its level will increase in response to inflammation (acute phase reactant). ESR is an indirect measure of acute phase reactants and is also a positive inflammatory marker. Both are raised in anemia due to chronic inflammation and normal in other conditions [28].

The biochemical tests for liver, kidney, thyroid, pancreas, and bone are helpful if a patient is suffering from chronic inflammation/ infections of these organs.

Q16. This patient has deranged iron profile. What is the role of transferrin, transferrin saturation, and ferritin in evaluation and differential diagnosis of microcytic hypochromic anemia?

Answer: Transferrin is a glycoprotein produced from liver and is responsible for transport of iron to various organs like liver, spleen, and bone marrow. It binds to transferrin receptors on target cells and delivers iron to them. Its synthesis is decreased in ACD but increased in iron deficiency. Values are usually normal in thalassemia. Its saturation is decreased in iron deficiency [7, 26].

Ferritin is storage form of iron in circulation (blood). It is water soluble and is composed of apoprotein enclosing iron molecules. It is a marker of total iron store in body. Liver, spleen, muscles, reticuloendothelial cells, and bone marrow have highest concentration. Low ferritin is a sensitive marker for diagnosis of early IDA. It is also an acute phase reactant with increased levels seen in chronic inflammations and infections [29].

Q17. How is hemosiderin different from ferritin and what is its significance?

Answer: Hemosiderin is composed of partially degraded ferritin molecules, proteins, and lipids. It contains ferric iron. Major site of storage is macrophages in bone marrow, reticuloendothelial cells of liver, spleen, etc. Prussian blue stain on bone marrow smears shows a blue colored pigment in macrophages and erythroid precursors. This pigment is ferri-ferrocyanide formed by combination of acidic ferrocyanide with ferric ions [30].

In normal bone marrow, siderotic granules are seen in erythroid precursors. Their number is usually less than 15 per cell and are randomly distributed. No ring sideroblasts are seen. However, they are either absent or their number is significantly reduced in IDA depending on severity. In case of sideroblastic anemia, increased number of granules are seen and these are arranged in form of ring around the nucleus [31]. In ACD, increased hemosiderin is noted in macrophages. ([32] Given below are representative images of iron in normal bone marrow (Fig. 1.8), iron overload anemia (Fig. 1.9), anemia of chronic disorder (Fig. 1.10), and sideroblastic anemia (Fig. 1.11).

Fig. 1.8 BM aspirate. Normal iron stores. Prussian blue stain ×40

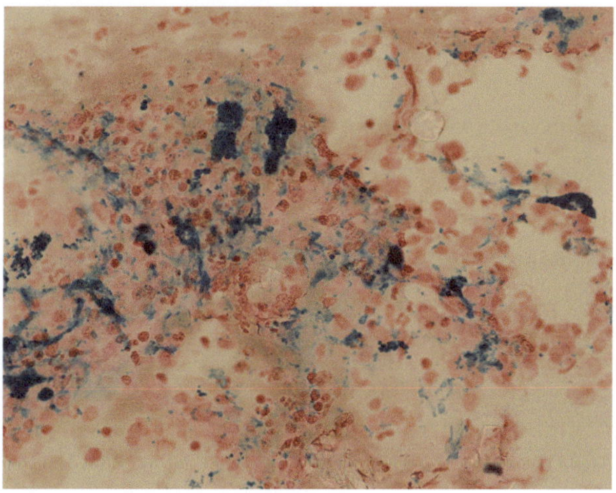

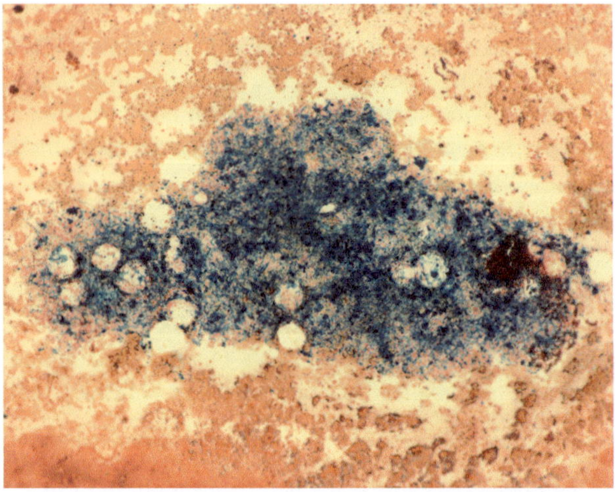

Fig. 1.9 BM aspirate. Markedly increased iron stores (iron overload anemia). Prussian blue stain ×40

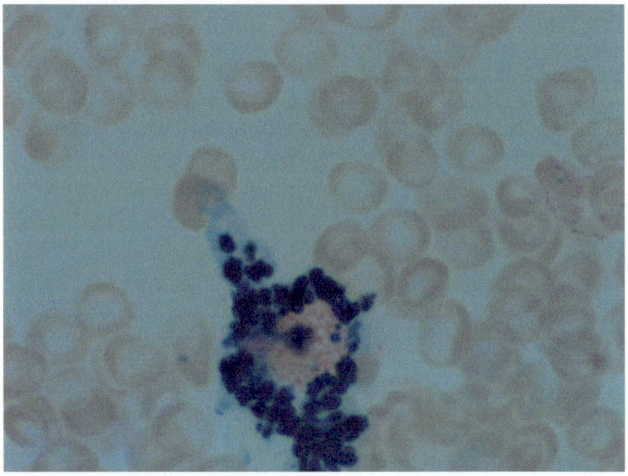

Fig. 1.10 BM aspirate. A macrophage loaded with iron (ACD) Prussian blue stain ×100

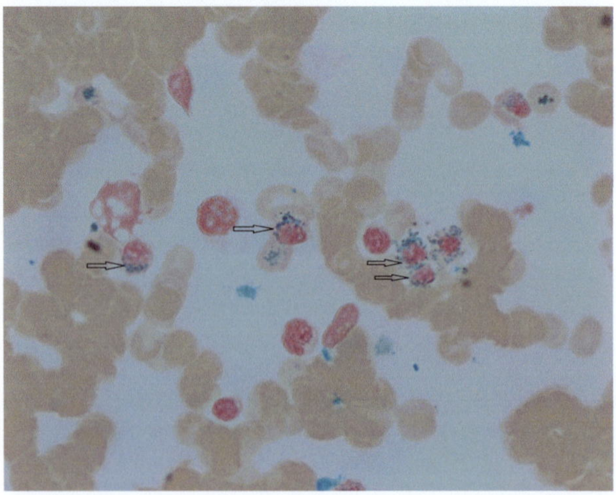

Fig. 1.11 BM aspirate. Ring sideroblasts (sideroblastic anemia) Prussian blue stain ×100

Q18. How is bone marrow graded for iron status?

Answer: A fairly used system of grading iron status in bone marrow has been in practice for a long time. It is graded from zero (0) to 6+ based on the size and quantity of iron granules. For practical purposes, content less than 2+ is considered a deficient state. More details are in reference [33].

Q19. Which foods are rich in iron?

Answer: Foods which are rich in iron include chicken, turkey, duck meat, pork, lamb, beef, fish, green leafy vegetables such as broccoli, kale, legumes, pasta, etc.

Q20. What is the mechanism of absorption of iron.

Answer: Food contains two forms of iron—one is heme and the other nonheme. Heme iron is present in products of animal origin such as fish, meat, and poultry. The nonheme iron is found in vegetables, fruits, nuts, beans, grains, and meat [34]. In intestine, the heme iron has better absorption than nonheme iron [35]. Iron absorption occurs mainly in the duodenum and the proximal jejunum [36].

Most of the non-heme iron in the diet is in the ferric form. For its absorption, it needs to be reduced to Fe^{2+} form. This is achieved by the actions of the membrane bound duodenal cytochrome B, a ferric reductase enzyme expressed on brush border membrane of intestinal epithelial cells [37]. Ferrous iron moves across the apical membrane of enterocytes by a protein known as divalent metal transporter 1 (DMT1) [38].

To enter the systemic circulation from intestinal cells, iron has to cross the basolateral membrane of intestinal enterocytes. This is helped by another protein called ferroportin [39].

The release of ferrous iron into the blood by ferroportin is assisted by hephaestin. These enzymes oxidize Fe^{2+} to Fe^{3+} before the iron binds to the iron-transport protein transferrin in circulation [40].

Heme iron is more readily absorbed than non-heme iron derived from vegetables and grain. Most heme is absorbed in the proximal intestine, with absorptive capacity decreasing distally [40].

Q21. What are rare and refractory causes of IDA?

Answer: Refractoriness is considered when there is no response after the patient has received at least 100 mg of elemental iron per day for 4 to 6 weeks. There are numerous causes of iron deficiency anemia refractory to treatment. Among them are H. pylori infection, autoimmune gastritis, and celiac disease which will require additional specialized investigation [4]. Mutations in the TMPRSS6 gene have been identified as cause of iron-refractory iron deficiency anemia (IRIDA) [40]. Several other reasons can result in poor response to treatment with iron. Some of them are poor compliance, malabsorption, continuous bleeding, drug/food interaction, incorrect diagnosis, or more than one cause of anemia.

Some more rare causes include INH therapy, hereditary orotic aciduria, hypo- or atransferrinemia, nephritic syndrome, copper deficiency, and inborn errors of iron metabolism.

1.3 Quick Information for Practicing Clinicians and Students

References [1–7, 12, 24, 26, 29, 41, 42]:

1. Serum ferritin is the most accurate for diagnosis of IDA. A cutoff value of 30 ng per mL has more than 90% sensitivity and specificity. Since it is acute phase reactant, IDA should be considered when levels are below 50 ng per mL in presence of infection/ inflammation.
2. Normal red cell indices do not exclude iron deficiency as a cause of anemia.
3. Transferrin saturation (TSAT) of <16% can support the diagnosis of iron deficiency if initial tests are inconclusive.
4. The total iron-binding capacity (TIBC) is a functional measurement of the level of transferrin in circulation.
5. Decreased serum iron, decreased transferrin saturation with increased total iron-binding capacity (TIBC), and reduced ferritin levels are most helpful for diagnosis of IDA.
6. Mean reticulocyte Hb content of <29 pg can support diagnosis of iron deficiency.
7. The reticulocyte count should start increasing within 5 to 10 days of beginning of iron therapy and the hemoglobin should increase by about 2 g/dL within 3 to 4 weeks. Anemia is considered refractory if the response is not satisfactory.
8. The sTfR assay, zinc protoporphyrin, and hepcidin tests are not currently recommended for investigating iron deficiency.
9. Increased red cell count with decreased Hb, MCV MCH, target cells, and basophilic stippling suggest possibility of thalassemia. Hb electrophoresis should be done.
10. Microcytic hypochromic cells with basophilic stippling on the peripheral blood smear and presence of ring sideroblasts in bone marrow should raise suspicion of lead (Pb) poisoning. Lead levels should be considered.
11. Microcytic hypochromic cells with raised serum iron and transferrin along with elevated LDH, and sideroblasts more than 15% in the bone marrow strongly suggest sideroblastic anemia.

To acquire further knowledge on the subject, the following sources are recommended:

1. BCSH guidelines
2. Br Jr Hematology
3. ASH education book
4. Blood
5. NEJM
6. Int Jr Lab Hematology

References

1. Matos JF, Dusse LMS, Borges KBG, et al. A new index to discriminate between iron deficiency anemia and thalassemia trait. Rev Bras Hematol Hemoter. 2016;38(3):214–9. https://doi.org/10.1016/j.bjhh.2016.05.011.
2. Camaschella C. Iron-deficiency anemia. N Engl J Med. 2015;372(19):1832–43.
3. Lopez A, Cacoub P, Macdougall IC, Peyrin-Biroulet L. Iron deficiency anaemia. Lancet. 2016;387:907–16.
4. Hershko C, Camaschella C. How I treat unexplained refractory iron deficiency anemia. Blood. 2014;123:326–33.
5. Yamada H. Characterization of serum and red cell ferritin in haematological disorders. Acta Haematol. 1978;41:1334–7.
6. Pfeiffer CM, Looker AC. Laboratory methodologies for indicators of iron status: strengths, limitations, and analytical challenges. Am J Clin Nutr. 2017;106(Suppl 6):1606S–14S.
7. Archer NM, Brugnara C. Diagnosis of iron-deficient states. Crit Rev Clin Lab Sci. 2015;52(5):256–72.
8. Crichton RR, Charloteaux-Wauters M. Iron transport and storage. Eur J Biochem. 1987;164(3):485–506.
9. Schifman RB, Thomasson JE, Evers JM. Red blood cell zinc protoporphyrin testing for iron deficiency anemia in pregnancy. Am J Obstet Gynecol. 1987;157:304–7. https://doi.org/10.1016/S0002-9378(87)80157-6.
10. Scholnick P, Marver HS, Schmid R. Erythropoietic protoporphyria: evidence for multiple sites of excess protoporphyrin formation. J Clin Invest. 1971;50:203–8.
11. Watson CJ. The erythrocyte coproporphyrin. Arch Intern Med. 1950;86:797–809.
12. Watson CJ, Decker E, Lichtman HC. Hematologic studies of children with lead poisoning. Pediatrics. 1968;2:40–6.
13. Wang RH, Li C, Xu X, et al. A role of SMAD4 in iron metabolism through the positive regulation of hepcidin expression. Cell Metab. 2005;2:399–409.
14. Girelli D, Nemeth E, Swinkels DW. Hepcidin in the diagnosis of iron disorders. Blood. 2016;127(23):2809–13.
15. Donovan A, Lima CA, Pinkus JL, et al. The iron exporter ferroportin/Slc40a1 is essential for iron homeostasis. Cell Metab. 2005;1:191–200.
16. Vulpe CD, et al. Hephaestin, a ceruloplasmin homologue implicated in intestinal iron transport, is defective in the SLA mouse. NAT Genet. 1999;21:195–9.
17. John LB. Iron biology in immune function, muscle metabolism and neuronal functioning. J Nutr. 2001;131:5685–805.
18. Kettaneh A, Eclache V, Sontaq C, et al. Pica and food craving in patients with iron-deficiency anemia: a case-control study in France. Am J Med. 2005;118:185–8.
19. Trost L, Bergfeld W, Calogeras E. The diagnosis and treatment of iron deficiency and its potential relationship to hair loss. J Am Acad Dermatol. 2006;54:824–44.
20. Howell J, Monto R. Syndrome of anemia, dysphagia and glossitis (Plummer Vinson syndrome). N Engl J Med. 1953;249:1009–12.
21. Allen RP, Auerbach S, Bahrain H, Auerbach M, Earley CJ. The prevalence and impact of restless legs syndrome on patients with iron deficiency anemia. Am J Hematol. 2013;88(4):261–4.
22. Nagwan R, Ahmd El-abd A, Mohammed H, Maha EM. Hematological indices in differentiation between iron deficiency anemia and beta-thalassemia trait. Int J Pediatr. 2022;10(1):15285–95. https://doi.org/10.22038/ijp.2021.59644.4644.
23. Palmer L, Briggs C, McFadden S, Zini G, et al. ICSH recommendations for the standardization of nomenclature and grading of peripheral blood cell morphological features. Int J Lab Hem. 2015;37:287–3032.
24. Piva E, Brugnara C, Spolaore F, Plebani M. Clinical utility of reticulocyte parameters. Clin Lab Med. 2015;2015(35):133–63.

25. Archer NM, Brugnara C. Diagnosis of iron-deficient states. Crit Rev Clin Lab Sci. 2015;52:256–76.
26. Brugnara C, Adamson J, Auerbach M, Kane R, Macdougall I, Mast A. Iron deficiency: what are the future trends in diagnostics and therapeutics? Clin Chem. 2013;59:740–5.
27. Rayko E, Adam B, Kristine J, et al. Iron deficiency alters megakaryopoiesis and platelet phenotype independent of thrombopoietin. Am J Hematol. 2014;89(5):524–9.
28. Harrison M. Erythrocyte sedimentation rate and C-reactive protein. Aust Prescr. 2015;38(3):93–4.
29. Goddard AF, James MW, McIntyre AS, Scott BB, British Society of Gastroenterology. Guidelines for the management of iron deficiency anemia. Gut. 2011;60(10):1309–16.
30. Hiroshi S. Metabolism of iron stores. Nagoya J. Med Sci. 2014;76:235–54.
31. Mufti GJ, Bennett JM, Goasguen J, et al. Diagnosis and classification of myelodysplastic syndrome: international Working Group on Morphology of myelodysplastic syndrome (IWGM-MDS) consensus proposals for the definition and enumeration of myeloblasts and ring sideroblasts. Haematologica. 2008;93(11):1712–7.
32. Pujara KM, Bhalara RV, Dhruva GA. A study of bone marrow iron storage in hematological disorder. Int J Health Allied Sci. 2014;3:2214.
33. Phiri KS, Calis JCJ, Kachala D, et al. Improved method for assessing iron stores in the bone marrow. J Clin Pathol. 2009;62(8):685–9.
34. Roughead ZK, Zito CA, Hunt JR. Initial uptake and absorption of nonheme iron and absorption of heme iron in humans are unaffected by the addition of calcium as cheese to a meal with high iron bioavailability. Am J Clin Nutr. 2002;76(2):419–25.
35. Fuqua BK, Vulpe CD, Anderson GJ. Intestinal iron absorption. J Trace Elem Med Biol. 2012;26:115–9.
36. McKie AT, Barrow D, Latunde-Dada GO, Rolfs A, Sager G, Mudaly E, et al. An iron-regulated ferric reductase associated with the absorption of dietary iron. Science. 2001;291:1755–9.
37. Gunshin H, Mackenzie B, Berger UV, Gunshin Y, Romero MF, Boron WF, et al. Cloning and characterization of a mammalian proton-coupled metal-ion transporter. Nature. 1997;388:482–8.
38. Donovan A, Brownlie A, Zhou Y, Shepard J, Pratt SJ, Moynihan J, et al. Positional cloning of zebrafish ferroportin1 identifies a conserved vertebrate iron exporter. Nature. 2000;403:776–81.
39. Vulpe CD, Kuo YM, Murphy TL, Cowley L, Askwith C, Libina N, et al. Hephaestin, a ceruloplasmin homologue implicated in intestinal iron transport, is defective in the sla mouse. Nat Genet. 1999;21:195–9.
40. Le Blanc S, Garrick MD, Arredondo M. Heme carrier protein 1 transports heme and is involved in heme-Fe metabolism. Am J Physiol Cell Physiol. 2012;302:C1780–5.
41. Matthew MH, Karin EF. Iron-refractory iron deficiency anemia (IRIDA). Hematol Oncol Clin North Am. 2014;28(4):637–52.
42. Fletcher A, Forbes A, Svenson N, Thomas D. A British Society for Haematology good practice paper. Br J Haematol. 2022;196:523–9.

Chapter 2
Megaloblastic Anemia

A 38-year-old lady presents with progressive generalized weakness, lethargy, and dyspnea on exertion for the preceding 2 months. She also gives history of soreness of tongue, numbness, and tingling in the feet and hands (stocking–glove distribution). There is no history of bleeding or any other significant past history except for diabetic status for the last 2 years. She is not compliant to antidiabetic medications. There is no history of intake of drugs or alcoholism. Her social history is unremarkable. She was on restricted diet for weight control and had turned pure vegetarian for the last 2 years. Physical examination showed pallor, mild icterus, and glossitis. There is no palpable organomegaly. Table 2.1 shows result of CBC done at presentation.

Table 2.1 CBC

CBC parameter	Patient's result	Ref range
WBC	3.0	3.7–10 × 10^9/L
RBC	1.62	4.5–5.5 × 10^{12}/L
Hb	74	130–170 g/L
Hct	0.211	0.4–0.5 L/L
MCV	130.1	83–100 fL
MCH	35.6	27–32 pg
MCHC	345	315–345 g/L
RDW	30.0	11.6–14.6%
NRBCs	0	0
PLT	88	130–430 × 10^9/L
MPV	9.9	7–11 fL
POLY#	1.5	1.7–6 × 10^9/L
LYM#	1.3	1–3 × 10^9/L
MONO#	0.1	0.2–1.0 × 10^9/L
EO#	0.0	0.02–0.5 × 10^9/L
BAS#O	0	0.02–0.1 × 10^9/L
Ret%	0.5	0.5–1.5%

A. Gupta, *Decision Making Through Problem Based Learning in Hematology*, https://doi.org/10.1007/978-981-99-8933-1_2

2.1 Questions

Q1. Interpret the CBC result given above and suggest investigations for further evaluation in such case.

Answer: The CBC result shows pancytopenia (low values for white cells, red cells, hemoglobin, hematocrit, and platelets) and borderline reticulocytopenia. MCV, MCH, and RDW values are high. So, she has pancytopenia with reticulocytopenia. Anemia is macrocytic.

Macrocytosis (MCV more than 100 fL) can result from:

1. Megaloblastic anemia: Deficiency or impaired utilization of B12/ folic acid.
2. Non-megaloblastic pathologies: Myelodysplasia, liver disease, hypothyroidism, aplastic anemia, congenital dyserythropoietic anemia (CDA-I and III), erythroleukemia, reticulocytosis, alcoholism, certain drugs, and some inherited disorders of DNA synthesis (e.g., inherited orotic aciduria and Lesch-Nyhan syndrome). In addition, pseudo-macrocytosis (falsely high MCV) also needs to be excluded [1–3].

The next best tests will be to examine a blood film and do biochemical tests for liver, thyroid, renal, and pancreatic functions.

Q2. Given are images from peripheral blood film (Figs. 2.1, 2.2, 2.3, 2.4, 2.5, 2.6) and results of biochemical tests (Table 2.2). What is the interpretation and possible differential diagnosis? What further investigations will be required to exclude various possibilities? Suggest a final diagnosis.

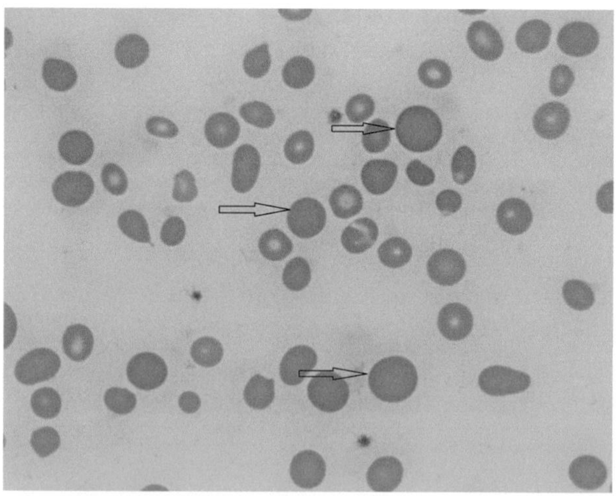

Fig. 2.1 PBF. Macrocytes. Leishman stain ×100

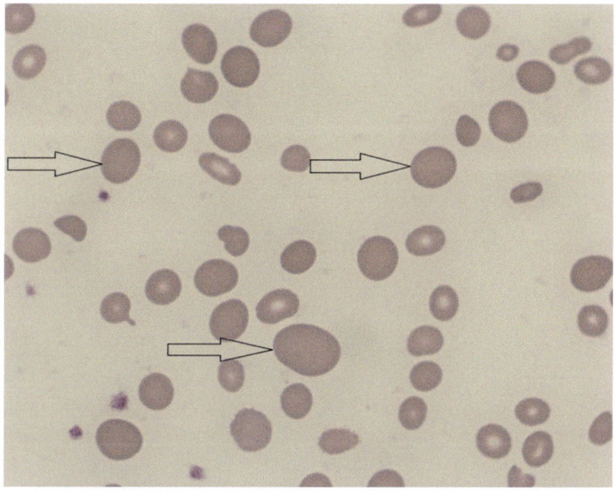

Fig. 2.2 PBF. Macro-ovalocytes. Leishman stain ×100

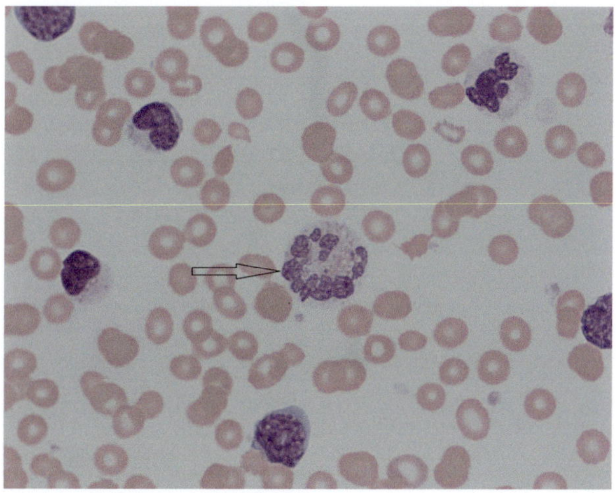

Fig. 2.3 PBF. Hypersegmented neutrophil. Leishman stain ×100

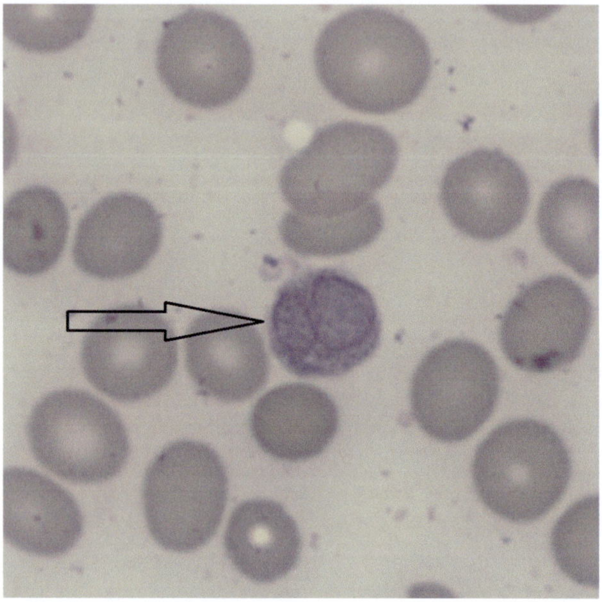

Fig. 2.4 PBF. Cabot ring. Leishman stain ×100

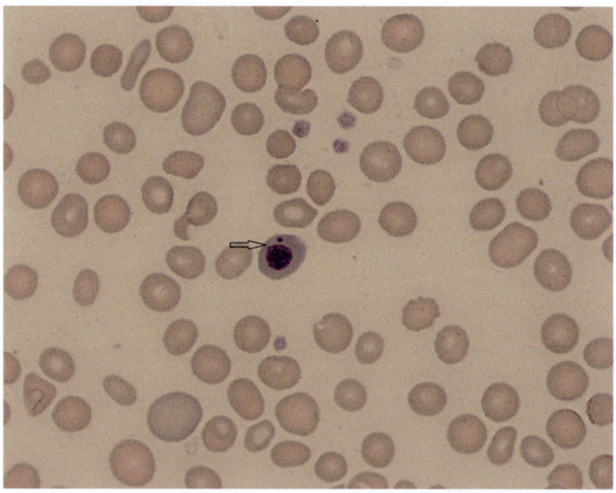

Fig. 2.5 PBF. Howell-Jolly body. Leishman stain ×100

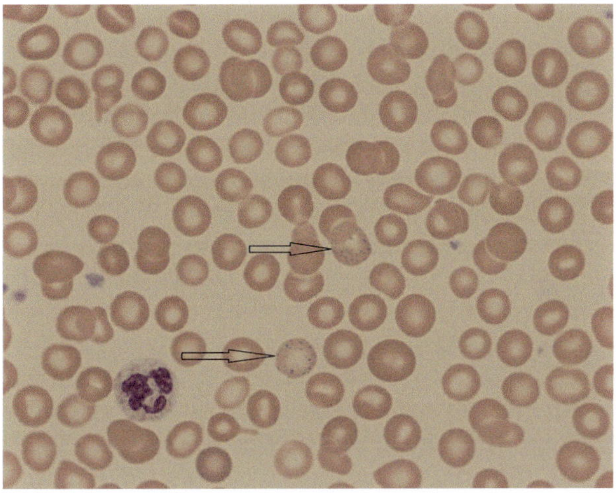

Fig. 2.6 PBF. Basophilic stippling. Leishman ×100

Table 2.2 Biochemical tests

Test	Patient's result	Ref range
Glu (F)	8.0	3.9–6.1 mmol/L
Urea	2.9	2.5–6.6 mmol/L
Creat	90	60–120 μmol/L
Na^+	139	136–146 mmol/L
K^+	4.5	3.7–5.0 mmol/L
Ca^+	2.3	2.2–2.6 mmol/L
Mg^+	1.0	0.08–1.1 mmol/L
T. Prot	68	63–80 mmol/L
Alb	39	35–47 mmol/L
Choles	2.5	1.5–5.2 mmol/L
TG	0.9	0.4–1.7 mmol/L
Urates	300	150–400 mmol/L
T Bil	52	3–20 μmol/L
Indirect Bil	45	5–20 μmol/L
D. Bil	7	0–5 μmol/L
Alk Ph	80	26–88 IU/L
ALT	55	10–60 IU/L
AST	32	10–42 IU/L
GGT	20	7–64 IU/L
LDH	1800	90–180 IU/L
Hapto	0.3	0.2–2.0 g/L
T4	10.6	7.8–16 pmol/L
TSH	3.99	0.27–4.2 μlU/mL
Amylase	20	28–100 IU/L
Lipase	30	0–160 U/L

Answer: The blood film images show red cell changes. There is variation in size (anisocytosis) and shape (poikilocytosis). Macrocytes (Fig. 2.1), macro-ovalocytes (Fig. 2.2), and hyper-segmented neutrophil are also seen (Fig. 2.3). In addition, Cabot ring (Fig. 2.4), Howell-Jolly body (Fig. 2.5), and basophilic stippling (Fig. 2.6) are also observed. The biochemical tests (Table 2.2) show high values for total bilirubin, indirect bilirubin, and LDH. Rest of the tests for liver, kidney, thyroid, and pancreatic functions are within normal range except for slightly high fasting blood glucose which indicates diabetic status. All these findings suggest megaloblastic anemia and exclude conditions like MDS, liver disease, and hypothyroidism as a cause of macrocytosis. High values for indirect bilirubin and LDH are indicators of hemolysis. For confirmation of megaloblastic anemia, estimations of serum B12, folic acid, and red cell folate are required.

Cabot rings are thin thread-like strands seen as loop in Fig. 2.8. These are microtubules which are remnants of mitotic spindle and indicate disturbed erythropoiesis. ***Howell-Jolly bodies*** *are small round dark purple to red colored inclusions often located peripherally in red cells. These are residual fragments of nuclear* material. ***Basophilic stippling*** is precipitated rRNA. This indicates disturbed erythropoiesis and is also seen in lead poisoning, nutritional deficiencies, myelodysplasia etc. ***Hyper-segmented neutrophils*** are polymorph neutrophils with 6 or more nuclear lobes. Also hyper-segmentation is diagnosed when more than 5% neutrophils are seen with 5 lobes in a blood film.

Q3. Given are results of serum B12, folic acid, and red cell folate (Table 2.3). Interpret the results and suggest final diagnosis.

Table 2.3 Results of serum B12, folic acid, and red cell folate

Test	Patient's result	Reference value
Serum B12	58	150–700 pmol/L
Serum FA	31.7	10–42 nmol/L
RBC folate	1959	1187–2854 nmol/L

Answer: Serum B12 is low. Serum folate and red cell folate levels are normal. Diagnosis of megaloblastic anemia secondary to B12 deficiency is confirmed.

Q4. Which more tests are required to be done to exclude other possible non-megaloblastic causes of macrocytic anemia?

Answer: Non-megaloblastic macrocytic anemia is also seen in myelodysplasia, aplastic anemia, CDA, and erythroleukemia. Although not indicated in this case, a bone marrow examination may be considered for excluding these conditions and looking at morphological abnormalities. Inherited orotic aciduria and Lesch-Nyhan syndrome are inherited disorders of DNA synthesis where macrocytic anemia is observed. However, their presentation and diagnosis are in pediatric age-group [4, 5].

Q5. Given are the images of bone marrow aspirate smears and biopsy (Figs. 2.7, 2.8, 2.9, 2.10, 2.11). What are the main findings?

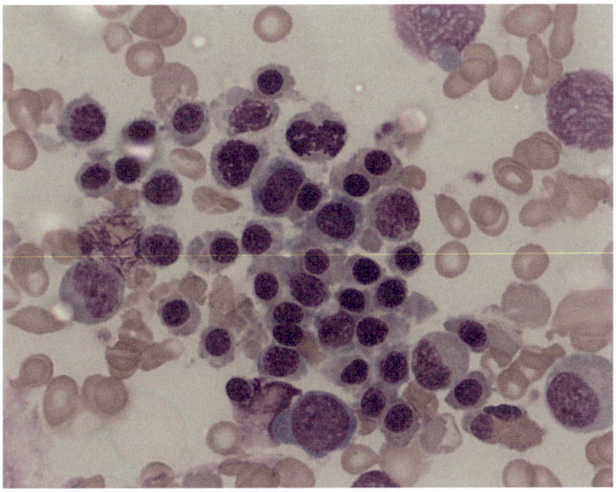

Fig. 2.7 BM aspirate. Erythroid hyperplasia. Leishman stain ×100

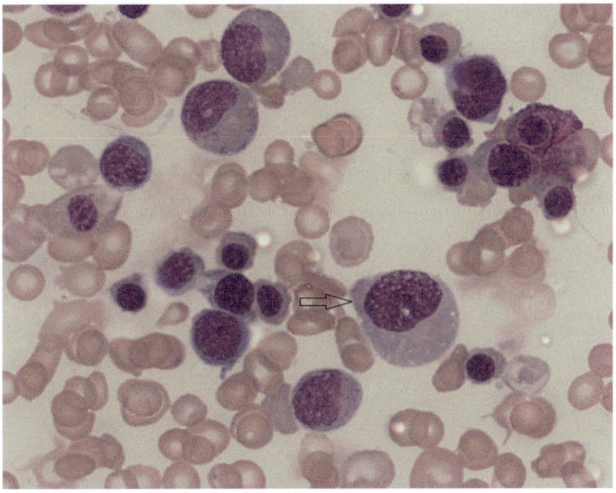

Fig. 2.8 BM aspirate. Giant myelocyte. Leishman stain ×100

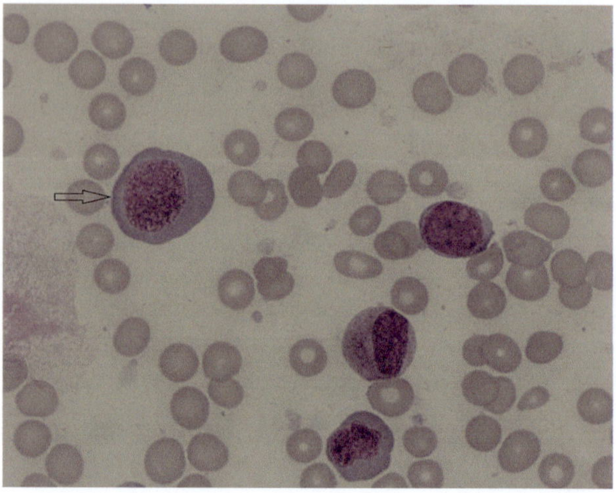

Fig. 2.9 BM aspirate. Intermediate megaloblast. Leishman stain ×100

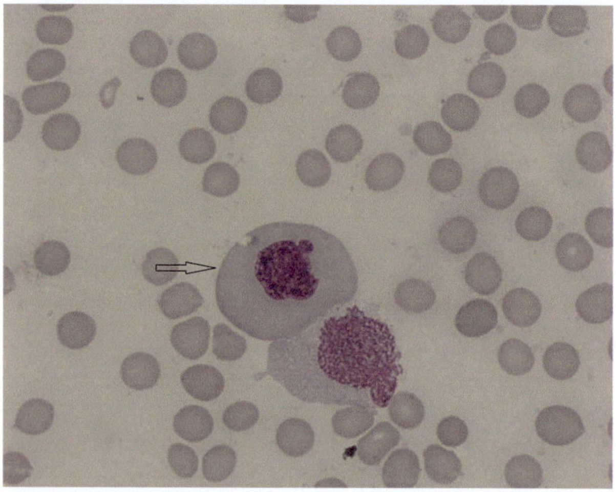

Fig. 2.10 BM aspirate. Late megaloblast. Leishman stain ×100

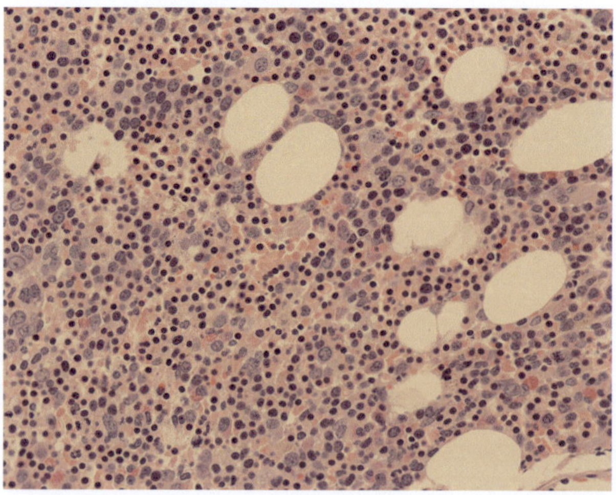

Fig. 2.11 Bone marrow biopsy. Erythroid hyperplasia. H/E stain ×40

Answer: The bone marrow smears show erythroid hyperplasia (Fig. 2.7) along with giant myelocytes (Fig. 2.8) and megaloblastic changes in intermediate (Fig. 2.9) and late erythroid precursors (Fig. 2.10). The bone marrow biopsy (Fig. 2.11) shows erythroid hyperplasia. There is no evidence of leukemia or any other pathology. These observations confirm a diagnosis of megaloblastic anemia and exclude possibilities of myelodysplasia, aplastic anemia, CDA, and erythroleukemia.

Megaloblasts are structurally abnormal, immature red cell precursors which show nuclear immaturity (lag due to impaired DNA synthesis) in relation to cytoplasmic maturity (which remains normal for the stage of development). This is called nucleo-cytoplasmic asynchronization.

Q6. Once Megaloblastic anemia is diagnosed, next step is to explore cause of this disease. What are the causes and which tests are recommended for its evaluation?

Answer: B12 deficiency can result from a number of causes, some of which are inadequate nutrition, people on vegetarian diet, malabsorption due to gastric causes like pernicious anemia, atrophic gastritis, gastric bypass, Zollinger-Ellison syndrome, pancreatic insufficiency, disorders of terminal ileum like tropical sprue, inflammatory bowel disease, lymphoma and ileal resection, bacterial colonization, worm infestations (e.g., fish tape worm), exposure to nitrous oxide, etc. [1, 2]

So, further specialized tests are required to detect antibodies to intrinsic factor (IF) and gastric parietal cells, tissue transglutaminase, examination of stools for parasites, upper GI endoscopy and duodenal biopsy, estimation of serum gastrin levels, serum MMA, and plasma homocysteine levels. Bone marrow examination is rarely done now due to widely and easily available blood tests. Estimation of serum transcobalamin can be considered in rare situations where transcobalamin-II deficiency is suspected. However, the availability of this test is limited [6–8].

Schilling test is now almost obsolete.

Q7. Given are the results of immunological investigations (Table 2.4). What is the significance of anti-IF and anti-parietal antibodies?

Table 2.4 Immunological investigations

Test	Result	Ref range
Anti-nuclear antibodies- screen	Negative	Negative
Anti-dsDNA antibodies	Negative	0–20
Anti-intrinsic factor Ab	Positive 9.7 EU/mL	0–6 EU/mL
Anti-gastric parietal Ab	Positive 34 EU/mL	0–25 EU/mL
Anti-tissue transglutaminase IgA	Negative	0–20 CU
Anti-tissue transglutaminase IgG	Negative	0–20 CU

Answer: Both anti-IF antibodies and anti-parietal cell antibodies are positive. Tests for screening of celiac disease (anti-TTG IgG and IgA) are negative. Tests for other immunological disorders (ANA, dsDNA) are also negative.

Anti-IF antibodies are seen in 50–60% cases of pernicious anemia (PA) and are specific for this disease. Anti-parietal cell antibodies are seen in 90% of the patients of PA but are not specific. They are also seen in some patients with non-specific gastritis, thyroiditis, and other autoimmune disorders [9].

IF antibodies are of two types—Type I–which blocks binding of IF to B12 and Type II–which prevent IF-B12 complex to attach to ileal receptors. Patients of PA can have either of the two. So, in this patient cause of megaloblastic anemia is secondary to anti-IF antibodies and anti-parietal antibodies [10].

Q8. Under which situations are methylmalonyl-CoA (MMA) and homocysteine (HC) tested? What is their importance?

Answer: Methylmalonyl-CoA increases in cobalamin deficiency. Homocysteine is increased in both folate and B12 deficiency. If both MMA and homocysteine are increased and B12 is only mildly decreased, it suggests an early or mild B12 deficiency. If only homocysteine is elevated, and MMA is normal, it indicates folate deficiency. The distinction is important because giving folate to someone who is B12 deficient will treat anemia but will not revert neurological damage [11].

Q9. How does estimation of serum B12, serum folate, red cell folate, MMA, and homocysteine help in differentiating B12 deficiency from folate deficiency?

Answer: Some of the salient points which help to evaluate differences between cobalamin and folate deficiency are summarized in Table 2.5 [11–13].

Table 2.5 Differentiation between cobalamin and folate deficiency

Test	Cobalamin deficiency	Folate deficiency
Serum cobalamin	Decreased	Usually normal
Serum folate	Normal to increased	Decreased
Red cell folate	Decreased	Decreased
Serum MMA	Increased	Normal
Serum homocysteine	Increased	Increased (moderately)

Cobalamin is necessary for pushing methyltetrahydrofolate from plasma into RBCs. So in approximately 60% patients with cobalamin deficiency, red cell folate is also expected to be low.

Q10. What is the role of Schilling test and how is it interpreted?

Answer: Schilling test is done in two parts. In part I—an oral dose of radioactive B12 (RA B12) is given along with intramuscular non-radioactive cobalamin. Urine is collected for 24 h, and RA B12 is measured. In part II, oral IF is added along with RAB12 and its excretion is measured in urine over next 24 h. Interpretation [14–16]:

1. Under normal circumstances, >10% excretion is observed.
2. Less than 5% excretion in both parts indicates intestinal malabsorption.
3. Less than 5% excretion in Part-I but more than 10% excretion in part-II, indicates pernicious anemia.

Schilling test is now almost obsolete.

In healthy people and those whose dietary intake is not adequate, 10% and above excretion is seen in both parts of test. However, in cobalamin deficiency, only part-I is abnormal. In malabsorption, both part-I and part-II are abnormal.

Q11. What is the role of transcobalamin in B12 metabolism and how is it related to megaloblastic anemia?

Answer: Transcobalamins are carrier proteins for cobalamin (B12). There are 3 types of transcobalamins—TC-I, TC-II, and TC-III. TC-I binds 80% of the total serum B12. TC-II binds to 5–25% of B12 and is the main carrier protein crucial for delivery of B12 to tissues.

In absence of TC-II, severe megaloblastic anemia occurs but if serum B12 is tested, its levels are normal because most of the cobalamin tested in serum will detect cobalamin bound to TC-I.

In myeloproliferative disorders such as chronic myeloid leukemia, there is increase in TC-I and an increase in total serum B12 is noted. Congenital deficiency of TC-I and TC-III results in low serum B12. TC-I and TC-III are derived primarily from the specific granules in neutrophils [17].

**B12-TC-I complex is called Holohaptocorrin*

**The TCII-B12 complex is called Holotranscobalamin*

Q12. What are the steps in Vitamin B12 absorption?

Answer: The steps involved in absorption of B12 are as follows:

In stomach, B12 is separated from the food protein by pepsin and gastric acid. The released B12 binds to B12-binding proteins (R proteins) produced by the salivary glands (which blocks binding of IF to B12 in stomach).

In duodenum, the B12 is released from the R proteins by pancreatic enzymes, allowing IF to bind to the B12 in duodenum.

When the IF–cobalamin complex reaches terminal ileum, IF attaches to a specific receptor (cubilin) and helps B12 to get absorbed. Cobalamin enters the portal blood, attached to transcobalamin (TC-II), which is probably synthesized in the ileum [9, 18].

Q13. What is the mechanism of commonly encountered causes of megaloblastic anemia?

Answer: Megaloblastic changes and anemia are seen in a number of conditions with different mechanisms of action. Few examples of commonly encountered conditions are summarized [6, 19]:

(a) Pregnancy, lactation, hemolytic anemia, hyperthyroidism, and exfoliative dermatitis: mechanism-increased folate consumption.
(b) HIV infection and myelodysplastic disorders: Mechanism—direct DNA changes.
(c) Intestinal disorders like tropical sprue, inflammatory bowel disease, ileal resection, etc.: Mechanism—folate malabsorption.
(d) Pancreatic insufficiency: Mechanism—release of cobalamins from R-proteins doesn't occur, so cobalamins are not absorbed.
(e) Zollinger-Ellison syndrome: Mechanism—gastric acid in large quantity inactivates pancreatic enzymes.
(f) Fish tapeworm: Mechanism—competition for absorption with host for ingested cobalamin.
(g) Alcohol: Mechanism—reduced bioavailability of folate.
(h) Nitrous oxide exposure: Mechanism—oxidative inactivation of cobalamin.

Q14. What is the pathogenesis of anemia and neurological impairment in megaloblastic anemia?

Answer: Vitamin B12 and FA are coenzymes required for synthesis of thymidine (DNA). Deficiency of these vitamins results in defective maturation due to inadequate DNA synthesis resulting in impaired cell division which affects development of hemopoietic precursors. Mature red cell precursors are destroyed in bone marrow prior to entering the blood stream (intramedullary hemolysis) resulting in anemia. All nucleated cells will be morphologically abnormal. Intramedullary hemolysis results in low peripheral blood reticulocyte count. When there is deficiency of cobalamin, 5 methyltetrahydrofolate is not converted to tetrahydrofolate (which is required for DNA synthesis) and less of methionine is formed from homocysteine. Reduced active form of methionine S-adenosyl methionine (SAM) affects myelination of nerves. Similarly in absence of cobalamin, MMA is not converted to succinyl CoA. The MMA accumulates and enters the nerves and produces conduction defects resulting in neuropathy [19, 20]. The mechanism is explained in simplified way in Fig. 2.12.

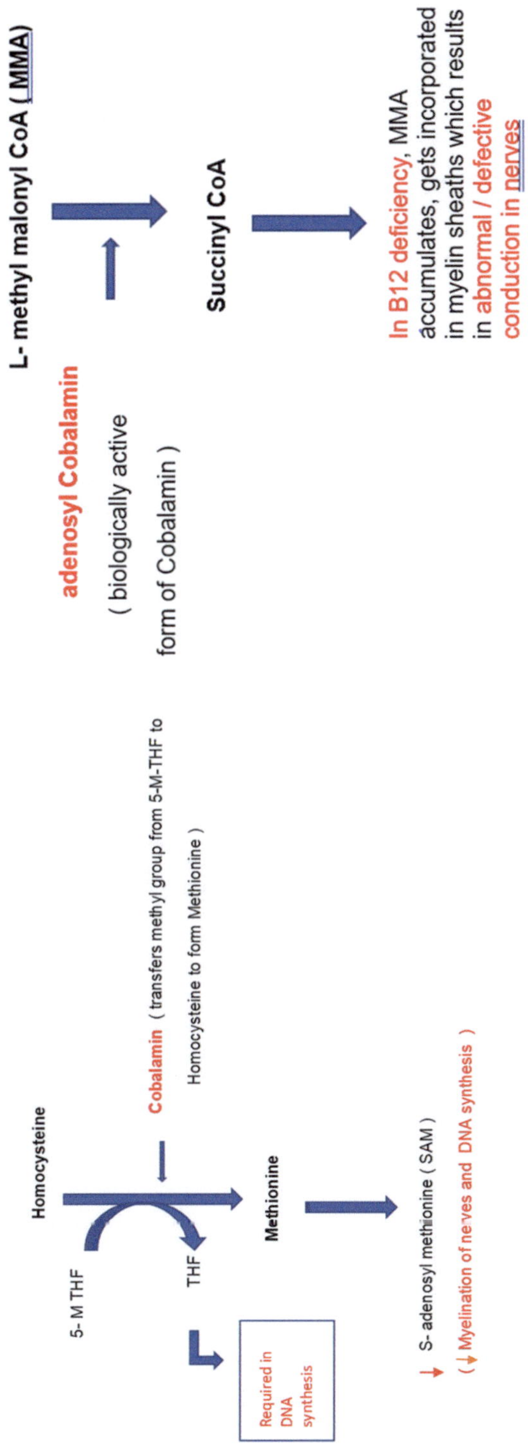

Fig. 2.12 Pathogenesis of neuropathy in megaloblastic anemia

2.2 Correlation of Results of Preliminary Investigations with Symptom and Signs in Megaloblastic Anemia

Q15. What are the main clinical symptoms of megaloblastic anemia and how do they corelate with our patient?

Answer: Depending on number of cell lines involved, the presentation can be with anemia, bicytopenia, or pancytopenia. Invariably, the patients have symptoms of anemia like fatigue, muscular weakness, loss of appetite and weight, pale skin, hair loss, numbness and tingling sensation in hand and feet, impaired memory, depression, recurrent headache, dizziness, tremors, and palpitations. If thrombocytopenia is present, symptoms of bleeding such as bruising, purpura, etc. are noted. In case of neutropenia, recurrent infections can occur. These are some of the clinical features of megaloblastic anemia [3].

Our patient had generalized weakness, lethargy, and dyspnea on exertion which are the indicators of anemia. She also had numbness and tingling in the feet and hands (stocking–glove distribution) suggesting neuropathy. Physical examination showed pallor and mild icterus, the later indicated possibility of hemolysis.

Q16. CBC shows pancytopenia. What is the cause of cytopenia in megaloblastic anemia?

Answer: Most commonly, megaloblastic anemia presents as macrocytic anemia without leukopenia or thrombocytopenia. However, severe megaloblastic anemia can produce pancytopenia. This is due to abnormal maturation of all nucleated hemopoietic precursor cells resulting from inadequate DNA synthesis. This culminates into intramedullary cell death and reflects as peripheral blood pancytopenia.

All nucleated cells will be morphologically abnormal. In addition, the compensatory high proliferative rate of the marrow requires adequate nutritional supply, particularly vitamin B12 and folic acid. So there is decreased production of all hemopoietic cells in deficiency states [3, 6, 10].

Q17. What are the causes of macrocytosis seen in peripheral blood?

Answer: Major causes of macrocytosis include:

Megaloblastic anemia (B12/FA deficiency).

Non-megaloblastic causes: Liver disease, hypothyroidism, multiple myeloma, MDS, aplastic anemia, acute leukemia, CDA (type II), myeloproliferative neoplasms, alcohol intake, and in conditions with increased reticulocytes [3, 6].

Drugs: Cyclophosphamide, hydroxyurea, MTX, azathioprine, 6MP, cladribine, cytosine arabinoside, 5 FU, pyrimethamine, sulfamethoxazole, trimethoprim, valacyclovir, triamterene, zidovudine, phenytoin, primidone, valproic acid, metformin nitrous oxide, sulfasalazine [21].

Q18. What are the causes of false positive macrocytosis?

Answer: Pre-analytical causes which can result in false elevations of the MCV (pseudo-macrocytosis) are agglutination of the red cells as in cold agglutinin disease, hyperglycemia, marked leukocytosis, or if the blood sample is left outside at room temperature for long time.

Analytical errors due to partial occlusion of aperture in automated analyzer may also result in false elevations [22, 23].

Q19. What is the cause of low reticulocyte count in megaloblastic anemia?
Answer: Intramedullary death of cells occurs in bone marrow due to lack of vit B12 and/or folic acid which are required for synthesis of DNA. So, lack of production results in inappropriately low reticulocyte count. It is called ineffective erythropoiesis.

Q20. This patient has high indirect bilirubin and LDH. How do they corelate with diagnosis of megaloblastic anemia?
Answer: High LDH and high indirect bilirubin are main indicators of ineffective erythropoiesis seen in megaloblastic anemia. High LDH results from accelerated turnover of bone marrow cells during which this enzyme is released from dividing and dying cells.

High indirect bilirubin comes from metabolism of hemoglobin released from dead cells. Other indicators which can be associated with ineffective erythropoiesis and hemolysis are reduced haptoglobins, raised urine urobilinogen, positive urine hemosiderin, and raised serum iron and ferritin.

Q21. What is the triad of symptoms and signs in pernicious anemia?
Answer: Megaloblastic anemia, glossitis (recurrent sore tongue and mouth with progressive atrophy of papillae), and CNS changes are considered classical triad of pernicious anemia [24].

Q22. In which conditions B12 is elevated in blood?
Answer: Myeloproliferative diseases especially chronic myeloid leukemia, myelosclerosis, polycythemia vera, hepatoma, increased granulocyte production (e.g., inflammatory bowel disease, liver abscess), and eosinophilia due to hypereosinophilic syndrome are some of the causes in which serum B12 is elevated in blood [25].

Q23. What are the main causes of folate deficiency? How is interpretation of red cell folate and serum folate correlate in megaloblastic anemia?
Answer: The main causes of folate deficiency are poor nutritional intake, chronic alcoholism, malabsorption due to celiac disease (Non tropical sprue), intestinal resection, increased demand in pregnancy, lactation, skin disorders, hemodialysis, hemoglobinopathies, certain drugs, and rare hereditary disorders like hereditary hyperhomocysteinemia.

Red cell folate is low both in B12 and folate deficiency. But serum folate may be normal/ increased in B12 deficiency [6, 18, 26].

Q 24. How is folate absorbed and transported?
Answer: Folate absorption is receptor mediated which occurs throughout the small intestine. Folate is transported in plasma—about one-third is loosely bound to albumin and two-thirds is unbound. In all body fluids (plasma, cerebrospinal fluid, milk, bile), folate is mainly in form of 5-methyl-THF [6, 18, 26].

Q25. What are some of the common diseases which produce folate deficiency?
Answer: Some common diseases which produce folate deficiency are as follows:

1. Chronic hemolytic anemia such as autoimmune hemolytic anemia, sickle cell anemia, and congenital spherocytosis.
2. Chronic inflammatory diseases, like exfoliative dermatitis, tuberculosis, Crohn's disease, psoriasis, rheumatoid arthritis, bacterial endocarditis, and chronic bacterial infections. These may cause deficiency by reducing the appetite and by increasing the demand for folate [6, 18, 26].

Q26. What are some of the richest sources of folates?
Answer: Spinach, lettuce, asparagus, lemons, broccoli, mushrooms, melons, liver, and banana are rich in folate. To prevent loss of folate, foods should not be cooked excessively and should not be diluted in large amount of water [26].

Q27. What additional diagnostic studies are indicated in suspected folate deficiency?
Answer: In addition to serum folate estimation, red cell folate may be done in presence of normal serum B12 levels. Plasma homocysteine level helps to confirm folate deficiency in special circumstances. Studies to detect malnutrition, sprue, chronic hemolysis, and exfoliative dermatitis are also recommended [6–8, 11, 12].

Q28. What are some of the rare tests which may be required in establishing diagnosis of megaloblastic anemia?
Answer: Anti-thyroid antibodies, tests for malabsorption including celiac disease (anti-gliadin and anti-endomysial), and endoscopy with gastric biopsy. Measurement of IF in gastric juice after maximal stimulation may be considered under appropriate circumstances (obsolete now) [6–8, 11, 12].

Q29. How do we monitor response to therapy in this patient?
Answer: A common treatment modality is giving Cobalamin (100–1000 μg) parenterally daily for 2 weeks, then weekly until the hematocrit value is normal. This is followed by maintenance injections monthly for whole life (depending on cause) [6–8, 11, 12, 26].

1. Reticulocytosis is seen within 3–5 days, and it peaks in 4–10 days.
2. The hemoglobin increment is approximately 1 g/dL each week. If it is not normalized within 2 months, other causes of anemia, such as iron deficiency, should be considered.
3. Leukocyte and platelets counts return to normal within days after therapy but hyper-segmented neutrophils may persist for 10–14 days.
4. Elevated levels of lactate dehydrogenase (LDH) and indirect bilirubin fall rapidly. If prolonged, it may indicate failure of therapy.
5. Serum potassium level should be monitored as it can fall during treatment.
6. Megaloblastic changes start getting reversed within 12 h after starting treatment. The bone marrow morphology becomes almost normal within 2–3 days.
7. During recovery, iron is also consumed quickly, it may produce iron deficiency.

2.3 Quick Information for Practicing Clinicians and Students

References [1–24]:

1. Anemia, bicytopenia, or pancytopenia with high MCV and inappropriately low reticulocyte response should raise suspicion of megaloblastic anemia. MCV more than 100 is highly suggestive of this entity.
2. Blood film should be examined in all cases for exclusion of pseudo-macrocytosis.
3. It is very important to distinguish between cobalamin and folate deficiencies since the treatment of the former with folate but not cobalamin can lead to the progression of neurological impairment.
4. Body stores of vitamin B12 are 2–3 mg enough to last 3–4 years.
5. Vitamin B12 is required in small amounts (1–2 μg daily) and since adequate B12 is found in all foods of animal origin, it is extremely rare for anyone other than a strict vegetarian to become B12 deficient on a dietary basis.
6. B12 deficiency is usually seen after 10–15 years of decreased intake. Folate deficiency is observed after 4 months of decreased intake.
7. The parietal cell antibodies are present in 90% of patients with pernicious anemia, but it can also found in thyroid disease and other autoimmune disorders. Anti-intrinsic factor antibodies (type I and II) are highly specific for pernicious anemia.
8. MMA is more sensitive for identifying non-anemic cobalamin deficiency patients than homocysteine.
9. Peripheral neuritis is common, and subacute combined degeneration is unique to B12 deficiency (it does not occur with folate deficiency).
10. If there is folic acid deficiency during pregnancy, neural tube defects can develop.

To acquire further knowledge on the subject, following sources are advised:

1. BCSH guidelines
2. Br Jr. Hematology
3. ASH education book
4. Blood
5. NEJM
6. Int Jr. Lab Hematology

References

1. Savage DG, Ogundipe A, Allen RH, Stabler SP, Lindenbaum J. Etiology and diagnostic evaluation of macrocytosis. Am J Med Sci. 2000;319(6):343–52.
2. Aslinia F, Mazza JJ, Yale SH. Megaloblastic anemia and other causes of macrocytosis. Clin Med Res. 2006;4(3):236–41.

3. Dali-Youcef N, Andres E. An update on cobalamin deficiency in adults. QJM. 2009;102(1):17–28.
4. Al Absi HS, Sacharow S, Al Zein N, et al. Hereditary orotic aciduria (HOA): a novel uridine-5-monophosphate synthase (*UMPS*) mutation. Mol Genet Metab Rep. 2021;26:100703. https://doi.org/10.1016/j.ymgmr.2020.100703.
5. Cakmakli HF, Torres RJ, Menendez A, et al. Macrocytic anemia in Lesch-Nyhan disease and its variants. Genet Med. 2019 Feb;21(2):353–60. https://doi.org/10.1038/s41436-018-0053-1.
6. Torrez M, Chabot-Richards D, Babu D, Lockhart E, Foucar K. How I investigate acquired megaloblastic anemia. Int J Lab Hematol. 2022;44:236–47.
7. Khera S, Pramanik SK, Patnaik SK. Transcobalamin deficiency: vitamin B_{12} deficiency with normal serum B_{12} levels. BMJ Case Rep. 2019;30:12.
8. Lindenbaum J, Savage DG, Stabler SP, Allen RH. Diagnosis of cobalamin deficiency: II. Relative sensitivities of serum cobalamin, methylmalonic acid, and total homocysteine concentrations. Am J Hematol. 1990;34(2):99–107.
9. Devalia V, Hamilton MS, Molloy AM, British Committee for Standards in Haematology. Guidelines for the diagnosis and treatment of cobalamin and folate disorders. Br J Haematol. 2014;166(4):496–513. https://doi.org/10.1111/bjh.12959.
10. Kundrapu S, Noguez J. Laboratory assessment of anemia. Adv Clin Chem. 2018;83:97–225.
11. Carmel R. Biomarkers of cobalamin (vitamin B-12) status in the epidemiologic setting: a critical overview of context, applications, and performance characteristics of cobalamin, methylmalonic acid, and holotranscobalamin II. Am J Clin Nutr. 2011;94:348S–58S.
12. Lee S-M, Jongwon O, Chun M-R, Lee S-Y. Methylmalonic acid and homocysteine as indicators of vitamin B12 deficiency in patients with gastric cancer after gastrectomy. Nutrients. 2019;11(2):450. https://doi.org/10.3390/nu11020450.
13. Varela-Moreiras G, Murphy MM, Scott JM. Cobalamin, folic acid, and homocysteine. Nutr Rev. 2009;67(1):S 69-72.
14. Höegenauer C, Hammer HF. Maldigestion and malabsorption. In: Feldman M, Friedman LS, Brandt LJ, editors. Sleisenger and Fordtran's gastrointestinal and liver disease. 11th ed. Philadelphia: Elsevier; 2021: chap 104.
15. Nickoloff E. Schilling test: physiologic basis for and use as a diagnostic test. Crit Rev Clin Lab Sci. 1988;26(4):263–76.
16. Zuckier LS, Chervu LR. Schilling evaluation of pernicious anemia: current status. J Nucl Med. 1984;25(9):1032–9.
17. Das B, Bhatia SY, Pal BM. Comparison of diagnostic accuracy of active B12 (holotranscobalamin) and total vitamin B12 (cobalamin) and verification of active B12 test. Ind J Med Biochem. 2020;24(1):25–31.
18. Stabler SP. Vitamin B12. In: Marriott BP, Birt DF, Stallings VA, Yates AA, editors. Present knowledge in nutrition. 11th ed. Washington, DC: Elsevier; 2020. p. 257–71.
19. Green R. Vitamin B12 deficiency from the perspective of a practicing hematologist. Blood. 2017;129(19):2603–11.
20. Hoffbrand AV, Jackson BF. Correction of the DNA synthesis defect in vitamin B12 deficiency by tetrahydrofolate: evidence in favour of the methyl-folate trap hypothesis as the cause of megaloblastic anaemia in vitamin B12 deficiency. Br J Haematol. 1993;83(4):643–7.
21. Hesdorffer CS, Longo DL. Drug-induced megaloblastic anemia. N Engl J Med. 2015;373(17):1649–58.
22. Van Duijnhoven HL, Treskes M. Marked interference of hyperglycemia in measurements of mean (red) cell volume by Technicon H analyzers. Clin Chem. 1996;42(1):76–80.
23. Francis DA, Francis JL, Roath OS. Improved assessment of haemoglobin and red cell indices in blood samples with high white cell counts. Med Lab Sci. 1985;42(3):285–6.
24. Mohamed M, Thio J, Thomas RS, Philips J. Pernicious anemia. BMJ. 2020;369:m1319.
25. Andrès E, Serraj K. The pathophysiology of elevated vitamin B12 in clinical practice. QJM. 2013;106(6):505–15.
26. Carmel R. How I treat cobalamin (vitamin B12) deficiency. Blood. 2008;112(6):2214–21. https://doi.org/10.1182/blood-2008-03-040253.

Chapter 3
Thalassemia Major

A one-and-a-half-year-old male child was referred to hematology OPD. The main complaints of the mother were the observation of pale skin and passing of high-colored urine by the child during the previous 1 month. She also complained about the child developing irritable behavior, being less active, and more lethargic in comparison to earlier phase of infancy. A followup by a general pediatrician had recorded slightly delayed developmental milestones. There was no history of recent illness, chronic disease, or drug intake. His appetite and bowel habits were normal. Child was receiving oral food supplements. The socio-economic status of the family was satisfactory. There was no significant family history except that the mother of the child revealed episodes of extreme weakness during menstrual period and rarely during episodes of infections. Both parents were never investigated for any hematological illness.

Examination of the child revealed pallor and mild jaundice. Mild hepatomegaly and splenomegaly were observed. Table 3.1 shows CBC result done at presentation.

A. Gupta, *Decision Making Through Problem Based Learning in Hematology*, https://doi.org/10.1007/978-981-99-8933-1_3

Table 3.1 CBC

CBC parameter	Patient's result	Reference range
WBC	7.24	3.7–10 × 10^9/L
RBC	5.7	4.2–5.4 × 10^{12}/L
HB	80	130–170 g/L
Hct	0.24	0.36–0.46 L/L
MCV	66.5	83–101 fL
MCH	22.2	27–32 pg
MCHC	333	315–345 g/L
RDW	20	11.6–14.6%
PLT	196	130–430 × 10^9/L
MPV	10	7–11 fL
Poly #	2.9	1.7–6 × 10^9/L
Lymp#	3.6	1–3 × 10^9/L
Mono#	0.6	0.2–1.0 × 10^9/L
EO#	0.1	0.02–0.5 × 10^9/L
BASO#	0	0.02–0.1 × 10^9/L
NRBC	0.4	0
RETIC%	4.9	0.5–1.5%
ESR	32	0–20 mm 1st h Westergren

3.1 Questions

Q1. Interpret the CBC result given above and suggest investigations for further evaluation in such case.

Answer: The CBC shows low values for hemoglobin, hematocrit, MCV, and MCH. The red cell count is slightly increased. RDW is slightly high. Nucleated red cells (NRBCs) are present. Reticulocyte percentage is raised. ESR is slightly high. These findings indicate microcytic hypochromic anemia with erythrocytosis and reticulocytosis.

Microcytic hypochromic red cells are seen in:

1. Iron deficiency anemia (IDA),
2. Thalassemia,
3. Sideroblastic anemia,
4. Anemia of chronic disorders,
5. Lead poisoning and
6. Some cases with dual deficiency anemia (combined iron and B_{12}/folic acid deficiency).

Reticulocytosis indicate rapid response of bone marrow as seen in hemolytic anemia, anemia due to blood loss, or when patients with nutritional deficiency receive supplements of vitamins. NRBCs are seen when there is a rapid release of immature red cells from bone marrow due to quick reduction of hemoglobin in peripheral blood and increased production of red cells as seen in hemolytic anemias.

Further evaluation of microcytic hypochromic anemia requires examination of peripheral blood film, estimation of serum iron, ferritin, transferrin, transferrin saturation, serum B_{12}, folic acid, and CRP. Also required are biochemical tests for functions of liver, kidney, thyroid, pancreas, and bone as well as routine examination of stools and urine. Presence of NRBCs and reticulocytosis indicates possibility of hemolytic anemia. To confirm the presence of hemolysis, estimation of LDH, indirect bilirubin, and haptoglobin should be included in biochemical tests.

Q2. Given are images from blood film (Figs. 3.1, 3.2, 3.3 and 3.4), serum levels of iron, ferritin, transferrin, percentage of transferrin saturation, serum B_{12}/folic acid, and CRP (Table 3.2), results of liver, kidney, thyroid, pancreas, and bone profiles (Table 3.3), and urine + stool examination (Table 3.4). Interpret these investigations and suggest provisional diagnosis. What further investigations should be done to confirm this provisional diagnosis?

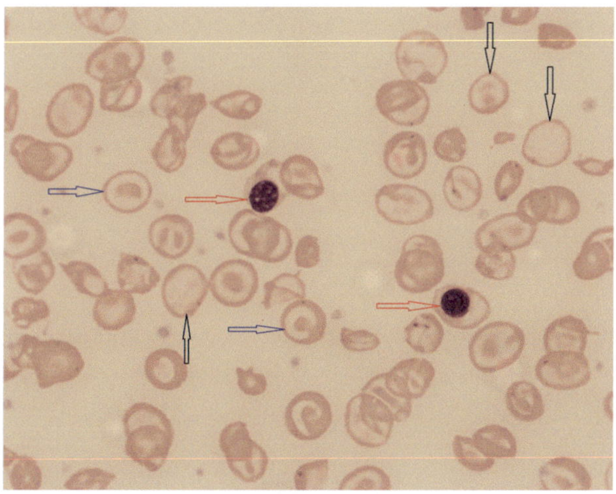

Fig. 3.1 PBF. Microcytic hypochromic red cells (black arrows), NRBCs (red arrows), and target cells (blue arrows). Leishman stain ×100

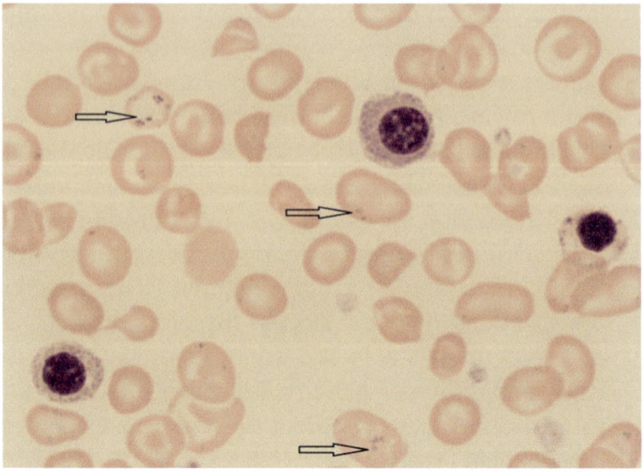

Fig. 3.2 PBF. Siderotic granules (black arrows). Leishman stain ×100

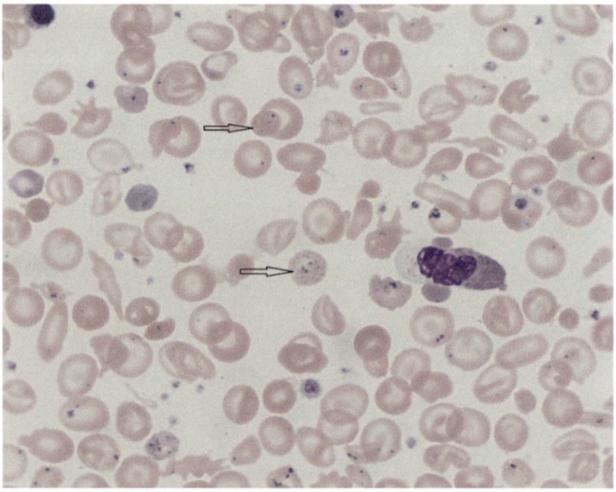

Fig. 3.3 PBF. Basophilic stippling (black arrows). Leishman stain ×100

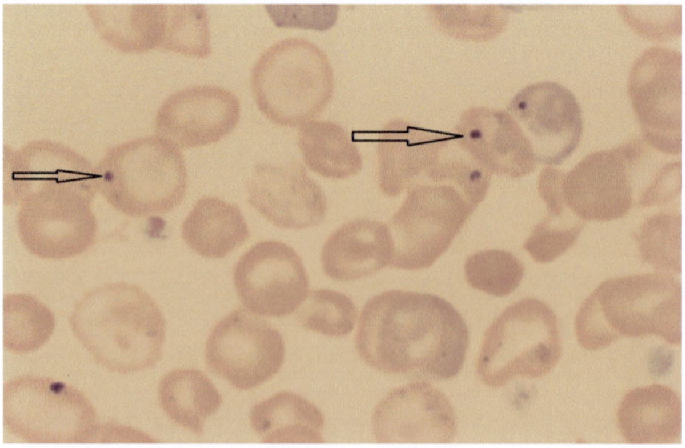

Fig. 3.4 PBF. Howell Jolly bodies (black arrows). Leishman stain ×100

Table 3.2 Serum iron profile, B_{12}, folic acid, and CRP

Test	Patient's result	Ref range
S. iron	35	11–31 μol/L
Transferrin	2.9	2.1–3.6 g/L
Trans. sat %	45	20–40%
Ferritin	450	11–307 ng/mL
S. B_{12}	665	150–700 pmol/L
S. folate	31.7	10–42 nmol/L
RBC folate	2554	1187–2854 nmol/L
CRP	3	0–10 mg/L

Table 3.3 Biochemical tests

Test	Patient's result	Ref range
Glu	4.5	3.9–6.1 mmol/L
Urea	2.9	2.5–6.6 mmol/L
Creat	90	60–120 μmol/L
Na+	139	136–146 mmol/L
K^+	4.5	3.7–5.0 mmol/L
Ca+	2.3	2.2–2.6 mmol/L
Mg+	1.0	0.08–1.1 mmol/L
T. Prot	68	63–80 mmol/L
Alb	25	35–47 mmol/L
Choles	2.5	1.5–5.2 mmol/L
TG	0.9	0.4–1.7 mmol/L
Urates	370	150–400 mmol/L
T Bil	38	3–20 μmol/L
D. Bil	5	0–5 μmol/L
I Bil	33	5–15 μmol/L
Alk Ph	41	26–88 IU/L
ALT	54	10–60 IU/L
AST	32	10–42 IU/L
GGT	20	7–64 IU/L
LDH	250	90–180 IU/L
Hapto	0.1	0.2–2.0 g/L
T4	10.6	7.8–16 pmol/L
TSH	3.99	0.27–4.2 μIU/ml
Amylase	20	28–100 IU/L
Lipase	30	0–160 U/L

Table 3.4 Urine and stool examination

Urine examination	Patient's result	Reference range
SG	1.020	1.005–1.030
Ph	6	5–7
Leu	Neg	Neg
Nit	Neg	Neg
Pro	Neg	Neg
Glu	Neg	Neg
Ket	Neg	Neg
Uro	Positive	Neg
Bil	Neg	Neg
Hemosiderin	Positive	Neg
Stool examination		
Occult blood	Neg	Neg
Ova/cysts	Neg	Neg

Answer: The blood films show anisopoikilocytosis, microcytic hypochromic red cells, target cells, few fragmented cells, Pappenheimer bodies (siderotic granules), basophilic stippling, and Howell jolly bodies. Serum iron, transferrin saturation, and ferritin are high. Vitamin B_{12} and folic acid are within normal limits. The biochemical tests show increased total bilirubin (with increased fraction of indirect bilirubin), raised values for LDH, and reduced haptoglobin. Examination of urine shows the presence of urobilinogen and hemosiderin. Examination of stools is normal.

Anemia with reticulocytosis, blood film findings, indirect hyperbilirubinemia, reduced haptoglobin, and presence of urobilinogen and hemosiderin in urine suggest hemolytic anemia. High values of serum iron, transferrin saturation, and ferritin negate the diagnosis of IDA, and a normal CRP excludes the possibility of chronic infections/inflammatory disorders. The remaining important possibilities are thalassemia and sideroblastic anemia. Since there is evidence of hemolysis in this patient, thalassemia becomes most likely possibility and should be confirmed first. Due to the presence of anisopoikilocytosis, rare possibilities like hereditary pyropoikilocytosis (HPP) and congenital dyserythropoietic anemia (CDA) should also be considered in this age group.

Next best investigation will be to exclude thalassemia by performing hemoglobin electrophoresis. Quantitation of hemoglobin A2 and hemoglobin F are important. Bone marrow examination is an invasive investigation. It should be done in the end if sideroblastic anemia and congenital dyserythropoietic anemia still remain possibilities.

Q3. Given is result of hemoglobin analysis (HPLC) done on Bio-Rad Variant-II (Fig. 3.5). Interpret the result and suggest final diagnosis.

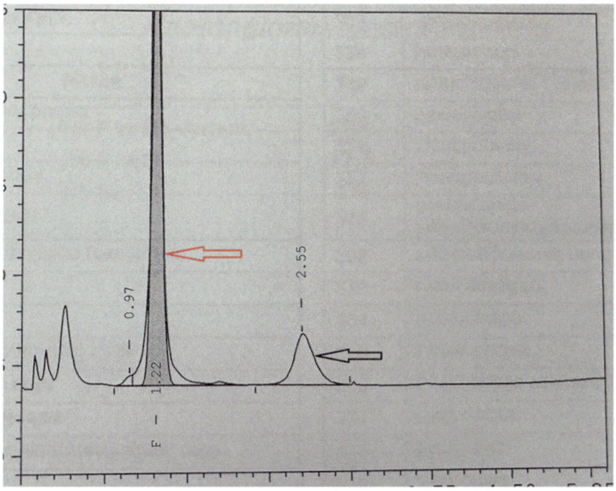

Fig. 3.5 HPLC (Bio-Rad Variant II), HbF: 95.5% (red arrow), Hb A2: 4.2% (black arrow)

Answer: The HPLC result of hemoglobin analysis shows peak in the region of HbF (quantified at 95.5%).

This confirms the final diagnosis of beta thalassemia major in this child.

Q4. Final diagnosis in this patient is based on high HbF. Which other conditions can have raised fetal hemoglobin?

Answer: HbF constitutes about 75–80% of total hemoglobin in neonates. It gradually decreases to reach around 1% by the age of 2 years. An increase up to 10% can be seen in normal pregnancies [1]. Table 3.5 shows common pathological conditions associated with high HbF.

A rough guide to interpret high HbF (expected values):

1. HbF between 90 and 100%: Beta thalassemia major, thalassemia intermedia, delta-beta thalassemia.
2. HbF between 2% and 10%: Beta thalassemia trait.
3. HbF between 20% and 30%: Hereditary persistence of fetal hemoglobin (HPFH).

Table 3.5 Pathological conditions with raised HbF

Conditions with hemoglobinopathy	Conditions without hemoglobinopathy
1. Beta thalassemia major 2. Delta-beta thalassemia 3. HPFH	1. Aplastic anemia 2. Hereditary spherocytosis 3. Acute leukemia 4. Myeloproliferative diseases as JMML 5. Medications as hydroxyurea/lenalidomide

Q5. How to differentiate beta thalassemia major from delta-beta thalassemia and HPFH?

Answer: In beta thalassemia major, HbF as well as Hb A2 are raised.

In delta/beta thalassemia, hemoglobin F will be high (5–15% if heterozygous and 100% if homozygous), but the hemoglobin A2 level will be absent/low or normal (<3.5%).

In HPFH, HbF is increased to 20–30% and Hb A2 levels are normal. It can be differentiated from delta-beta thalassemia by examining the distribution of hemoglobin F in red cells. Kleihauer-Betke acid elution test is useful. It shows a uniform (pancellular) distribution in HPFH, whereas it is heterogeneously distributed in delta-beta thalassemia. The distribution of hemoglobin F can also be assessed by flow cytometry using a fluorescence labeled anti-hemoglobin F antibody [2].

Q6. What additional investigations should be considered in such patients?

Answer:

1. X-ray of skull: In thalassemia major, due to severe hemolysis, the bone marrow responds by erythroid hyperplasia. There is expansion of bone marrow spaces, resulting in thinning of cortex and widening of diploic spaces. This gives the appearance of "hair on end" on plain X-rays of skull [3].

   Similarly, there is an expansion and prominence of maxillary bone resulting in typical appearance called "Chipmunk" facies [4].
2. Hb electrophoresis on the parent's blood: It can be helpful in assessing undiagnosed hemoglobinopathies in parents. It should be part of family screening (refer to genetics below).
3. Globin chain analysis: This test identifies impaired production of certain globin chains that confirm the diagnosis of thalassemia.
4. PCR assay techniques: The affected neonates and individuals with carrier state can be diagnosed accurately and quickly [5].

Q7. How is thalassemia classified?

Answer: Thalassemia is classified into beta, alfa, gamma, delta/beta, and gamma/delta/beta types. Of these, only alfa and beta thalassemias are common and will be discussed here [6].

Adult hemoglobin is composed of two alfa and two beta chains. These pair with each other in the ratio of 1:1. Thalassemia results from either reduced production or absence of one of these chains. Based on the involvement of beta or alfa globin chains, it is classified as beta or alfa thalassemia, respectively. Beta chain production is controlled by two genes on chromosome 11 and alfa chain production is controlled by four genes on chromosome 16 [7].

1. β-Thalassemia is classified into three categories:

   (a) β-Thalassemia trait (also called minor): when patients have one defective gene and one normal gene. Patients have mild anemia but usually do not require transfusion.

(b) β-Thalassemia intermedia: patients have two defective genes, but some β-globin production is still possible. In such patients transfusions may be required intermittently.
(c) β-Thalassemia major: Such patients have both defective genes resulting in no synthesis of β-globin chains. These patients have severe disease and require lifelong transfusion support.

If beta gene is completely abnormal with no potential of chain production, it is designated as $Beta^0$.

If beta gene is mutated but retains some potential of chain production, it is designated as $Beta^+$.

2. Alfa thalassemia is classified into four categories based on the number of genes involved. As there are four genes for alfa thalassemia, abnormality in one or more genes is designated as follows:

(a) Alfa thalassemia trait with one abnormal gene.
(b) Alfa thalassemia trait with two abnormal genes.
(c) Hb-H disease with three gene abnormalities.
(d) Hydrops fetalis with all four gene abnormalities.

In addition to these, beta thalassemia can be seen in association with other hemoglobinopathies such as HbC (HbC + beta Thal), Hb E (HbE + beta Thal), and HbS (HbS + beta Thal). Similarly, alfa thalassemia can also be seen in association of other hemoglobinopathies such as sickle cell anemia.

Q8. what is genotype-phenotype correlation in thalassemia?

Answer: The phenotypic expression of disease is based on alterations in genome. The clinical symptoms are also variable depending on the **combination** of defects in genes [8, 9].

A. Normal to mild phenotype: (1) alfa-Thal with one or two gene deletions (2) $beta^N$/Hemoglobin Lepore.
B. Mild to moderate phenotype: (1) $Beta^N/beta^0$ (2) $Beta^N/beta^+$.
C. Moderate to severe phenotype: (1) $Beta^0$/delta + beta (2) $Beta^+$/delta+beta (3) $Beta^+$/HbE.
D. Severe phenotype: (1) $Beta^0/beta^0$ (2) $Beta^+/beta^0$ (3) $Beta^+/beta^+$ (3) $beta^0$/Hb Lepore (4) $beta^0$/Hb E.

* $beta^N$—Normal gene; $Beta^+$—Some functional gene; $beta^o$—No production.

Q9. What is molecular basis of thalassemia? What is the pathophysiology of ineffective erythropoiesis in thalassemia?

Answer: Beta thalassemia results from point mutations in the genes. Deletions are not common. Mutation results in reduced or absent production of beta chains. If there is no beta globin chain production, the phenotype is $Beta^0$, and if reduced production is seen, the phenotype is labeled as $Beta^+$ [10].

Normally the alfa and beta chains pair with each other in the ratio of 1:1. In the absence or deficiency of beta chains, excess of alfa chains are formed, which accumulate in red cells and affect the functional properties of cells like stability and deformability. This results in cell death in bone marrow. This is the basis of ineffective erythropoiesis. This is also contributed by apoptosis (programmed cell death). In response to anemia, there is the production of erythropoietin which stimulates extramedullary hematopoiesis in the skull, thorax, and paraspinal region. Chronic anemia and hypoxia cause increased iron absorption from GIT. Excess of free iron is seen when saturation exceeds 70%. This free iron produces oxygen free radicals and further damage to organs [11].

3.2 Correlation of Results of Investigations with Symptoms and Signs in Thalassemia Major

Q10. Correlate symptoms and signs with the diagnosis of thalassemia in this patient. Also indicate how CBC parameters are helpful in this patient.

Answer: The observations of irritable behavior, less activity, lethargy, and pale skin are suggestive of anemia. Pallor, high-colored urine, and jaundice are suggestive of hemolytic anemia, and the presence of hepatosplenomegaly indicates extramedullary hematopoiesis and may point to the possibility of hereditary cause of hemolytic anemia.

The CBC shows high values for red cell count, low hemoglobin, Hct, MCV, and MCH. Nucleated red cells are present. Reticulocyte percentage is raised. Thus a microcytic hypochromic anemia with reticulocytosis, nucleated red cells, target cells, basophilic stippling, and Pappenheimer bodies suggest the diagnosis of thalassemia [12].

Q11. What are indicators of hemolysis in this patient?

Answer:

1. Reticulocytosis in CBC. It indicates the response of bone marrow due to peripheral reduction of hemoglobin. Causes of reticulocytosis are mainly hemolytic anemia, hemorrhage, and recovery from anemia treated with iron, B_{12}, or folic acid. These conditions may have to be excluded while investigating thalassemia.
2. Polychromasia, red cell fragments, and NRBCs in peripheral blood are strong indicators of hemolytic anemia.
3. High indirect bilirubin, decreased haptoglobin in serum, and the presence of urobilinogen and hemosiderin in urine confirm intravascular hemolysis.
4. Others indicators which can be tested for the presence of hemolysis are serum hemopexin (decreased) and serum potassium (high values in acute hemolysis) [13].

Q12. What is the cause of high values for ferritin, transferrin saturation, and iron in this patient?

Answer: Chronic anemia and hypoxia cause increased iron absorption from GIT. Iron stores (ferritin) are increased, and transferrin gets saturated. Once the saturation exceeds 70%, free iron is seen in serum. Excess of free iron is toxic as it induces oxygen free radical production. There is paradoxical suppression of hepcidin. Iron is also released from intramedullary hemolysis.

Q13. What are Pappenheimer bodies, and how these can be differentiated from basophilic stippling?

Answer: Pappenheimer bodies are also called siderocytes. They appear as abnormal basophilic granules inside red blood cells on a Romanowsky stain. They are composed of ferritin aggregates or phagosomes containing aggregated ferritin. Ribosomes are co-precipitated with the iron-containing organelles. They are usually observed in sideroblastic anemia, hemolytic anemia, lead poisoning, and following splenectomy.

In contrast to it, basophilic stippling is due to aggregation of ribosomes or ribosomal RNA indicating impaired protein synthesis. The granules are diffusely and evenly scattered throughout the cell. These are seen in thalassemia; megaloblastic anemia; myelodysplasia; heavy metal poisoning as lead, arsenic, and mercury poisoning; unstable hemoglobin; and in rare condition like hereditary pyrimidine 5′-nucleotidase deficiency [14].

Prussian blue stain (for iron) will stain the Pappenheimer bodies blue but not granules associated with basophilic stippling.

Q14. What is the type of hemolysis in thalassemia? What is the difference between intravascular and extravascular hemolysis?

Answer: Hemolysis in thalassemia is both intra- as well as extravascular in nature. The fragile red blood cell (RBC) precursors are destroyed in the bone marrow prior to release into the circulation. This is intramedullary hemolysis and is associated with a release of RBC lactate dehydrogenase (LDH). Hemoglobin released from damaged RBCs leads to an increase in indirect bilirubin and urobilinogen levels. Reticuloendothelial cells in liver and spleen remove abnormal poikilocytes from circulation, resulting in extravascular hemolysis. This also contributes to hepatosplenomegaly [15].

Few common differences between intravascular and extravascular hemolysis are summarized in Table 3.6.

Table 3.6 Differences between extravascular and intravascular hemolysis

Test	Extravascular hemolysis	Intravascular hemolysis
CBC	Decreased (−)	Decreased (−)
Hb	Increased (+++)	Increased (+++)
Reticulocyte%		
Blood film	Present (+++)	Absent/present (0/+)
Spherocytes	Present/absent (+/0)	Present (+++)
Schistocytes	Present (+++)	Present (+++)
Polychromasia		
Serum chemistry	Present (++)	Present (+++)
LDH	Decreased (−)	Absent (0)
Haptoglobin	Increased (++)	Increased (+++)
Unconjugated bilirubin	Normal/decreased	Decreased (−)
Methemalbumin	(N/−)	Increased (+++)
Plasma Hb	Normal/increased (N/+)	
Urine analysis:	Absent (0)	Present (++)
Hemoglobinuria	Absent (−)	Present (++)
Hemosiderinuria	Present (+)	Present (++)
Urinary urobilinogen		

Q15. This child will require regular transfusion support in future. What lab investigations may be required in the followup, and what complications can occur in such patients?

Answer: Complete RBC phenotypic assessment, a hepatitis screen, folic acid levels, and human leukocyte antigen (HLA) typing are recommended before initiation of blood transfusion therapy.

During the course of management, for the assessment of iron overload, liver iron concentration and cardiac T2* are usually required based on clinical situation. Serum levels of zinc, ascorbic acid, and folate are required to be estimated as their levels usually fall. Hepcidin measurement may be helpful in future [16].

Serum ferritin should be measured at least every 3 months. Levels >2000 ng/mL pose increased risk of complications. Liver function tests should be done at least every 6 months. T2*-based MRI or liver biopsy should be done every 1–2 years starting from the age of 5 years. Echocardiography and cardiac T2*-weighted MRI should be started by the age of 10 years. Ophthalmologic and audiologic testing are recommended every year, especially if on chelation therapy [17, 18].

Q16. How does alfa thalassemia present clinically. What is the pathophysiology of Hb-H disease?

Answer: The production of alfa chain is controlled by four genes on chromosome 16. Deletions of one gene does not produce symptoms and are, thus, clinically asymptomatic, and patients are silent carriers. Deletion of two genes is also a carrier state and clinically asymptomatic (Trait). Both are labeled as alfa thalassemia trait. For the classification of alfa thalassemia, refer to Q 7. A deficiency of α chain leads to the production of excess β chains, which form Hb Bart's and Hb H, respectively. These soluble tetramers do not precipitate in the bone marrow, and hence erythropoiesis is more effective than in β thalassemia [17, 19, 20].

Symptoms may be more overt in individuals that are pregnant, under stress, or malnourished. Deletion of three genes results in hemoglobin H disease. These patients have severe thalassemic signs and symptoms. Usually, they present within the first 2 years of life. Symptoms are of severe anemia such as pale and listless appearance, poor appetite, and dark urine. Deletion of all four genes results in hydrops fetalis. This is recognized by the finding of a hydropic infant with a severe anemia and a thalassemic blood picture. Presence of 80% or more of Hb Bart's on hemoglobin electrophoresis confirms the diagnosis [17, 19, 20].

In alfa thalassemia trait, the red cells are microcytic, hypochromic with elevated amount of Hb Bart's (usually 3–8%). Hemoglobin H disease can be diagnosed from the observation of Hb-H inclusions (also known as golf holes) on supravital staining of blood film. Leishman-stained (Fig. 3.6) and reticulin-stained

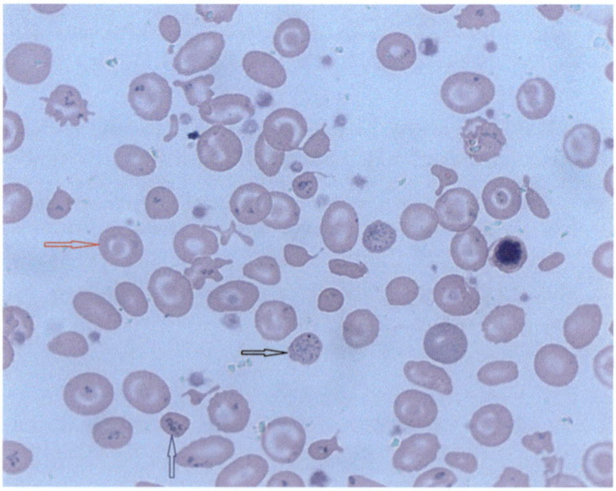

Fig. 3.6 PBF. Hemoglobin H disease. Basophilic stippling (black arrow), Pappenheimer bodies (blue arrow), target cells (red arrow). Leishman stain ×100

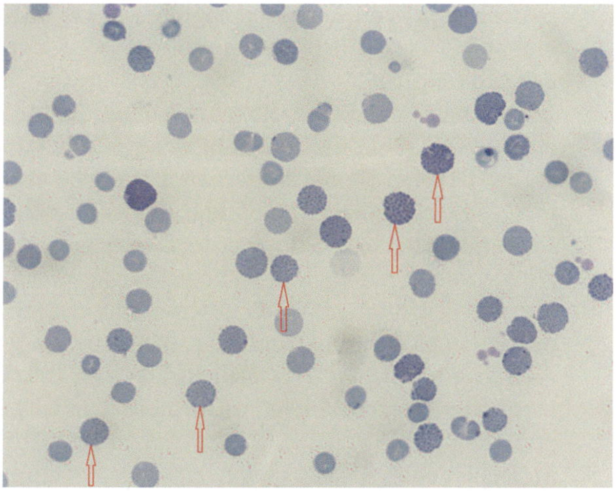

Fig. 3.7 PBF. Hemoglobin H inclusions (red arrows). New methylene blue stain ×100

(Fig. 3.7) blood film images from a patient of hemoglobin H disease are provided. DNA analysis tests are used to help confirm mutations in the alfa genes. DNA testing is not routinely done but is used to help confirm thalassemia [17, 19, 20].

3.3 Quick Information for Practicing Clinicians and Students

References[6, 7, 10–12, 17–22]:

1. IDA is the most common cause of microcytic hypochromic anemia. Rule out IDA first if CBC shows low MCV and MCH. To check iron status, iron profile should include serum iron, transferrin levels, total iron-binding capacity (TIBC)/transferrin saturation %, and ferritin.
2. Interpretation of red cell indices is helpful if the patient has thalassemia. Patients with low hemoglobin but disproportionally increased red cell count (erythrocytosis) and microcytosis are suspected to have thalassemia. If the MCV/RBC ratio is less than 13, further tests for thalassemia should be carried out. It is also known as Mentzer index.
3. If the MCV and MCH are low with normal iron levels, a provisional diagnosis of a thalassemia trait should be considered. Ferritin or zinc protoporphyrin (ZPP) values can help in differentiating IDA from thalassemia.
4. HPLC (Bio-Rad V-II or Sebia) should be done to measure hemoglobin A2 and hemoglobin F levels. Both of these are raised in beta thalassemia but not in alfa thalassemia.

5. In delta-beta thalassemia, hemoglobin F will be high (5–15%), but the hemoglobin A2 level will be low to normal (<3.5%) as a result of deletion of the delta chain gene.
6. In alfa thalassemia trait, HbA2 is reduced. HbA2 is also reduced in iron deficiency. So iron profile should be done in all cases if MCV, MCH, and MCHC are low. HPLC should be repeated after the correction of iron deficiency if there is no clear diagnosis of thalassemia at initial HPLC test.
7. Hb variants like HbS, HbC, or HbD may present with normal parameters and remain undetected by routine hematologic investigations.
8. For the detection of Hb-H disease (three gene deletions), examination of peripheral blood using supravital stains, such as Brilliant cresyl blue, is useful. As a rough guide, Hb-H inclusions less than 10% suggest alfa thalassemia trait (one or two gene deletions) while more than 10% suggest Hb-H disease (three gene deletions).
9. Molecular analysis may not be required to confirm the diagnosis of a beta thalassemia trait, but it is required to confirm alfa thalassemia carrier state.
10. Family screening should be done in all newly diagnosed cases.
11. Genetic screening for the confirmation and prognosis of offspring is highly recommended.
12. Tests for iron overload should be considered in all patients on treatment. Serum ferritin (every 3 months), liver function tests (every 6 months), liver iron content estimation (every 1–2 years), and ophthalmic and auditory function tests (every year) should be considered.
13. It has been observed that each 1 mg/g dry weight increase in liver iron content is associated with thrombosis, pulmonary hypertension, and hypogonadism in non-transfusion-dependent thalassemia.

To acquire further knowledge on the subject, following sources are advised:

1. BCSH guidelines
2. Br Jr. Hematology
3. ASH education book
4. Blood
5. NEJM
6. Int Jr. Lab Hematology

References

1. Amato A, Cappabianca MP, Perri M, Zaghis I, et al. Interpreting elevated fetal hemoglobin in pathology and health at the basic laboratory level: new and known c- gene mutations associated with hereditary persistence of fetal hemoglobin. Int Jnl Lab Hem. 2014;36:13–9.
2. Trent RJ, Webster B, Bowden DK, Gilbert A, Joy HP, et al. Complex phenotypes in the haemoglobinopathies: recommendations on screening and DNA testing. Pathology. 2006;38:507–19. https://doi.org/10.1080/00313020601027634).

3. Basu S, Kumar A. Hair-on-end appearance in radiograph of skull and facial bones in a case of beta thalassaemia. Br J Haematol. 2009;144:807.
4. Helmi N, Bashir M, Shireen A, Ahmed IM. Thalassemia review: features, dental considerations and management. Electron Physician. 2017;9(3):4003–8.
5. Origa R, Baldan A, Marsella M, Borgna-Pignatti C. A complicated disease: what can be done to manage thalassemia major more effectively? Expert Rev Hematol. 2015;8:851–62.
6. Munkongdee T, Chen P, Winichagoon P, Fucharoen S, Paiboonsukwong K. Update in laboratory diagnosis of thalassemia. Front Mol Biosci. 2020;7:74. https://doi.org/10.3389/fmolb.2020.00074.
7. Viprakasit V, Ekwattanakit S. Clinical classification, screening and diagnosis for thalassemia. Hematol Oncol Clin North Am. 2018;32(2):237–45. https://doi.org/10.1016/j.hoc.2017.11.006).
8. Weatherall DJ. Phenotype–genotype relationships in monogenic disease: lessons from the thalassemias. Nat Rev Genet. 2001;2:245–55.
9. Danjou F, Anni F, Galanello R. Beta-thalassemia: from genotype to phenotype. Haematologica. 2011;96(11):1573–5.
10. Lee JS, Cho SI, Park SS, et al. Molecular basis and diagnosis of thalassemia. Blood Res. 2021;56(Suppl 1):39–43.
11. Arthur WN, David GN. Pathophysiology and clinical manifestations of the β-Thalassemias. Cold Spring Harb Perspect Med. 2012;2(12):a011726. https://doi.org/10.1101/cshperspect.a011726.
12. Brancaleoni V, Di Pierro E, Motta I, Cappellini MD. Laboratory diagnosis of thalassemia. Int Jnl Lab Hem. 2016;38:32–40. https://doi.org/10.1111/ijlh.12527.
13. Barcellini W, Fattizzo B. Clinical applications of hemolytic markers in the differential diagnosis and management of hemolytic anemia. Dis Markers. 2015;2015:635670. https://doi.org/10.1155/2015/635670.
14. Cheson BD, Rom WN, Webber RC. Basophilic stippling of red blood cells: a nonspecific finding of multiple etiology. Am J Ind Med. 1984;5(4):327–34. https://doi.org/10.1002/ajim.4700050409.
15. Phillips J, Henderson AC. Hemolytic anemia: evaluation and differential diagnosis. Am Fam Physician. 2018;98(6):354–61.
16. Venée NT, Ellen BF, Maria V, et al. Guidelines for the standard monitoring of patients with thalassemia: report of the thalassemia longitudinal cohort. J Pediatr Hematol Oncol. 2015;37(3):e162–9. https://doi.org/10.1097/MPH.0000000000000307.
17. Sharma DC, Arya A, Kishor P. Overview on thalassemias: a review article. Med Res Chron. 2017;4(3):325–37.
18. Taher AT, Saliba AN. Iron overload in thalassemia: different organs at different rates. Hematology Am Soc Hematol Educ Program. 2017;8(1):265–71. https://doi.org/10.1182/asheducation-2017.1.265.
19. Mentzer WC. Differentiation of iron deficiency from thalassaemia trait. Lancet. 1973;1(7808):882. https://doi.org/10.1016/S0140-6736(73)91446-3.
20. Cornelis HL, Ahlem Achour A, Sandra JG, et al. The hemoglobinopathies, molecular disease mechanisms and diagnostics. Int J Lab Hematol. 2022;44(Suppl 1):28–36. https://doi.org/10.1111/ijlh.13885.
21. Farmakis D, Porter J, Taher A, et al. Thalassaemia International Federation guidelines for the management of transfusion-dependent thalassemia. Hemasphere. 2021;6(8):e732. https://doi.org/10.1097/HS9.0000000000000732.
22. Taher AT, Musallam KM, Wood JC, Cappellini MD. Magnetic resonance evaluation of hepatic and myocardial iron deposition in transfusion-independent thalassemia intermedia compared to regularly transfused thalassemia major patients. Am J Hematol. 2010;85(4):288–90.

Chapter 4
Thalassemia Trait

A 10-year-old girl was referred to hematology OPD with complaints of weakness, lethargy, and easy fatigability reported by her mother. There was no recent illness, history of chronic disease, or drug intake. Her appetite and bowel habits were normal. The socio-economic status was satisfactory. The mother of the child revealed similar episodes of weakness and lethargy during menstrual period and rarely excessive weakness during episodes of infections.

Examination of child revealed pallor without jaundice. No organomegaly was detected. There was nothing significant in general physical examination. Table 4.1 shows CBC result done at presentation.

Table 4.1 CBC

CBC parameter	Patient's result	Reference range
WBC	6.4	3.7–10 × 10^9/L
RBC	5.9	4.5–5.4 × 10^{12}/L
HB	9	130–170 g/L
Hct	0.27	0.36–0.46 L/L
MCV	62	83–101 fL
MCH	22	27–32 pg
MCHC	319	315–345 g/L
RDW	14.2	11.6–14.6%
PLT	256	130–430 × 10^9/L
MPV	10	7–11 fL
Poly #	2.1	1.7–6 × 10^9/L
Lymp#	2.9	1–3 × 10^9/L
Mono#	0.9	0.2–1.0 × 10^9/L
EO#	0.5	0.02–0.5 × 10^9/L
BASO#	0	0.02–0.1 × 10^9/L
RETIC%	2.9	0.5–1.5%
ESR	32	0–20 mm 1st h Westergren

A. Gupta, *Decision Making Through Problem Based Learning in Hematology*, https://doi.org/10.1007/978-981-99-8933-1_4

4.1 Questions

Q1. Interpret the CBC result given above and suggest investigations for further evaluation in such case

Answer: The CBC shows high values for red cell count and low values for hemoglobin, Hct, MCV, and MCH. Reticulocyte percentage is mildly raised. ESR is slightly high. Thus, there is microcytic hypochromic anemia with erythrocytosis and mild reticulocytosis. Microcytic hypochromic red cells are seen in the following conditions [1]:

1. Iron deficiency anemia (IDA),
2. Thalassemia,
3. Sideroblastic anemia,
4. Anemia of chronic disorders,
5. Lead poisoning, and
6. Some cases with dual deficiency anemia (combined iron and B_{12}/folic acid deficiency).

Reticulocytosis indicate rapid response of bone marrow or when patients with nutritional deficiency receive supplements of vitamins.

For evaluation of microcytic hypochromic anemia, further tests should include examination of peripheral blood film, estimation of serum iron, ferritin, transferrin, transferrin saturation, serum B_{12}, folic acid, and CRP. Also required are biochemical tests for functions of liver, kidney, thyroid, pancreas, and bone, as well as routine examination of stools and urine.

To confirm the presence of hemolysis, estimation of LDH, indirect bilirubin, and haptoglobin should be included in biochemical tests.

Q2. Given are images from blood film (Figs. 4.1 and 4.2), serum levels of iron, ferritin, transferrin, percentage of transferrin saturation (Table 4.2), results of liver, kidney, thyroid, pancreas, and bone profiles (Table 4.3), and urine + stool examination (Table 4.4). Interpret these results and suggest a provisional diagnosis. What further investigations should be done to exclude various possibilities?

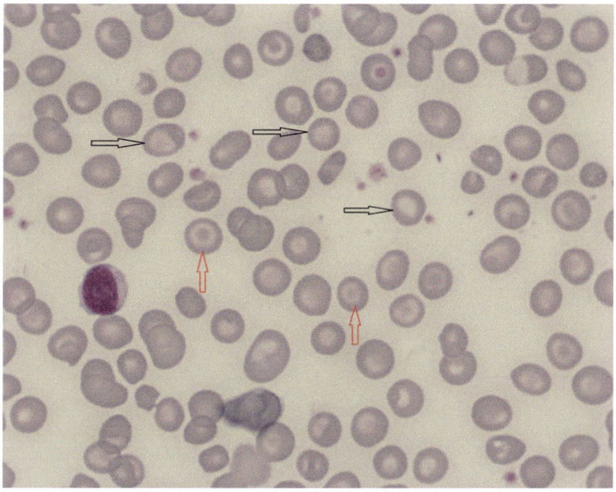

Fig. 4.1 PBF. Microcytic hypochromic cells (black arrows) and target cells (red arrows). Leisman stain ×100

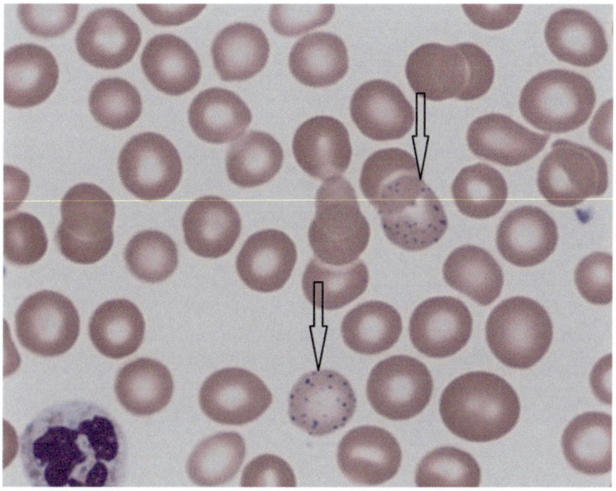

Fig. 4.2 PBF. Basophilic stippling (black arrows). Leishman stain ×100

Table 4.2 Serum iron profile, vitamin B_{12}, folate, and CRP

Test	Patient's result	Ref range
S. Iron	15	11–31 µmol/L
Transferrin	2.9	2.1–3.6 g/L
Trans. Sat%	25	20–40%
Ferritin	450	11–307 ng/mL
S. B_{12}	565	150–700 pmol/L
S. folate	31.7	10–42 nmol/L
RBC folate	2554	1187–2854 nmol/L
CRP	3	0–10 mg/L

Table 4.3 Biochemical tests

Test	Patient's result	Ref range
Glu	4.5	3.9–6.1 mmol/L
Urea	2.9	2.5–6.6 mmol/L
Creat	90	60–120 μmol/L
Na+	139	136–146 mmol/L
Ca+	2.3	2.2–2.6 mmol/L
Mg+	1.0	0.08–1.1 mmol/L
T. Prot	68	63–80 mmol/L
Alb	25	35–47 mmol/L
Choles	2.5	1.5–5.2 mmol/L
TG	0.9	0.4–1.7 mmol/L
Urates	370	150–400 mmol/L
T Bil	18	3–20 μmol/L
D. Bil	5	0–5 μmol/L
Alk Ph	41	26–88 IU/L
ALT	40	10–60 IU/L
AST	32	10–42 IU/L
GGT	20	7–64 IU/L
LDH	120	90–180 IU/L
Hapto	0.5	0.2–2.0 g/L
T4	10.6	7.8–16 pmol/L
TSH	3.99	0.27–4.2 μIU/ml
Amylase	20	28–100 IU/L
Lipase	30	0–160 U/L

Table 4.4 Urine and stool examination

Urine examination	Patient's result	Reference range
SG	1.020	1.005–1.030
Ph	6	5–7
Leu	Neg	Neg
Nit	Neg	Neg
Pro	Neg	Neg
Glu	Neg	Neg
Ket	Neg	Neg
Uro	Neg	Neg
Bil	Neg	Neg
Stool examination		
Occult blood	Neg	Neg
Ova/cysts	Neg	Neg

Answer: The blood film shows microcytic hypochromic red cells, target cells, and few cells with basophilic stippling. Serum iron, transferrin, transferrin saturation, B_{12}, and folic acid are within normal limits. Serum ferritin is increased. The biochemical tests and CRP are within normal range. Examination of urine and stools are also normal.

CBC findings of low Hb with disproportionately high red cell count, low MCV, low MCH, mild reticulocytosis, microcytic hypochromic red cells on blood film, along with target cells and basophilic stippling suggest a possibility of hemoglobinopathy, most likely thalassemia trait. For confirmation, hemoglobin analysis is required. Quantitation of hemoglobin A2 and hemoglobin F are important.

Q3. Given is the result from hemoglobin analysis by electrophoresis (Bio-Rad Variant II (Fig. 4.3)). Interpret the results and suggest final diagnosis.

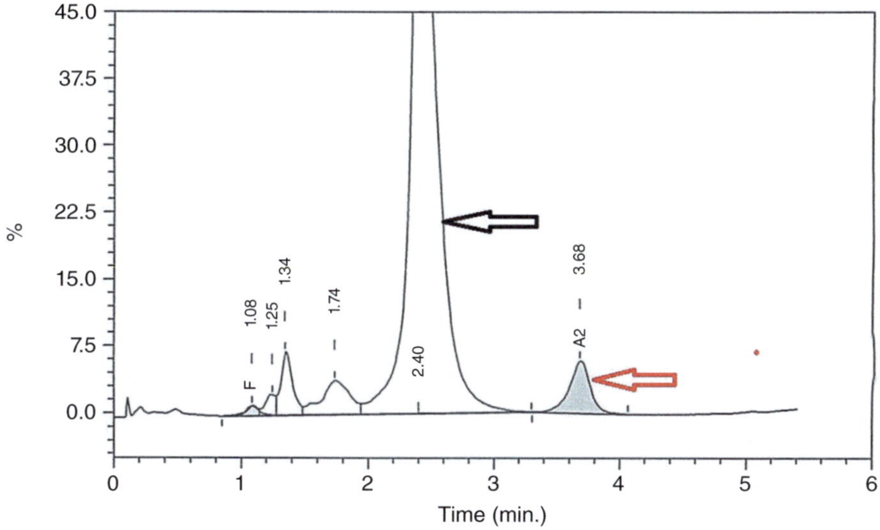

Fig. 4.3 HPLC–Bio-Rad Variant II. HbA (black arrow) 94.3%, HbA2 (red arrow) 4.5%

Answer: The high-performance liquid chromatography (HPLC) graph shows bands in the position of HB A and Hb A2 (quantified as 94.3% and 4.5% respectively). Levels of Hb F are within normal range. Presence of high HbA2 (more than normal of 3.5%) confirms diagnosis of beta thalassemia trait in this patient.

Q4. Based on the CBC result of microcytic hypochromic anemia with erythrocytosis, what differential diagnosis should be considered?

Answer: Microcytic hypochromic anemia with erythrocytosis also suggests alfa thalassemia trait. However, in alfa thalassemia trait, HbA2 is either normal or reduced. Beta thalassemia in some patients may be associated with iron deficiency. In such situation, iron deficiency reduces HbA2 [2], and the value of HbA2 may not be elevated above the upper limit of normal. So all patients who have iron deficiency and have normal HbA2 with abnormal indices (suggesting thalassemia) must undergo a repeat HPLC analysis after the correction of iron deficiency. Calculation of Mentzer index is helpful. An index of more than 13 suggests iron deficiency while below 13 indicates thalassemia [3]. In literature, the commonest cause mentioned for reduced HbA2 is the presence of alfa or delta chain variants, which are not recognized or quantified by routine diagnostic methods. The presence of delta thalassemia will also show reduced HbA2 [4].

In clinical practice, alfa thalassemia trait is a diagnosis by exclusion of other causes of anemia and observation of reduced HbA2. Genetic analysis may be considered for its confirmation. In beta thalassemia, diagnosis is usually done by HPLC, and genetic studies are not required unless it forms a part of genetic counseling for family screening or premarital assessment.

Q5. Which type of chains are found in normal hemoglobin? What is the pathophysiology of beta thalassemia trait?

Answer: Normal adult hemoglobin contains

1. Hemoglobin A: 95% to 98% (composed of two alpha and two beta chains).
2. Hemoglobin A2: 2% to 3% (composed of two alpha and two delta chains).
3. Hemoglobin F: <1% to absent (composed of two alpha and two gamma chains).

Adult hemoglobin is composed of two alfa and two beta chains. These pair with each other in the ratio of 1:1. Beta thalassemia results from either reduced production or the absence of beta chains.

Formation of beta chain is controlled by two genes. A point mutation in one beta gene results in either reduced or no production of beta chains. However, the second unaffected gene functions normally and produces sufficient beta chain protein. There will be relative excess of alpha chains. These excess alpha chains get precipitated on inner surface of red cell membrane and lead to only mild hemolysis and ineffective hematopoiesis. This results in milder form of beta thalassemia (trait/minor). Patient will have less clinical symptoms because the degree of anemia is not severe, although red blood cells are microcytic hypochromic. Thus, as a compensatory mechanism in such patients, there is an increased production of red cells that contains the delta chain (hemoglobin A2). So in electrophoresis, an increased amount of hemoglobin A2 fraction is seen [5, 6].

4.2 Correlation of investigations with symptoms and signs in Thalassemia Trait

Q6. Correlate symptoms, signs, and CBC parameters with the diagnosis of beta thalassemia trait in this patient.

Answer: This child has symptoms and signs of anemia (complaints of weakness, lethargy, easy fatigability, and pallor). Reduced hemoglobin with lowered values of MCV and MCH but disproportionally high red cells count is typical of thalassemia trait. Mildly raised reticulocyte count indicates bone marrow response to anemia. Normal RDW is also a feature of thalassemia trait which may help differentiating it from IDA (High RDW).

Q7. How CBC parameters are helpful in differentiating IDA from beta thalassemia trait?

Answer: A number of indices are mentioned in the literature which help in distinguishing IDA from beta thalassemia trait, such as the Mentzer index, Shine and Lal index, and Srivastava index. Out of all these, the Mentzer index provides the highest sensitivity (98.7%) and specificity (82.3%). Mentzer index (MCV/RBC) more than 13 indicates iron deficiency anemia and less than 13 indicates thalassemia [3, 7].

Q8. What is the cause of basophilic stippling and target cells in thalassemic trait patients?

Answer: Basophilic stippling is due to aggregation of ribosomes or ribosomal RNA indicating impaired protein synthesis. The granules are diffusely and evenly scattered throughout the cell. In addition to thalassemia, these are also seen in megaloblastic anemia, myelodysplasia, heavy metal poisoning (lead, arsenic, and mercury), unstable hemoglobin, and in rare condition like hereditary pyrimidine 5′-nucleotidase deficiency [8].

Target cells are formed when there is a disproportional increase in the ratio of surface membrane area to volume of red cells. In thalassemia, it is due to decreased volume resulting from reduced intracellular hemoglobin content. In addition to thalassemia, target cells are also seen in hemoglobinopathies as hemoglobin E and SC disease [9].

Q9. In addition to beta thalassemia trait, which other conditions are associated with raised Hb A2?

Answer: Raised Hb A2 can be seen in association with sickle cell trait, sickle cell anemia, unstable hemoglobin, and Hb S/beta^0 thalassemia. Thyrotoxicosis, megaloblastic anemia, HIV infection, and zidovudine therapy are also some of the acquired conditions which can result in mild increase in Hb A2 [4, 10].

Q10. Which other diseases can mimic signs and symptoms of beta thalassemia trait?

Answer: Beta thalassemia trait can be associated with other hemoglobinopathies such as hemoglobin E (HbE/beta thalassemia), hemoglobin C (HbC/beta thalassemia), and hemoglobin S (HbS/beta thalassemia). All these conditions can clinically resemble beta thalassemia. Analysis of hemoglobin through HPLC by Bio-Rad Variant II or Sebia capillary electrophoresis is used to identify such compound states. Sometimes, sideroblastic anemias and congenital dyserythropoietic anemias (CDA) can mimic beta thalassemia trait clinically [11].

Q11. Do all cases of beta thalassemia have raised Hb A2?

Answer: Very rarely beta thalassemia trait is not associated with elevated Hb A2 and may present with values within normal range. Also when beta thalassemia trait is associated with iron deficiency or alfa thalassemia, the overall value of HbA2 may not reach 3.5%. Under such circumstances, interpretation has to be done carefully, and a repeat HPLC after correction of iron deficiency (if IDA is suspected) or help of genetic studies may be required (if alfa thalassemia is thought to be the associated factor) [12].

Q12. What are commonly used methods for hemoglobin A2 estimation and analysis of globin chain?

Answer: Various methods have been used for the estimation of fractions of the hemoglobin A2. Some of these include cellulose acetate electrophoresis, micro-column chromatography, alkaline denaturation test, cation-exchange high-performance liquid chromatography (HPLC), capillary zone electrophoresis, flow cytometric methods, and beta globin gene mutational analysis by polymerase chain reaction, ARMS technique, etc. Most of these tests are available only in specialized laboratories [13–18].

Q13. What is the importance of detecting thalassemia trait?

Answer: Patients with thalassemia trait have lifelong mild anemia and usually do not require treatment. However, diagnosis is required because it is a carrier state, and genetic counseling is required to determine the risk of developing major disease in offsprings if both parents are carriers. Family screening is usually advised [19].

4.3 Quick Information for Practicing Clinicians and Students

References[1–19]:

1. IDA is the most common cause of microcytic hypochromic anemia. Rule out IDA first if CBC shows low MCV and MCH. To check iron status, iron profile should include serum iron, transferrin levels, total iron-binding capacity (TIBC)/transferrin saturation %, and ferritin.

2. Anemia, with disproportionately high red cell count, is a pointer to thalassemia trait. HPLC (Bio-Rad Variant II) or Sebia capillary electrophoresis is used to confirm the presence of high HbA2, which is a diagnostic of beta thalassemia trait.
3. Beta thalassemia in some patients may be associated with iron deficiency. The presence of iron deficiency reduces HbA2. In such case, HbA2 may not be elevated above the upper limit of normal. So all patients who have iron deficiency and have normal HbA2 with abnormal indices (suggesting thalassemia) must undergo a repeat HPLC analysis after the correction of iron deficiency. Alfa thalassemia and hereditary persistence of fetal hemoglobin are also associated with low HbA2.
4. High HbA2 is also seen when beta thalassemia trait occurs in association with sickle cell disease or unstable hemoglobin.
5. Calculation of Mentzer index is helpful in differentiating thalassemia trait from IDA. An index of more than 13 suggests iron deficiency while below 13 indicates thalassemia.
6. Alfa thalassemia trait with microcytic hypochromic anemia, reticulocytosis, and erythrocytosis is a diagnosis by exclusion of other causes of anemia and requires genetic studies for exact categorization of gene status.
7. Genetic analysis is not required for the diagnosis of beta thalassemia trait. It is considered necessary for the assessment of premarital status and as a part of family screening in cases of family planning.
8. Very rarely beta thalassemia trait is not associated with elevated Hb A2 and may present with values within normal range. However, red cell indices are abnormal. A clinical suspicion and family screening may be helpful.
9. In literature, the commonest cause mentioned for reduced HbA2 is presence of alfa or delta chain variants. These variants cannot be recognized or quantified by routine diagnostic methods.

To acquire further knowledge on the subject, following sources are advised:

1. BCSH guidelines
2. Br Jr. Hematology
3. ASH education book
4. Blood
5. NEJM
6. Int Jr. Lab Hematology

References

1. Ford J. Red blood cell morphology. Int J Lab Hematol. 2013;35(3):351–7. https://doi.org/10.1111/ijlh.12082.
2. Mosca A, Paleari R, Ivaldi G, Galanello R, Giordano PC. The role of haemoglobin A2 testing in the diagnosis of thalassaemias and related haemoglobinopathies. J Clin Pathol. 2009;62:13–7. https://doi.org/10.1136/jcp.2008.056945.

3. Mentzer WC. Differentiation of iron deficiency from thalassaemia trait. Lancet. 1973;1(7808):882. https://doi.org/10.1016/S0140-6736(73)91446-3.
4. Stephens AD, Angastiniotis M, Baysal E, et al. ICSH recommendations for the measurement of haemoglobin A_2. Int J Lab Hematol. 2012;34(1):1–13.
5. Lee JS, Cho SI, Park SS, et al. Molecular basis and diagnosis of thalassemia. Blood Res. 2021;56(Suppl 1):39–43.
6. Arthur WN, David GN. Pathophysiology and clinical manifestations of the β-thalassemias. Cold Spring Harb Perspect Med. 2012;2(12):a011726. https://doi.org/10.1101/cshperspect.a011726.
7. Okanv V, Cigiloglu A, Cifci S, Yilmaz M, Pehlivan M. Red cell indices and functions differentiating patients with the β-thalassaemia trait from those with iron deficiency anaemia. J Int Med Res. 2009;37:25–30.
8. Cheson BD, Rom WN, Webber RC. Basophilic stippling of red blood cells: a nonspecific finding of multiple etiology. Am J Ind Med. 1984;5(4):327–34. https://doi.org/10.1002/ajim.4700050409.
9. Bunyaratvej A, Sahaphong SV, Bhamarapravati N, Prawase WP. Quantitative changes of red blood cell shapes in relation to clinical features in *β*-thalassemia/HbE disease. Am J Clin Pathol. 1985;83(5):555–9. https://doi.org/10.1093/ajcp/83.5.555.
10. Steinberg MH, Rodgers GP. HbA_2: biology, clinical relevance and a possible target for ameliorating sickle cell disease. Br J Haematol. 2015;170(6):781–7.
11. Saha S, Ghosh S, Basu K, Bhattacharyya M. Prevalence of β-haemoglobinopathies in Eastern India and development of a novel formula for carrier detection. J Hematopathol. 2020;13:159–64.
12. Maria SF. The importance of hemoglobin A2 determination. Rev Bras Hematol Hemoter. 2015;37(5):287–9.
13. Sanguansermsri T, Thanarattanakorn P, Steger HF, Tongsong T, Chanprapaph P, Wanpirak C, et al. Prenatal diagnosis of beta-thalassemia major by high-performance liquid chromatography analysis of hemoglobins in fetal blood samples. Hemoglobin. 2001;25(1):19–27.
14. Pornprasert S, Kongthai K, Waneesorn J, Jaiping K, Treesuwan K. Development of control material for hemoglobin analysis. Clin Chem Lab Med. 2011;50(2):351–6.
15. Tayapiwatana C, Kuntaruk S, Tatu T, Chiampanichayakul S, Munkongdee T, Winichagoon P, et al. Simple method for screening of alpha-thalassaemia 1 carriers. Int J Hematol. 2009;89(5):559–67.
16. Thorpe SJ, Thein SL, Sampietro M, Craig JE, Mahon B, Huehns ER. Immunochemical estimation of haemoglobin types in red blood cells by FACS analysis. Br J Haematol. 1994;87(1):125–32.
17. Jenkins MA, Hendy J, Smith IL. Evaluation of hemoglobin A2 quantitation assay and hemoglobin variant screening by capillary electrophoresis. J Capillary Electrophor. 1997;4(3):137–43.
18. Tatu T, Kiewkarnkha T, Khuntarak S, Khamrin S, Suwannasin S, Kasinrerk W. Screening for co-existence of alpha-thalassemia in beta-thalassemia and in HbE heterozygotes via an enzyme-linked immunosorbent assay for Hb Bart's and embryonic zeta-globin chain. Int J Hematol. 2012;95(4):386–93.
19. Giambona A, Passarello C, Renda D, Maggio A. The significance of the hemoglobin A(2) value in screening for hemoglobinopathies. Clin Biochem. 2009;42(18):1786–96.

Chapter 5
Anemia of Chronic Disorders

A 47-year-old female patient was referred to hematology OPD with complaints of tiredness, dizziness, easy fatigability, and mild dyspnea on exertion of 2-month duration. She was also experiencing episodes of palpitations on brisk walking during this time. About 3 months back, she was diagnosed to have systemic lupus erythematosus (SLE), based on clinical symptoms of facial rash, mouth ulcers, joint pains, myalgias, and symptoms of anemia supported by laboratory investigations. She had been taking oral steroids which were temporarily stopped due to an increase in blood glucose level and mild hypertension. There was no history of bleeding or recent infection. Examination revealed pallor but no jaundice. Mild malar flush was observed. There was no lymphadenopathy or palpable organomegaly. Table 5.1 shows results of CBC done at presentation:

Table 5.1 CBC

CBC parameter	Patient's result	Reference range
WBC	5.6	3.7–10 × 10^9/L
RBC	3.08	4.5–5.4 × 10^{12}/L
HB	80	130–170 g/L
Hct	0.25	0.36–0.46 L/L
MCV	79.5	83–101 fL
MCH	25	27–32 pg
MCHC	315	315–345 g/L
RDW	18.2	11.6–14.6%
PLT	256	130–430 × 10^9/L
MPV	10	7–11 fL
Poly #	2.1	1.7–6 × 10^9/L
Lymp#	1.9	1–3 x10^9/L
Mono#	0.9	0.2–1.0 × 10^9/L
EO#	0.5	0.02–0.5 × 10^9/L
BASO#	0	0.02–0.1 × 10^9/L
RETIC%	0.5	0.5–1.5%
ESR	65	0–20 mm 1st h Westergren

A. Gupta, *Decision Making Through Problem Based Learning in Hematology*, https://doi.org/10.1007/978-981-99-8933-1_5

5.1 Questions

Q1. Interpret the CBC result given above and suggest investigations for further evaluation in such case.

Answer: The CBC shows low values for red cell count, hemoglobin, hematocrit (hct), and borderline decrease in MCV, MCH, and MCHC. The reticulocyte count percentage is on lower side of normal value. RDW and ESR are high.

So there is mild microcytic hypochromic anemia [1].

Microcytic hypochromic red cells are seen in the following conditions:

1. Iron deficiency anemia (IDA),
2. Thalassemia,
3. Sideroblastic anemia,
4. Anemia of chronic disorders,
5. Lead poisoning, and
6. Some cases with dual deficiency anemia (combined iron and B_{12}/folic acid deficiency).

The anemia in this patient is associated with reduced response of bone marrow for the production of red cells as indicated by reticulocyte count, which is on lower side of normal.

Based on the causes mentioned above, next best test should be the examination of peripheral blood film. Also estimation of serum iron, ferritin, transferrin, transferrin saturation, serum B_{12}, folic acid, and CRP should be done. In addition biochemical tests for functions of liver, kidney, thyroid, pancreas, and bone are also required. Routine stools and urine examination are also recommended.

Q2. Given are images from blood film (Figs. 5.1 and 5.2), serum levels of iron, ferritin, transferrin, percentage of transferrin saturation (Table 5.2), results of liver, kidney, thyroid, pancreas, and bone profiles (Table 5.3), and urine + stool examination (Table 5.4). Interpret these investigations and suggest a provisional diagnosis. What further investigations should be done to exclude various possibilities?

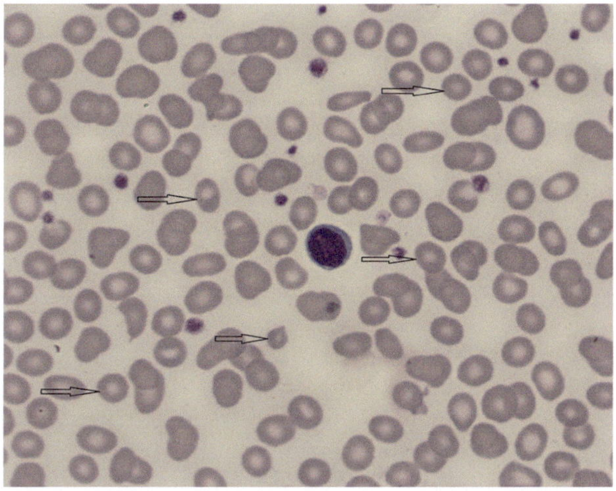

Fig. 5.1 PBF. Microcytic red cells (arrows). Leishman stain ×100

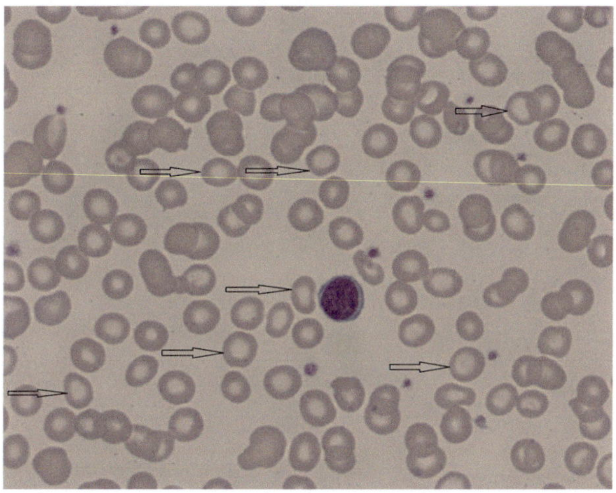

Fig. 5.2 PBF. Microcytic hypochromic cells (arrows) Leishman stain ×100

Table 5.2 Serum iron profile, vitamin B_{12}, folate, and CRP

Test	Patient's result	Ref range
S. iron	9	11–31 μmol/L
Transferrin	0.7	2.1–3.6 g/L
Trans. sat%	55.8	20–40%
Ferritin	521	11–307 ng/mL
S. B_{12}	565	150–700 pmol/L
S. folate	31.7	10–42 nmol/L
RBC folate	2554	1187–2854 nmol/L
CRP	79.5	0–10 mg/L

Table 5.3 Biochemical tests

Test	Patient's result	Ref range
Glu	6.7	3.9–6.1 mmol/L
Urea	2.9	2.5–6.6 mmol/L
Creat	90	60–120 μmol/L
Na+	139	136–146 mmol/L
Ca+	2.3	2.2–2.6 mmol/L
Mg+	1.0	0.08–1.1 mmol/L
T. Prot	68	63–80 mmol/L
Alb	25	35–47 mmol/L
Choles	2.5	1.5–5.2 mmol/L
TG	0.9	0.4–1.7 mmol/L
Urates	370	150–400 mmol/L
T Bil	18.1	3–20 μmol/L
D. Bil	5	0–5 μmol/L
Alk Ph	41	26–88 IU/L
ALT	29	10–60 IU/L
AST	32	10–42 IU/L
GGT	20	7–64 IU/L
LDH	210	90–180 IU/L
Hapto	0.5	0.2–2.0 g/L
T4	10.6	7.8–16 pmol/L
TSH	3.99	0.27–4.2 ulU/ml
Amylase	20	28–100 IU/L
Lipase	30	0–160 U/L

Table 5.4 Urine and stool examination

Urine examination	Patient's result	Reference range
SG	1.020	1.005–1.030
Ph	6	5–7
Leu	Neg	Neg
Nit	Neg	Neg
Pro	0.1 g/L	Neg
Glu	Neg	Neg
Ket	Neg	Neg
Uro	Neg	Neg
Bil	Neg	Neg
Stool examination		
Occult blood	Neg	Neg
Ova/cysts	Neg	Neg

Answer: The peripheral blood films show two populations of red cells. One is microcytic (long arrows) and the other is microcytic hypochromic (short arrows). These are seen along with normocytic normochromic red cells. It is also referred to as dimorphic population. A rough visual assessment of microcytosis on blood films can be done by comparing the size of red cell with the size of lymphocytes, and for hypochromia, central pale area should be more than one-third of the total diameter of the red cell.

The value for serum iron and transferrin are low and transferrin saturation is high. Ferritin level is also high. Serum folate and B_{12} levels are within normal range. CRP is elevated.

The blood glucose level is slightly high. Albumin is reduced. LDH shows borderline increase. Rest of the results for kidney, liver, thyroid, bone, and pancreatic functions are within normal range.

Urine examination shows mild proteinuria. There is no hematuria. The stool examination does not show occult or fresh blood.

So, a mildly microcytic hypochromic anemia, with dimorphic population of red cells, high ESR and CRP, low serum iron and transferrin, high transferrin saturation, and elevated ferritin, suggests anemia due to chronic disorder. The results of the serum iron, transferrin saturation, and high ferritin exclude the possibility of pure iron deficiency, and normal values for serum B_{12} and folate make the diagnosis of dual deficiency least likely. Red cell count is not raised, and there are no target cells or basophilic stippling. This excludes the possibility of thalassemia trait in this patient.

As the history of the patient indicates, she developed anemia few months after SLE was diagnosed. So this is most likely a cause of anemia in this case. She was being treated with steroids but could not continue with treatment as she had developed side effects. However, SLE needs to be reconfirmed for its activity.

Further evaluation will require screening panel for autoimmune diseases to check for disease activity. As the iron stores are high in blood (high ferritin), bone marrow examination to assess iron stores (hemosiderin) may be considered as part of evaluation for sideroblastic anemia.

Q3. Given are results of immunology screen and DCT (Table 5.5), and images from bone marrow aspirate (Figs. 5.3, 5.4, and 5.5). Interpret the results and suggest final diagnosis.

Table 5.5 Immunological tests and DCT

Test	Patient's result	Ref range
Anti ds-DNA antibody	More than 200	0–20 Iu/mL
ANA screen	Positive	Negative
ANA pattern	Homogeneous	Negative
ANA titer	1:160	Negative
Sm B	Positive	Negative
RNP A and C	Positive	Negative
SS-A	Negative	Negative
SS-B	Negative	Negative
Scl-70	Negative	Negative
Jo-1	Negative	Negative
Ribosomal P	Negative	Negative
Histone	Negative	Negative
MPO Ab	Negative	Negative
Proteinase Ab	Negative	Negative
DCT	Positive	Negative

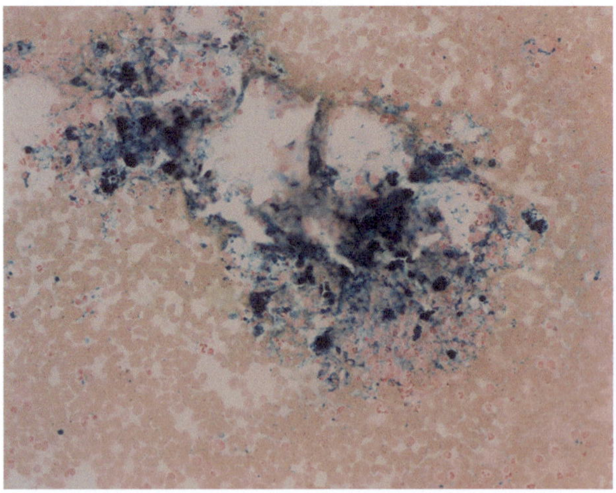

Fig. 5.3 BM aspirate. Increased iron stores. Prussian blue stain ×40

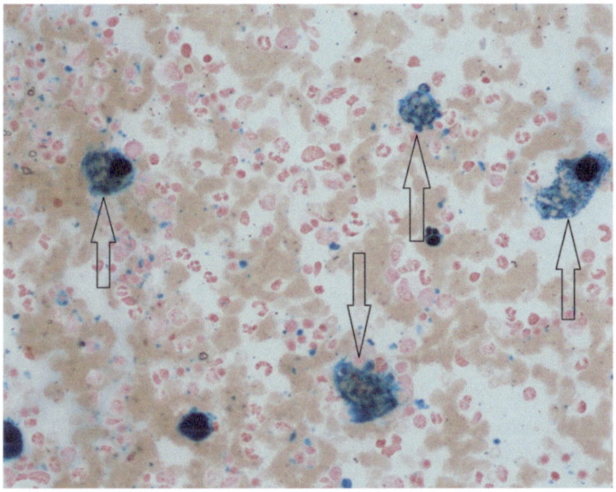

Fig. 5.4 BM aspirate. Hemosiderin-laden macrophages (arrows). Prussian blue stain ×40

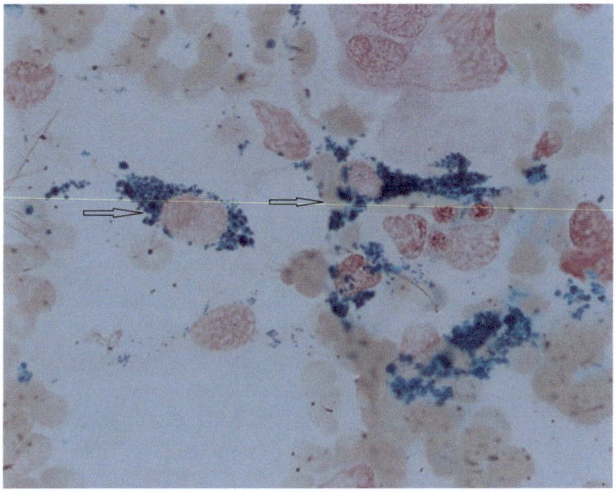

Fig. 5.5 BM aspirate. Hemosiderin-laden macrophages (arrows) from another patient of ACD. Prussian blue stain ×100

Answer: Immunological tests show positive results for ds-DNA, ANA, Sm B, and RNP antibodies. Direct Coombs test (DCT) is positive. These findings in association with high CRP and ESR indicate an active SLE. Bone marrow aspirate smears stained with Prussian blue stain show increased iron stores and hemosiderin-laden macrophages. No sideroblasts are seen. Thus, the possibility of sideroblastic anemia is also ruled out.

So, in this patient with active SLE, chronic inflammatory state is most likely a cause of anemia. Presence of proteinuria with resultant hypoalbuminemia (also a marker of disease activity) may have been an additional factor for anemia. Borderline increase in LDH and low positivity of direct Coombs test indicates an element of mild hemolysis. But main cause of anemia is due to chronic inflammatory state, and thus, a final diagnosis of anemia of chronic disease (ACD) due to chronic inflammation secondary to SLE is confirmed.

Q4. what are common diseases associated with anemia of chronic diseases?

Answer: Chronic infections and chronic inflammatory conditions result in ACD. Examples of chronic infections are osteomyelitis, bacterial endocarditis, tuberculosis, bronchiectasis, and chronic urinary tract infections. Examples of chronic inflammatory states are autoimmune diseases like systemic lupus erythematosus, rheumatoid arthritis, scleroderma, polymyalgia rheumatica, inflammatory bowel diseases, hepatitis, and HIV/AIDS. In addition, chronic renal failure, chronic liver disease, chronic heart failure, and cancers are important causes of ACD [2–4].

Q5. What are possible causes of anemia in a patient who is diagnosed with SLE?

Answer: ACD is the commonest cause of anemia in SLE and other associated immunological disorders. Other causes include blood loss (steroid induced), autoimmune hemolytic anemia, and nutritional deficiencies. In addition, urinary blood loss due to renal involvement, development of myelofibrosis, DIC, and red cell aplasia can produce anemia. Rarely, concomitant infections, hypersplenism, and myelodysplasia may accompany SLE resulting in anemia [5].

Q6. What is the pathogenesis of anemia in ACD?

Answer: During inflammations and infections, inflammatory cytokines such as interleukin 1 (IL-1), tumor necrosis factor (TNF-alfa), and interferons-beta are produced. These suppress erythropoiesis by the blunting response of erythropoietin and also through its decreased production. These cytokines act on Kupffer cells of liver to secrete IL-6, which stimulates hepcidin secretion from hepatocytes. Hepcidin blocks release of iron from macrophages and inhibits transfer of iron to erythroblasts in bone marrow also. It also impedes iron absorption from intestines. This results in decreased serum iron. In autoimmune disorders, there can be decreased survival of red cells due to the adsorption of immune complexes on the surface of red cells, leading to phagocytosis by macrophages of the reticuloendothelial system [5].

Q7. What are acute phase reactants and markers of chronic inflammation?

Answer: Acute phase reactants are inflammatory markers which are produced mostly from liver and indicate acute and chronic inflammatory states. Commonly measured markers are CRP, ferritin, fibrinogen, and haptoglobin. Indicators of chronic inflammation are hypoalbuminemia, persistent leukocytosis, and high ESR [6]. Some acute phase reactants which are not readily available and rarely assessed are IL-6, TNF-alfa, procalcitonin, amyloid A, alfa1-acid glycoprotein, ceruloplasmin, and hepcidin [7].

Q8. ACD can show microcytic hypochromic anemia or, in many cases, normocytic normochromic anemia. What are causes of normocytic normochromic anemia?

Answer: Causes of normocytic normochromic anemia include [8, 9]:

(a) *Decreased production from marrow (will have low reticulocyte count):* Chronic pathological conditions (such as chronic inflammations, neoplastic pathologies, and infections), chronic renal failure, chronic liver disease, endocrinopathies, marrow infiltration, and hypoplastic anemias.

(b) Increased destruction (will have increased reticulocytes with normal marrow):

1. Red cell defects: Defects of red cell membrane, enzymes, or hemoglobin.
2. Without any defect of red cells (defects lies outside red cells): Autoimmune hemolytic anemia and micro-angiopathic hemolytic anemia (DIC/TTP/HUS).

(c) *Sequestration: splenomegaly.*

(d) *Hemorrhage.*

Autoimmune disorders can show both low reticulocyte count (when autoantibodies are suppressing/destroying bone marrow cells also) and high reticulocyte count (when there is only peripheral blood destruction).

Q9. Why ESR is high in ACD?

Answer: Under normal conditions, RBCs have negative charge on their outer surface; that is why they don't stick to each other in circulation. Many plasma proteins have positive charge, and when their concentration increases in plasma, they neutralize the negative surface charge of the RBCs. This allows red cells to stick together in the form of stacks of coin; this is referred to as rouleaux formation. An increase in plasma proteins (seen in almost all conditions resulting in ACD) will increase rouleaux formation, which allows the RBCs to settle at a faster rate, thus increasing the ESR [10].

Q10. Which factors can alter the severity of anemia in ACD?

Answer: The anemia in ACD is normocytic normochromic or mildly microcytic hypochromic. Dimorphic appearance of red cells is a helpful pointer. However, the pathological changes occurring in primary disease producing ACD will change the appearance of typical ACD. Few example are [11, 12]:

(a) If associated with coexistent IDA due to bleeding: increased number of microcytic hypochromic cells may be noted resembling IDA.

(b) If associated with renal failure: reduced erythropoietin production with more normocytic cells.

(c) Specific medications as antiplatelet drugs: subclinical bleeding leading to IDA.

(d) Dietary habits: IDA or multivitamin deficiencies.

(e) Hematological malignancies: dyserythropoiesis.

(f) Viral infections as parvovirus, CMV, EBV, HIV, or HCV: impaired red cell proliferation.

Q11. How is ACD differentiated from IDA?

Answer: Red cell population in pure ACD is predominantly normocytic, mildly microcytic, or a mixture of normocytic and hypochromic cells (dimorphic population). IDA has microcytic hypochromic population of red cells. Both have reduced reticulocyte count. Transferrin levels are reduced in ACD but normal in IDA. Transferrin saturation is normal to high in ACD but reduced in IDA. Ferritin is high in ACD (also an acute phase reactant) but reduced in IDA [13].

Transferrin saturation is low initially, but subsequently as the quantity of transferrin decreases, its saturation increases till iron deficiency also develops.

Q12. Microcytic hypochromic cells are seen in ACD, IDA, and thalassemia trait. Which tests are helpful in differentiating these conditions?

Answer: Test which may be of help in differentiating these conditions are [14–16]:

(a) MCV and MCH: less decreased in anemia of chronic disorder as compared to iron deficiency anemia.
(b) Soluble transferrin receptors: normal in an ACD but increased in IDA.
(c) Red cell protoporphyrin: increases in both IDA and ACD but normal in thalassemia trait.
(d) Hepcidin: increases in an ACD.

Q13. The blood film of this patient shows dimorphic/dual morphology of red cells. In which other conditions dimorphic or dual population of red cells is seen?

Answer: In dimorphic morphology, there are two distinct red cell populations (e.g., hypochromic microcytic and normochromic normocytic red cells). The term dimorphic is more widely used because it can be used for multiple red cell populations. Thus, the dimorphic blood picture will look like a dual population of microcytic and normocytic red cells.

Dimorphic/dual populations are commonly seen following the treatment of IDA or dual deficiency anemia with iron supplements, sideroblastic anemia, hemolytic anemias such as AIHA, post erythropoietin therapy, homozygous hemoglobinopathies, and myelofibrosis.

Q14. How can be anemia of inflammation (AI) differentiated from combined anemia of inflammation and IDA (AI + iDA)?

Answer: Anemia of inflammation in the presence of IDA (combined AI + IDA) poses real difficulty in diagnosis. History and some investigations may be helpful. In literature, a combination of reticulocyte Hb content, red cell Hb, RDW ,along with iron profile has been used to differentiate these two situations. Also ferritin index, calculated by sTfR/log ferritin values, helps in differentiating these conditions. The index is <1 in ACD and >2 in combined AI + IDA. Hepcidin measurement may play a role in evaluation. Hepcidin levels are increased in AI but reduced in AI + IDA [4, 12, 17–19].

Q15. The bone marrow smears show increased hemosiderin in macrophages. How is this test helpful in evaluating anemias?

Answer:

(a) Lack of hemosiderin in BM macrophages suggests IDA.
(b) Presence of increased hemosiderin in macrophages suggests ACD.
(c) Presence of hemosiderin in normoblasts (sideroblasts and ring sideroblasts) suggests sideroblastic anemia.

Q16. What are important points in history and examination in patients suspected to have ACD?

Answer: Concurrent or past history of infections, inflammatory conditions, and cancers is most important. History of chronic bleeding, exposure to chemicals and radiation, intake of medications, major surgery, or trauma should be taken. A family history of any chronic illness is also important.

A history of undiagnosed fever, generalized weakness, bony pains, and loss of appetite can identify the presence of underlying infections, neoplasms, and collagen vascular diseases. Explore symptoms suggesting a disease of cardiac, hepatic, renal disease, or endocrinopathy.

5.2 Correlation of Results of Preliminary Investigations with Symptoms and Signs of Anemia of Chronic Disorder

Q17. How do symptoms and signs correlate with the diagnosis of ACD in this patient?

Answer: This patient had symptoms of anemia in the form of tiredness, dizziness, easy fatigability, and mild dyspnea on exertion of 2-month duration. She had pallor but no jaundice. She was diagnosed to have systemic lupus erythematosus (SLE), which is a chronic inflammatory state and is associated with hematological alterations including anemia. Thus the symptoms in this patient correlate well with diagnosis.

Q18. How do the preliminary investigations correlate with the diagnosis of ACD in this patient.

Answer: The CBC shows anemia which is dimorphic with inadequate response of bone marrow (reticulocyte % inappropriately low for the degree of anemia). This in conjunction with low serum iron and transferrin level, high transferrin saturation, and high iron stores (ferritin and hemosiderin) correlates well with the diagnosis of anemia of chronic infections/inflammation.

There is mild proteinuria and hypoproteinemia which can add to etiology of anemia. She has active SLE as indicated by immunological profile and CRP, confirming inflammation associated with SLE as a cause of anemia in this patient.

5.3 Quick Information for Practicing Clinicians and Students

References [1–19]:

1. In ideal conditions, ACD presents with mild to moderate anemia—usually Hb is =/> 8 G/dL with low serum iron, high ferritin, low transferrin levels, and normal-to-high transferrin saturation in a pretext of either chronic infection or inflammation.
2. It is necessary to rule out coexisting causes of anemia that may require specific interventions.
3. Sometimes ACD coexists with IDA. It is important to diagnose concomitant IDA especially in patients with chronic renal failure undergoing dialysis and those with congestive heart failure in whom iron deficiency impairs cardiovascular performance.
4. Laboratory evaluation must include ESR, CRP, renal, hepatic and thyroid function tests, markers of hemolysis, folic acid, and cobalamin levels.
5. Vitamin D is a negative regulator of hepcidin expression. Anemia gets improved if vitamin D supplements are given. It acts by decreasing hepcidin levels.
6. If combined ACD + IDA is suspected, a therapeutic trial of intravenous iron along with erythropoiesis-inducing agents may be tried keeping in mind the possibility of exacerbating an existing infection. Risk-benefit should be assessed.
7. Anemia-related symptoms in ACD are often attributed to the underlying disease. So treatment of underlying cause is mandatory.
8. Newer erythropoiesis-stimulating agents, anti-cytokine drugs, and medications targeting the hepcidin-ferroportin pathway are being explored.

To acquire further knowledge on the subject, following sources are advised:

1. BCSH guidelines
2. Br Jr. Hematology
3. ASH education book
4. Blood
5. NEJM
6. Int Jr. Lab Hematology

References

1. Ford J. Red blood cell morphology. Int J Lab Hematol. 2013;35(3):351–7. https://doi.org/10.1111/ijlh.12082.
2. Cullis J. Anaemia of chronic disease. Clin Med. 2013;13:193–6.
3. Tim Goodnough L, Comin-Colet J, Leal-Noval S, et al. Management of anemia in patients with congestive heart failure. Am J Hematol. 2017;92(1):88–93.
4. Ferrucci L, Semba RD, Guralnik JM, et al. Proinflammatory state, hepcidin, and anemia in older persons. Blood. 2010;115(18):3810–6.

5. Giannouli S, Voulgarelis M, Ziakas PD, Tzioufas AG. Anaemia in systemic lupus erythematosus: from pathophysiology to clinical assessment. Ann Rheum Dis. 2006;65(2):144–8.
6. Sollie S, Michaud DS, Sarker D, Karagiannis SN. Chronic inflammation markers are associated with risk of pancreatic cancer in the Swedish AMORIS cohort study. BMC Cancer. 2019;19:858.
7. Khalil RH, Nabil A-HN. Types of acute phase reactants and their importance in vaccination. Biomed Rep. 2020;12(4):143–52.
8. Ward PC. Investigation of nonpoikilocytic normochromic normocytic anemia. Postgrad Med 1979;65(3):233-5–241-3.
9. Bonnet JD. Normocytic normochromic anemia. Postgrad Med. 1977;61(6):139–42.
10. Taneja N. Erythrocyte sedimentation rate- is there need for fasting blood sample? Med J Armed Forces India. 1997;53(1):72–4.
11. Weiss G, Schett G. Anaemia in inflammatory rheumatic diseases. Nat Rev Rheumatol. 2013;9(4):205–15.
12. Guenter W, Tomas G, Lawrence TG. Anemia of inflammation. Blood. 2019;133(1):40–50.
13. Thomas C, Thomas L. Anemia of chronic disease: pathophysiology and laboratory diagnosis. Lab Hematol. 2005;11(1):14–23.
14. Camaschella C. Iron-deficiency anemia. N Engl J Med. 2015;372(19):1832–43.
15. Lopez A, Cacoub P, Macdougall IC, Peyrin-Biroulet L. Iron deficiency anaemia. Lancet. 2016;387:907–16.
16. Crichton RR, Charloteaux-Wauters M. Iron transport and storage. Eur J Biochem. 1987;164(3):485–506.
17. Punnonen K, Irjala K, Rajamäki A. Serum transferrin receptor and its ratio to serum ferritin in the diagnosis of iron deficiency. Blood. 1997;89(3):1052–7.
18. Busti F, Campostrini N, Martinelli N, Girelli D. Iron deficiency in the elderly population, revisited in the hepcidin era. Front Pharmacol. 2014;5:83.
19. Nemeth E, Ganz T. Anemia of inflammation. Hematol Oncol Clin North Am. 2014;28(4):671–81. https://doi.org/10.1016/j.hoc.2014.04.005.

Chapter 6
Congenital Dyserythropoietic Anemia

A two-year-old male child is referred to hematology clinic with complaints from mother that the child is becoming gradually pale with decreased appetite and poor weight gain for the last 3–4 months. There is no history of fever, drug intake, or recurrent infections. However, she complained that child is becoming irritable and less active than other children of his age. The child had neonatal jaundice for which phototherapy was given. He was breastfed and weaned at an age of 4 months. There is no significant family history. None of the family members had ever been diagnosed with hematological disorder.

On examination, the child looked pale with mild jaundice. Both liver and spleen were just palpable below costal margins. There was no lymphadenopathy or any other skeletal abnormality.

CBC done at presentation (Table 6.1) is given.

Table 6.1 CBC

CBC parameter	Patient's result	Reference range
WBC	5.3	3.7–10 × 10^9/L
RBC	3.5	4.5–5.4 × 10^{12}/L
HB	8.9	11–140 g/L
Hct	0.26	0.33–0.43 L/L
MCV	100	83–101 fL
MCH	27	27–32 pg
MCHC	320	315–345 g/L
RDW	21	11.6–14.6%
PLT	256	130–430 × 10^9/L
MPV	10	7–11 fL
Poly #	1.9	1.7–6 × 10^9/L
Lymp#	2.0	1–3 × 10^9/L
Mono#	0.9	0.2–1.0 × 10^9/L
EO#	0.5	0.02–0.5 × 10^9/L
BASO#	0	0.02–0.1 × 10^9/L
RETIC%	1.9	0.5–1.5%
ESR	35	0–20 mm 1st h Westergren

A. Gupta, *Decision Making Through Problem Based Learning in Hematology*, https://doi.org/10.1007/978-981-99-8933-1_6

6.1 Questions

Q1. Interpret the CBC result given above and suggest investigations for further evaluation in such case.

Answer: The CBC shows low values for red cell count, hemoglobin, and hematocrit (Hct). MCV is within normal limits, although on higher side of normal. RDW is high. Reticulocyte percentage is normal (there is inadequate response to the degree of anemia) . ESR is slightly high. Thus, there is predominantly normocytic normochromic anemia with high RDW and inadequate reticulocyte response.

Possible etiology of normocytic normochromic anemia in this age group includes both hereditary and acquired causes.

1. Hereditary causes: Diamond Blackfan anemia, Fanconi anemia, red blood cell membrane defects (including HS, HE, and hereditary pyropoikilocytosis), enzyme deficiencies (G6PD and PK deficiencies), hemoglobinopathies, and congenital dyserythropoietic anemia (CDA).
2. Acquired causes: Bleeding, infections, and nutritional deficiencies like iron deficiency, combined deficiency of iron and B_{12}/folic acid, vitamin E, and copper deficiency Rarely, MDS can present in this age group [1].

Next best test will be to examine a blood film. Further tests to evaluate the above mentioned differential diagnoses will be based on blood film findings.

Q2. Given are images from blood film (Figs. 6.1, 6.2, and 6.3). Interpret these findings and suggest a differential diagnosis. What further investigations should be done to exclude various possibilities?

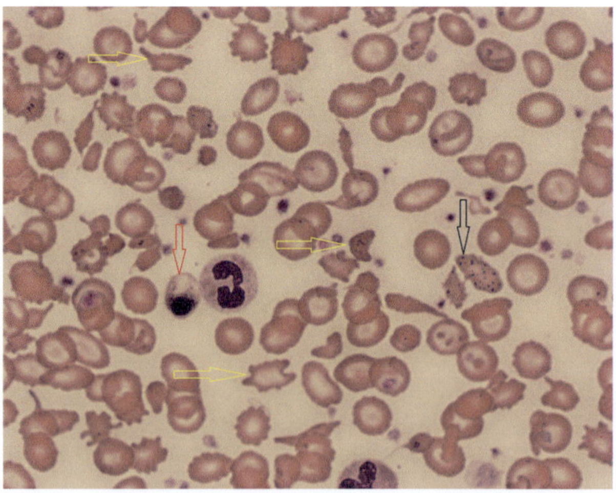

Fig. 6.1 PBF. Marked anisopoikilocytosis, basophilic stippling (black arrow), nucleated red cell (red arrow). Leishman ×100

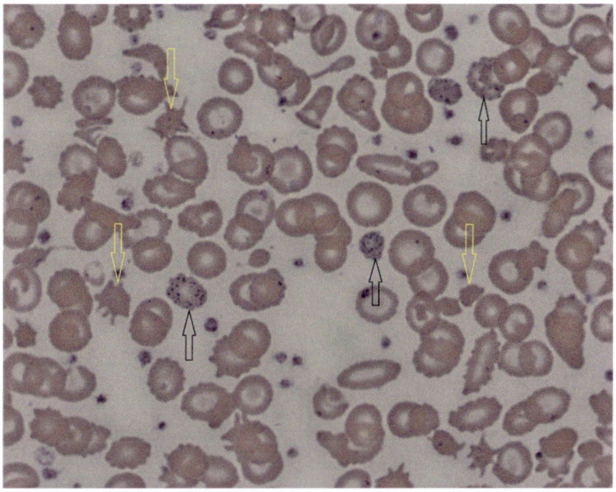

Fig. 6.2 PBF. Marked anisopoikilocytosis (yellow arrows), basophilic stippling (black arrows). Leishman ×100

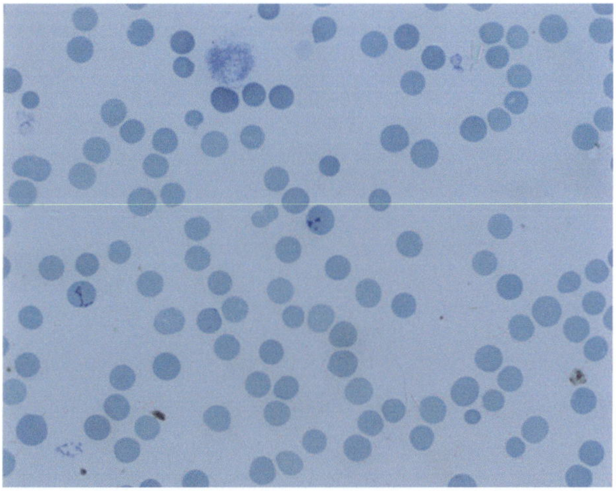

Fig. 6.3 PBF. Supravital stain (new methylene blue) ×100

Answer: The blood film shows marked anisopoikilocytosis with few macrocytes, normocytes, few microcytes, and some hypochromic cells, in addition to ovalocytes, irregularly contracted cells, teardrop poikilocytes, and a rare, fragmented cell. Also seen are nucleated red cells (red arrow) and basophilic stippling (black arrows). The blood film stained with supravital stain (NMB) does not show any evidence of Heinz bodies or golf holes (Hb-H inclusions).

The clinical presentation with hepatosplenomegaly, CBC, and blood film findings suggests the possibility of congenital/hereditary cause of anemia. Red cell enzyme (G6PD) deficiency is unlikely as there are no blister or bite cells in peripheral blood film. Also the absence of Heinz bodies and Hb-H inclusions exclude the diagnosis of unstable hemoglobin and Hb-H disease (alfa Thalassemia) respectively in this patient.

For further evaluation, next best investigations should include estimation of biochemical hemolytic markers (indirect bilirubin, LDH, and haptoglobin), analysis of hemoglobin by HPLC, and osmotic fragility test for exclusion of thalassemia and red cell membrane defects such as hereditary spherocytosis and hereditary elliptocytosis. Heat instability and autohemolysis tests may be done for further assessment of unstable hemoglobin and HPP.

Q3. Given are results of biochemical tests of functions of liver and kidney, including hemolytic markers (Table 6.2), analysis of hemoglobin by HPLC (Fig. 6.4), osmotic fragility test (Fig. 6.5), and tests for stability (Table 6.3). Analyze the results and suggest further investigations for most likely diagnosis in this patient.

Table 6.2 Biochemical tests

Test	Patient's result	Ref range
Glu	4.5	3.9–6.1 mmol/L
Urea	2.9	2.5–6.6 mmol/L
Creat	90	60–120 µmol/L
Na^+	139	136–146 mmol/L
K^+	4.5	3.7–5.0 mmol/L
Ca^+	2.3	2.2–2.6 mmol/L
Mg+	1.0	0.08–1.1 mmol/L
T. Prot	68	63–80 mmol/L
Alb	25	35–47 mmol/L
Choles	2.5	1.5–5.2 mmol/L
TG	0.9	0.4–1.7 mmol/L
Urates	370	150–400 mmol/L
T Bil	58	3–20 µmol/L
D. Bil	5	0–5 µmol/L
I Bil	53	5–15 µmol/L
Alk Ph	41	26–88 IU/L
ALT	54	10–60 IU/L
AST	32	10–42 IU/L
GGT	20	7–64 IU/L
LDH	290	90–180 IU/L
Hapto	0.1	0.2–2.0 g/L
T4	10.6	7.8–16 pmol/L
TSH	3.99	0.27–4.2 µlU/ml
Amylase	20	28–100 IU/L
Lipase	30	0–160 U/L

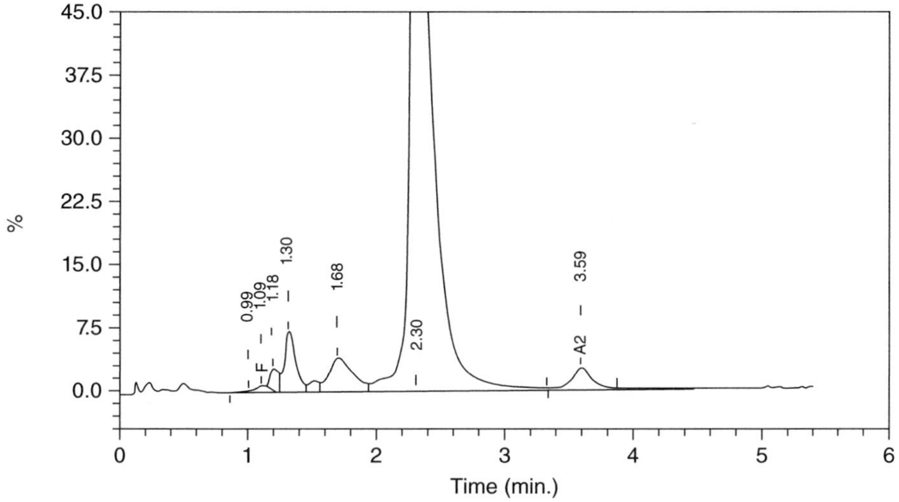

Fig. 6.4 HPLC: HbA –97%, HbA2–2.5%

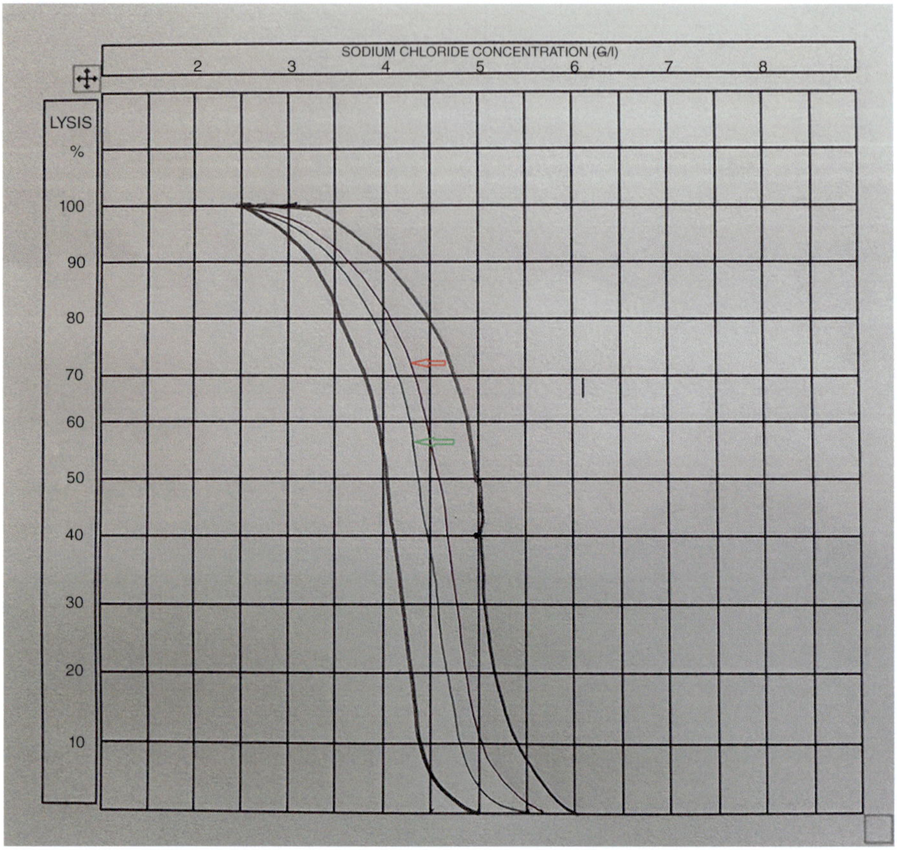

Fig. 6.5 Osmotic fragility test (OFT): Curve for control (red arrow) and patient (green arrow)

Table 6.3 Stability tests

Isopropanol stability test	Normal
Heat stability test	Normal

Answer: The biochemical tests show high total and indirect bilirubinemia, high LDH, and decreased haptoglobin indicating hemolytic process in this patient. Hemoglobin analysis by HPLC (Fig. 6.3), osmotic fragility test, heat stability, and isopropanol tests are normal. These findings confirm the hemolytic process and exclude the diagnosis of thalassemia, membrane defects including HPP, and unstable hemoglobin.

Next best investigation will be to perform bone marrow examination to diagnose possibilities like CDA, MDS, and myelofibrosis. Estimation of serum iron, ferritin, transferrin, transferrin saturation, and serum B_{12}/folic acid levels is optional.

Q4. Given are images from bone marrow aspirate (Figs. 6.6 and 6.7) and trephine biopsy (Fig. 6.8). Interpret the findings and suggest final diagnosis.

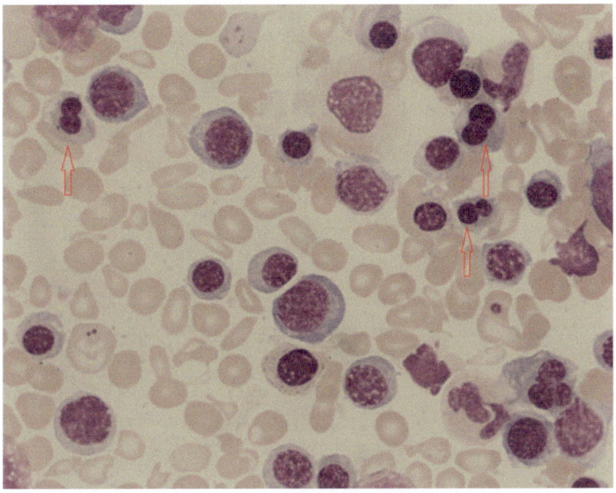

Fig. 6.6 Bone marrow aspirate. Binucleated erythroblasts (red arrows). Leishman stain ×100

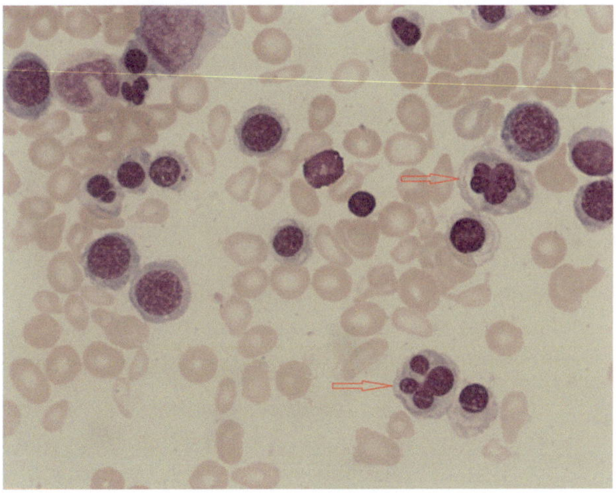

Fig. 6.7 Bone marrow aspirate. Tetra-nucleated erythroblasts (red arrows). Leishman stain ×100

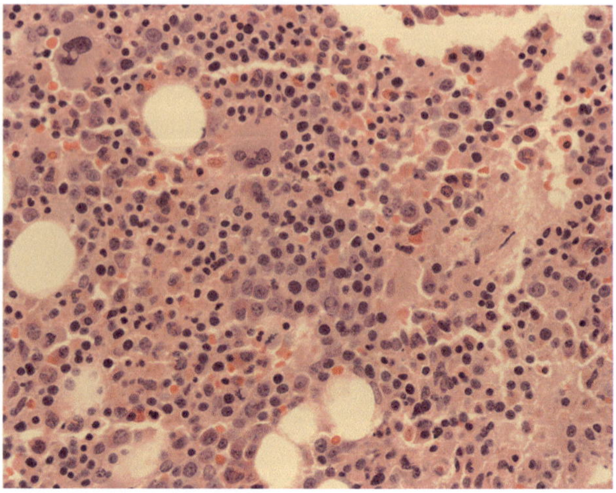

Fig. 6.8 Bone marrow biopsy. Erythroid hyperplasia. H/E stain ×100

Answer: The aspirate from bone marrow shows erythroid hyperplasia and evidence of dysplasia in erythroid series. Binucleate, trinucleate, and tetranucleated erythroid precursors are present. The other cell lines are unremarkable. The Prussian blue stain on aspirate smears did not show any sideroblasts. The trephine biopsy confirms erythroid hyperplasia with no evidence of fibrosis. These findings exclude the possibility of myelodysplasia and myelofibrosis in this case. Thus, based on morphological changes in bone marrow in association with earlier investigations, congenital dyserythropoietic anemia (CDA) is the most likely diagnosis in this patient.

Q5. What further tests can be done in such case to confirm the diagnosis of CDA?

Answer: Congenital dyserythropoietic anemia is classified into types I, II, III, and some variants based on the characteristic morphological, clinical, and genetic features. Types I and II are autosomal recessive, while type III is autosomal dominant. Type II is the most common type of CDA. The following tests help in the confirmation of the diagnosis [2–6]:

1. SDS-PAGE (sodium dodecyl sulfate polyacrylamide gel electrophoresis) of red cell membrane proteins shows a narrow and faster-migrating band 3.
2. A Western blot of red cell membrane proteins shows the presence of reticulum-endothelial proteins (calreticulin, glucose-regulated protein 78, protein disulfide isomerase) in CDA-II [2].
3. Eosin-5′-maleimide binding test by flow cytometry shows lower mean fluorescence intensity of EMA-tagged erythrocytes.
4. Cytogenetic studies of bone marrow cells and sequencing of the CDAN1 gene for mutational analysis for CDA-I and of the *SEC23B*-gene for CDA-II are confirmatory.

In general, examination of bone marrow aspirate for characteristic abnormalities is required for the diagnosis of CDA [4, 6]. Most of the tests mentioned above for confirmation of CDA are available only in specialized laboratories.

Q6. What is the defect in CDA, and how is it related to pathogenesis?

Answer: The congenital dyserythropoietic anemias (CDAs) are a group of hereditary disorders resulting from mutation in genes on chromosome 15 and chromosome 20. Three main types—types I, II, III—and some variants (including type IV and V) have been described. In types I, II, and III, mutations in CDAN1, SEC23B, and KIF23 genes have been identified, respectively. Additional genetic mutations in erythroid transcription factor genes (*GATA-1* and *KLF1*) have been mentioned in the literature. Erythrocyte membrane glycoproteins, such as band 3 and band 4.5, which are normally glycosylated with polylactosamines lack these carbohydrates especially in CDA-II (HEMPAS). In addition, mutations in codanin-1 induce increased proliferation in erythroid progenitors, and during this process assembly defects occur in chromatin [2, 6].

These molecular alterations induce abnormal cell maturation and division resulting in intramedullary death (ineffective erythropoiesis) and congenital anemia with characteristic morphologic features in bone marrow erythroblasts. CDA-I has abnormalities in chromatin structure, whereas CDA-II patients have increased bi- and multinucleated erythroblasts in bone marrow. CDA-III shows giant multinucleated erythroblasts in bone marrow [2, 6].

Due to intramedullary death of cells, there is inappropriately low reticulocyte response for the degree of anemia. Marked red cell anisopoikilocytosis results in hemolysis in peripheral blood with resultant increase in hemolytic parameters. Basophilic stippling is commonly observed in the peripheral blood smear [7].

Q7. What are clinical presentations of CDA?

Answer: Patients of CDA, in general, come to medical attention because of anemia combined with jaundice (90%), splenomegaly (70%), or hepatomegaly (45%). Hb is usually between 7 and 11 g/dL. Some cases are severe, requiring regular blood transfusions during childhood and adolescence [2, 4, 8].

Q8. What are characteristic bone marrow and EM changes in CDA?

Answer: In CDA-I, bone marrow shows incompletely divided erythroid cells with thin inter nuclear bridges. Electron microscopy depicts a "Swiss cheese" appearance. In CDA-II, hypercellular marrow with erythroid hyperplasia and large number of binucleate (10–35%) and rarely multinucleated erythroblasts are seen. The electron microscopy shows vesicles loaded with proteins beneath the plasma membrane. CDA-III is the rarest form. The bone marrow shows erythroid hyperplasia, with characteristic giant multinucleated erythroblasts. E/M shows autophagic vacuoles, iron-laden mitochondria, and myelin figures in the cytoplasm of the erythroblasts [2, 5–7].

6.2 Correlation of Results of Preliminary Investigations with Symptoms and Signs in Congenital Dyserythropoietic Anemia

Q9. Correlate symptoms, signs, and investigations done in this child with the clinical diagnosis of CDA.

Answer: This child has a history of becoming gradually pale with poor weight gain, being irritable and less active, and a history of recurrent infections. All these are symptoms of anemia. History of neonatal jaundice suggests the possibility of some congenital or hereditary cause of anemia. Examination showed anemia and jaundice (indirect hyperbilirubinemia) with hepatosplenomegaly, which indicates possible hemolysis with extramedullary hematopoiesis. Subsequent investigations revealed evidence of ineffective erythropoiesis with indication of intramedullary hemolysis (low reticulocyte response to the degree of anemia, high bilirubin, and low haptoglobin). The characteristic changes seen in erythroblasts in bone marrow confirmed the diagnosis of CDA.

Q10. What is the cause of marked anisopoikilocytosis in CDA?

Answer: The red cell membrane has abnormal band 3 protein. This protein is hydrophobic and tends to cluster and disrupts cytoskeleton, resulting in abnormal membrane architecture.

Q11. What are conditions with high RDW?

Answer: Early nutritional deficiency of iron, folate, or vitamin B_{12} can cause high RDW. In CDA, RDW becomes elevated earlier than abnormalities of other red cell parameters. RDW is also high in hereditary pyropoikilocytosis (HPP), thalassemia, myelofibrosis, some cases of MDS, red cell fragmentation, and agglutination [9].

Q12. Why is reticulocyte response inappropriately low to the degree of anemia in CDA, and what are other causes of such response?

Answer: The abnormal red cell precursors are destroyed in marrow resulting in low reticulocyte count in peripheral blood. Some of the other causes of hypoproliferative anemias (low reticulocyte response to the degree of anemia) are nutritional deficiencies, anemia of chronic inflammation, anemia secondary to endocrine diseases and CRF, BM failure syndromes, myelophthisic anemia, and anemia due to metastasis to BM. But none of these except megaloblastic anemia and CDA have intramedullary hemolysis resulting in ineffective erythropoiesis [2, 4, 7, 8].

Q13. Acidified serum test is positive in PNH as well as CDA II. How can we differentiate PNH from CDA?

Answer: In PNH, there is deficient expression of CD_{55} and CD_{59} on red cells. Sucrose lysis test is useful in differentiating these two conditions as this test is positive in PNH and negative in CDA type II. Analysis of red cell membrane protein is more helpful. Flow cytometric analysis of CD55 and CD59 on red cell membrane helps to confirm the diagnosis of PNH. Molecular analysis and EM are other methods of differentiation [2, 4].

6.3 Quick Information for Practicing Clinicians and Students

References [1–9]:

1. CDA is one of the rare causes of anemia in childhood.
2. Anemia, jaundice with hepatomegaly +/− splenomegaly should raise suspicion of CDA.
3. Blood film should be requested first. Presence of marked anisopoikilocytosis and basophilic stippling will exclude many acquired causes of anemia in children.
4. Anemia with inappropriate response of bone marrow (reticulocytopenia) indicates ineffective erythropoiesis-CDA remains a diagnostic possibility if other causes of hypo-proliferative anemias are ruled out (mentioned above).
5. Most of the times, in routine laboratories, diagnosis is based on characteristic bone marrow changes and exclusion of thalassemia (especially Hb-H disease), HPP, MDS, and myelofibrosis.
6. In specialized centers, SDS-PAGE of red cell membrane, electron microscopy, and molecular tests can be done for confirmation.
7. PNH is a close differential diagnosis in appropriate setting. CDA-II (HEMPAS) should be distinguished from PNH by HAM test, sucrose lysis test, flow cytometry for CD55 and CD59, and molecular analysis.
8. Complications include cholelithiasis, splenomegaly, and iron overload.

To acquire further knowledge on the subject, following sources are advised:

1. BCSH guidelines
2. Br Jr. Hematology
3. ASH education book
4. Blood
5. NEJM
6. Int Jr. Lab Hematology

References

1. Allali S, Brousse V, Sacri AS, et al. Anemia in children: prevalence, causes, diagnostic work-up, and long-term consequences. Expert Rev Hematol. 2017;10:1023–8.
2. Lolascon A, Esposito MR, Russo R. Clinical aspects and pathogenesis of congenital dyserythropoietic anemias: from morphology to molecular approach. Haemotologica. 2012;97:178–1794. https://doi.org/10.3324/haematol.2012.072207.
3. Heimpel H, Forteza-Vila J, Queisser W, Spiertz E. Electron and light microscopic study of the erythroblasts of patients with congenital dyserythropoietic anemia. Blood. 1971;37(3):299–310.
4. Crookston JH, Crookston MC, Burnie KL, Francombe WH, Dacie JV, Davis JA, et al. Hereditary erythroblastic multinuclearity associated with a positive acidified-serum test: a type of congenital dyserythropoietic anemia. Br J Haematol. 1969;17(1):11–26.
5. Anselstetter V, Horstmann K, Heimpel H. Congenital dyserythropoietic anaemia, types I and II: aberrant pattern of erythrocyte membrane proteins in CDA II, as revealed by two-dimensional polyacrylamide gel electrophoresis. Br J Haematol. 1977;35(2):209–15.
6. Wickramasinghe SN. Congenital dyserythropoietic anemias: clinical features, haematological morphology and new biochemical data. Blood Rev. 1998;12(3):178–200.
7. Verwilghen RL, Lewis SM, Dacie JV, Crookston JH, Crookston MC. Hempas: congenital dyserythropoietic anaemia (type II). Q J Med. 1973;42(166):257–78.
8. Heimpel H, Anselstetter V, Chrobak L, Denecke J, Einsiedler B, Gallmeier K, et al. Congenital dyserythropoietic anemia type II: epidemiology, clinical appearance, and prognosis based on long-term observation. Blood. 2003;102(13):4576–81.
9. Constantino BT. Red cell distribution width, revisited. Lab Med. 2013;44:e2–9.

Chapter 7
Hereditary Spherocytosis

A four-year-old male child was referred to hematology OPD. The main complaints by mother were observation of pale skin, development of irritable behavior, and child being less active and more lethargy in comparison to previous years of childhood. For the last 1 year, she had also observed repeated upper respiratory tract infections which required antibiotic therapy twice in the past 1 year.

Slightly delayed developmental milestones were recorded by general pediatrician, who had prescribed oral food supplements and multivitamins. His appetite and bowel habits were normal. The socio-economic status of the family was satisfactory. There was no significant family history except that the mother of the child revealed repeated episodes of extreme weakness especially during menstrual period. She was never investigated for anemia.

Examination of child revealed pallor and mild jaundice. Spleen was just palpable. There was no other organomegaly. Table 7.1 shows CBC result done at presentation.

A. Gupta, *Decision Making Through Problem Based Learning in Hematology*, https://doi.org/10.1007/978-981-99-8933-1_7

Table 7.1 CBC

CBC parameter	Patient's result	Reference range
WBC	7.4	3.7–10 × 10^9/L
RBC	3.9	4.2–5.4 × 10^{12}/L
HB	86	130–170 g/L
Hct	0.25	0.36–0.46 L/L
MCV	85	83–101 fL
MCH	28	27–32 pg
MCHC	390	315–345 g/L
RDW	12	11.6–14.6%
PLT	196	130–430 × 10^9/L
MPV	10	7–11 fL
Poly #	2.9	1.7–6 × 10^9/L
Lymp#	3.8	1–3 × 10^9/L
Mono#	0.5	0.2–1.0 × 10^9/L
EO#	0.2	0.02–0.5 × 10^9/L
BASO#	0	0.02–0.1 × 10^9/L
NRBC	0.3	0
RETIC%	4.2	0.5–1.5%
ESR	39	0–20 mm 1st h Westergren

7.1 Questions

Q1. Interpret the CBC result given above and suggest investigations for further evaluation in such case.

Answer: The CBC shows low hemoglobin, low RBC number, and reduced hematocrit (Hct). The MCV and MCH are within normal limits, but MCHC is high. There is reticulocytosis, and few NRBCs are also present. So, there is normocytic normochromic anemia with high MCHC and reticulocytosis.

Commonly observed causes of normocytic normochromic anemia include [1, 2]:

(a) *Decreased production from marrow (will have low reticulocyte count):* Early iron deficiency, transient erythroblastopenia of childhood, chronic pathological conditions (such as chronic inflammations, neoplastic pathologies, and infections), marrow infiltration, and hypoplastic anemias. Very rare conditions in this age include chronic renal failure, chronic liver disease, and endocrinopathies.

(b) *Increased destruction (will have high reticulocyte count with normal marrow):*

1. Red cell defects: Defects of red cell membrane, enzymes, or hemoglobin.
2. Without any defect of red cells (defects lies outside red cells): Autoimmune hemolytic anemia, micro-angiopathic hemolytic anemia (DIC/TTP/HUS).
3. PNH.

(c) *Sequestration: splenomegaly.*

(d) *Hemorrhage.*

Next best investigation would be to examine a blood film. Biochemical tests for liver and kidney including markers of hemolysis should also be done along with routine examination of urine and stools.

Q2. Given are images from blood film (Figs. 7.1 and 7.2), results of biochemical tests including hemolytic markers (Table 7.2), and routine examination of urine and stools (Table 7.3). Interpret the results and suggest investigations for further evaluation.

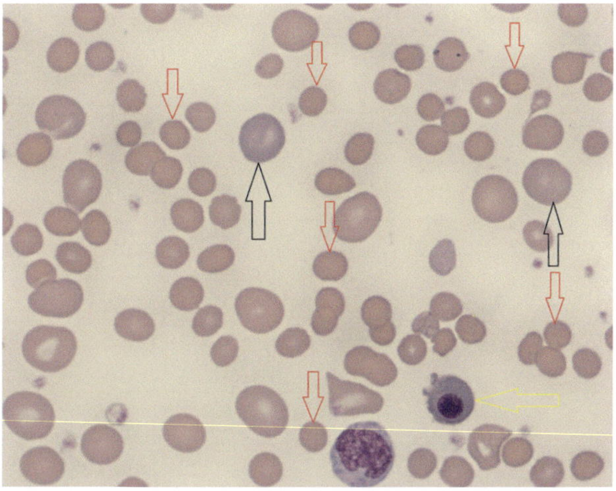

Fig. 7.1 PBF. Spherocytes (red arrows), polychromatic cell (black arrows), and nucleated red cell (yellow arow). Leishman stain ×100

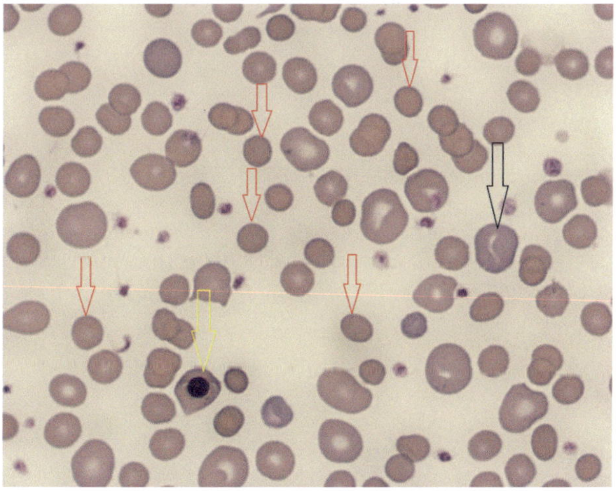

Fig. 7.2 PBF. Spherocytes (red arrows), polychromatic cell (black arrow), and nucleated red cell (yellow arow). Leishman stain ×100

Table 7.2 Biochemical tests

Test	Patient's result	Ref range
Glu	4.0	3.9–6.1 mmol/L
Urea	2.9	2.5–6.6 mmol/L
Creat	90	60–120 μmol/L
Na^+	138	136–146 mmol/L
Ca^+	2.3	2.2–2.6 mmol/L
Mg^+	1.0	0.08–1.1 mmol/L
T. Prot	68	63–80 mmol/L
Alb	42	35–47 mmol/L
Choles	2.5	1.5–5.2 mmol/L
TG	0.9	0.4–1.7 mmol/L
Urates	300	150–400 mmol/L
T Bil	46	3–20 μmol/L
Indirect Bil	40	5–20 μmol/L
D. Bil	6	0–5 μmol/L
Alk Ph	80	26–88 IU/L
ALT	54	10–60 IU/L
AST	30	10–42 IU/L
GGT	20	7–64 IU/L
LDH	250	90–180 IU/L
Hapto	0.2	0.2–2.0 g/L

Table 7.3 Urine and stool examination

Urine examination	Patient's result	Reference range
SG	1.020	1.005–1.030
Ph	6	5–7
Leu	Neg	Neg
Nit	Neg	Neg
Pro	Neg	Neg
Glu	Neg	Neg
Ket	Neg	Neg
Uro	Neg	Neg
Bil	Neg	Neg
Hemosiderin	Neg	Neg
Stool examination		
Occult blood	Neg	Neg
Ova/cysts	Neg	Neg

Answer: The blood films show low density of red cells. There are many microcytic cells, most of which are spherical in shape (arrows). Few cells appear little bluish in color—polychromatic cells (arrows). The microcytic spherical cells are hyperchromatic with no central area of pallor. Nucleated red cells are also seen (arrows). No red cell fragments are noted. The presence of polychromatic cells (reticulocytes) and nucleated red cells indicates increased bone marrow response to compensate for reduced number of red cells in peripheral blood—an indicator of hemolytic anemia.

The biochemical tests show high indirect hyperbilirubinemia, high LDH, and slightly decreased haptoglobin levels—all are markers of hemolytic anemia. Results of urine and stool examination are normal.

(Note: Spherocytes lack central pallor and have Increased density with high MCHC)

The conditions associated with spherocytes in peripheral blood are hereditary spherocytosis and autoimmune hemolytic anemia. Few spherocytes are also seen in G6PD deficiency and burns [3].

Further investigations should include direct Coombs test (DCT), osmotic fragility test, and auto-hemolysis test. As there are no bite or blister cells in peripheral blood film, possibility of G6PD is unlikely.

Q3. Given are results of osmotic fragility test (Fig. 7.3), auto-hemolysis test (Table 7.4), and DCT (Table 7.5). Interpret these results and suggest diagnosis. What confirmatory test is suggested for this diagnosis?

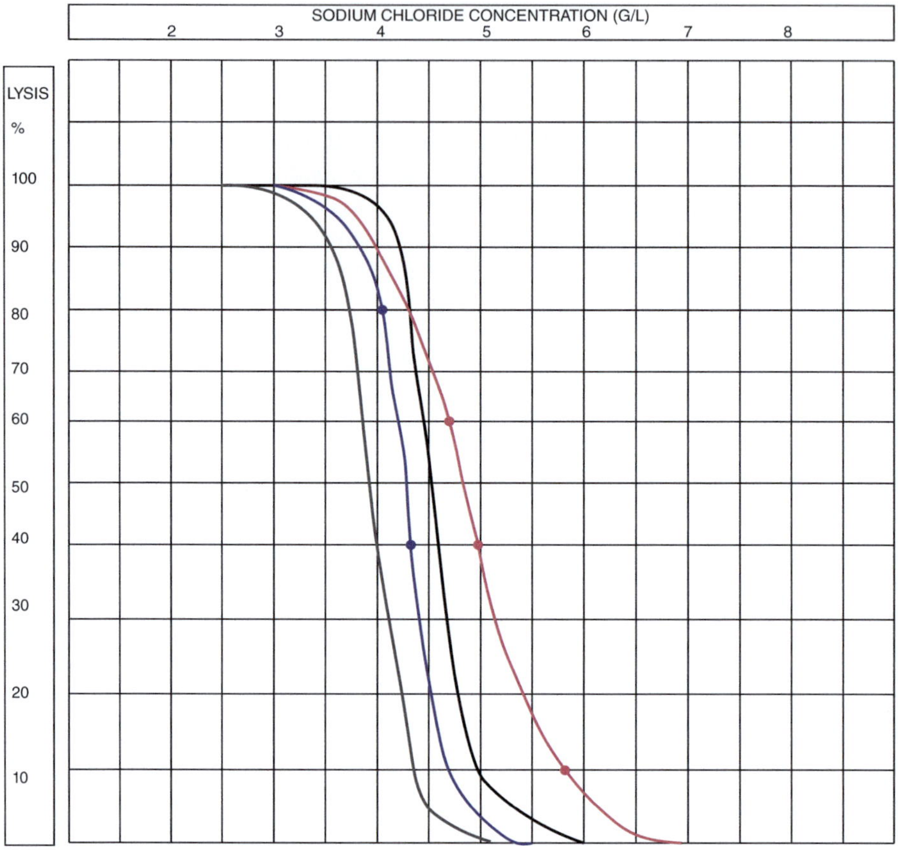

Fig. 7.3 Osmotic fragility test curve at 24 h. Shift of curve line to the right. Black lines indicate range of normal hemolysis. Blue line indicates control. Red line represents result of patient

Table 7.4 Auto-hemolysis test

Condition	Incubation at 37 °C for 48 h	Incubation with ATP	Incubation with glucose
Normal	0.4–2.0%	0.5–2.4%	0–0.8%
Patient	15%	2%	2%

Table 7.5 DCT

Direct Coombs test (DCT)	Negative

Answer: The OFT curve shows shift of curve (red line) to the right in comparison to blue line (control), which is within the normal reference range (two black lines). This positive result indicates the presence of osmotically fragile cells. The auto-hemolysis test shows 15% hemolysis at 37 °C for 48 h. This also suggests the presence of fragile cells undergoing hemolysis. Incubation of cells with glucose and ATP shows minimal hemolysis.

OFT can be positive in hereditary spherocytosis (HS), hereditary elliptocytosis (HE), and autoimmune hemolytic anemia (AIHA) [4]. Although positive OFT test and auto-hemolysis are sufficient for the diagnosis of hereditary spherocytosis in this patient with given clinical presentation, further confirmation can be done by analyzing red cell membrane proteins by sodium dodecyl sulfate-polyacrylamide gel electrophoresis (SDS-PAGE).

Q4. Given is the result of SDS-PAGE analysis (Fig. 7.4). Interpret the result and suggest final diagnosis.

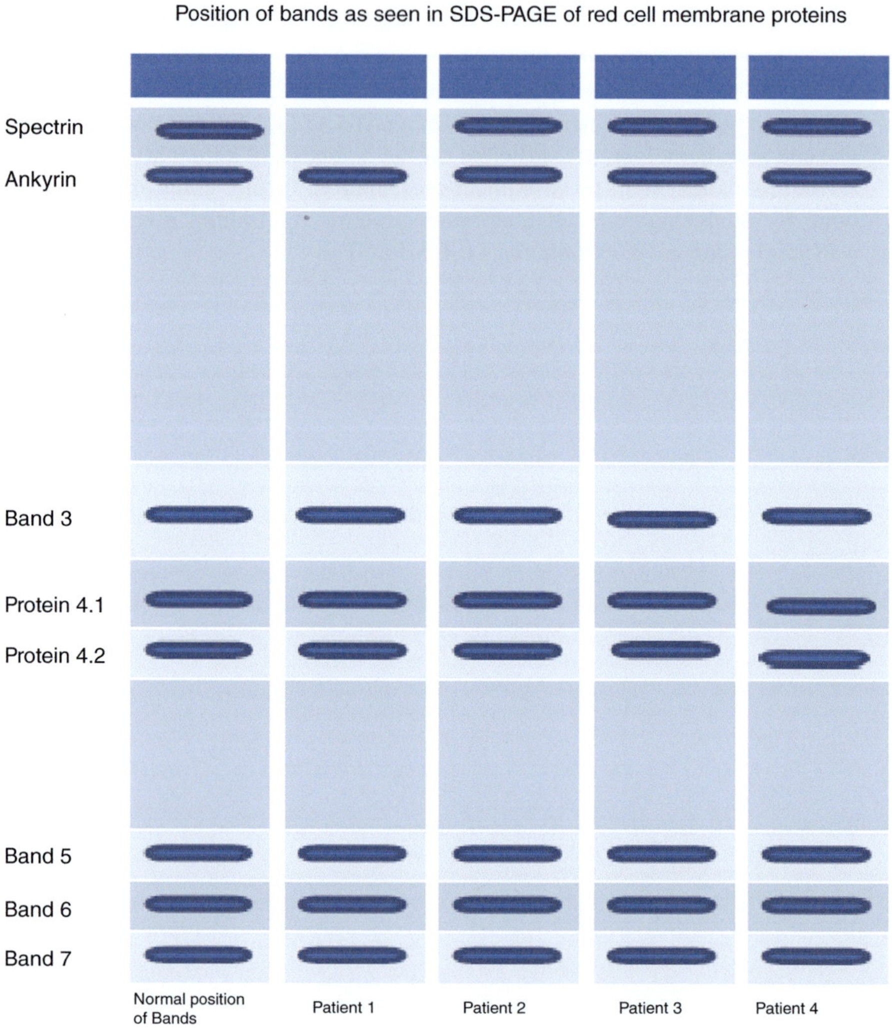

Fig. 7.4 SDS-PAGE

Answer: The SDS-PAGE shows various bands of red cell membrane proteins. The patient-1 (this patient) has absence of band in the position of spectrin, which indicates deficiency of this protein. The bands for other red cell membrane proteins are present. In other patients (control patients 2, 3, 4), all bands are present, indicating no deficiency of membrane proteins. Based on all these investigations, a final diagnosis of hereditary spherocytosis due to spectrin deficiency is confirmed.

The most sensitive test for HS is osmotic fragility testing (OFT), interpreted after incubating RBCs for 18–24 h under sterile conditions at 37 °C. However, it is laborious, requires expertise, and is time consuming. In hereditary spherocytosis, there is increased auto-hemolysis. This test is also abnormal in patients with red cell enzyme deficiencies and, therefore, has no advantage over osmotic fragility test.

SDS-PAGE can detect the defective gene mutation and helps to pinpoint the defective protein (spectrin, ankyrin, band 3 Protein 4.2, etc.). However, these studies are available only in advanced laboratories [5].

Q5. What other tests can be used for the diagnosis of HS? Which tests are currently recommended to confirm HS?

Answer: Following tests have been used for the diagnosis of HS [4, 6–8].

1. The acidified glycerol lysis test (AGLT).
2. The pink test.
3. Cryohemolysis test.
4. Osmotic gradient ektacytometry.
5. Flow cytometric analysis of eosin-5′-maleimide-labeled intact red blood cells (EMA-binding to band 3 protein, CD47, and Rh-associated glycoprotein).

Current guidelines suggest the use of flow cytometric analysis to screen patients for HS. This test has high sensitivity (92–93%) and specificity (99%) for hereditary spherocytosis.

Q6. Osmotic fragility test can show a tail of fragile cells toward right (Fig. 7.5) or shift of curve to left (Fig. 7.6). What do these changes signify? How does OFT helps to exclude other related hematological diseases?

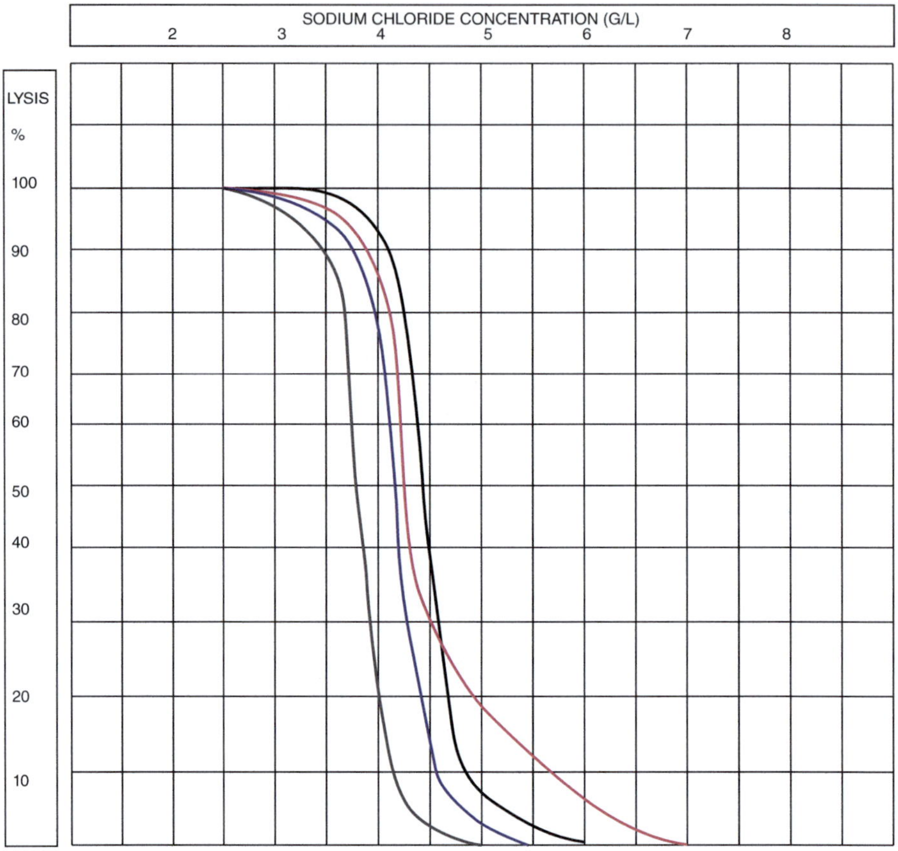

Fig. 7.5 OFT curve after 24 h incubation. Red line—tail of fragile cells. Black lines—range of normal hemolysis. Blue line—control

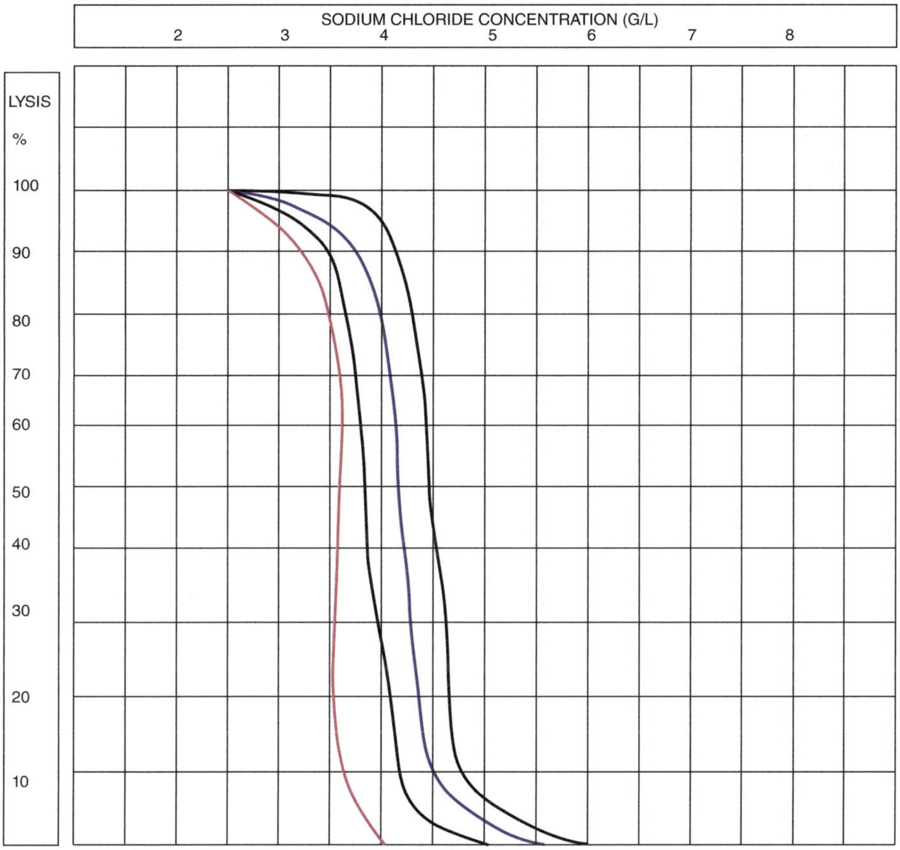

Fig. 7.6 OFT curve at 0 h. Shift of curve line to left. Black lines—range of normal hemolysis. Blue line—control. Red line—patient

Answer: A shift of tail toward right in curve signifies small number of fragile cells. Similar to HS, the curve shows shift to right in AIHA and following burns also. The position of curve in OFT can differentiate HS from other anemias. In iron-deficiency anemia (IDA), sickle cell anemia (SCA), and thalassemia, the curve is shifted to left [4].

Q7. What is the type of hemolysis in HS? What are other causes of extravascular hemolysis? What tests are helpful in differentiating extra- from intravascular hemolysis?

Answer: In HS, the hemolysis is extravascular. The spherocytic cells are non-deformable and get trapped while passing through spleen, where they undergo lysis following engulfment by splenic macrophages. Other conditions in which extravascular hemolysis is noted are autoimmune hemolytic anemia—both warm and cold type, hemoglobinopathies, red cell enzyme deficiencies, malaria, babesiosis, and some cases of

Table 7.6 Differences between extravascular and intravascular hemolysis

Test	Extravascular hemolysis	Intravascular hemolysis
CBC Hb Reticulocyte%	Decreased (−) Increased (+++)	Decreased (−) Increased (+++)
Blood film Spherocytes Schistocytes Polychromasia	Present (+++) Present/absent (+/0) Present (+++)	Absent/present (0/+) Present (+++) Present (+++)
Serum chemistry LDH Haptoglobin Unconjugated bilirubin Methemalbumin Plasma Hb	Present (++) Decreased (−) Increased (++) Normal/decreased (N/−) Normal/increased (N/+)	Present (+++) Absent (0) Increased (+++) Decreased (−) Increased (+++)
Urine analysis: Hemoglobinuria Hemosiderinuria Urinary urobilinogen	Absent (0) Absent (−) Present (+)	Present (++) Present (++) Present (++)

copper and lead poisoning. Also in hypersplenism extravascular hemolysis is noted. The intravascular hemolysis is seen mainly in micro-angiopathic hemolytic anemias, HELLP syndrome, PNH, and following transfusion reactions [9].

Laboratory tests which help to differentiate these two sites of hemolysis are presented in Table 7.6.

Q8. What is etiopathogenesis of hemolysis in HS?

Answer: Hereditary spherocytosis results from mutation in genes encoding for red cell membrane proteins. Most commonly, the defect is seen in genes for one of the four to five common types of proteins. These are spectrin, ankyrin, band 3, protein 4.1, and protein 4.2 (palladin). Of these, most common is spectrin-ankyrin complex defect. The disease is inherited in autosomal dominant fashion. Approximately 25% of the patients show autosomal-recessive inheritance.

Defective structural proteins result in loss of membrane surface area. The reduced surface-to-volume ratio gives rise to formation of spherocytes—the main characteristic of the HS [10].

The spherocytes are more rigid and less deformable than normal red cells. They get sequestrated and phagocytosed by the splenic macrophages, which results in anemia and splenomegaly. The extent of membrane surface area loss determines the severity of spherocytosis [11].

Q9. What are typical red cell indices in HS?

Answer: There is increased MCHC resulting from mild cellular dehydration. The mean cell volume (MCV) is actually low possibly resulting from membrane loss and cell dehydration.

Q10. what complications can arise in HS, and which test are recommended?

Answer: Patients with HS may develop aplastic and hemolytic crisis. During aplastic crises, testing for herpes simplex virus, parvovirus B19, and infectious mononucleosis may help identify an infectious etiology. Also vitamin B_{12} and folate levels should be measured to determine the nutritional stores during recovery from an aplastic crisis. Gallstones, growth retardation, delayed sexual maturation, and bony changes (thalassemic facies) are some of the common complications which are due to the effect of chronic hemolytic anemia [12].

Q11. Hereditary spherocytosis patients may require frequent blood transfusions. What tests may be required during the followup of patients on regular blood transfusion?

Answer: Complete red cell phenotypic assessment, a hepatitis screen, folic acid levels, and human leukocyte antigen (HLA) typing are recommended before initiation of blood transfusion therapy. During the course of management, assessment of iron overload (ferritin), serum levels of zinc, ascorbic acid, and folate are required to be estimated as their levels usually fall [13].

Q12. What are clinical presentations of hereditary spherocytosis?

Answer: Approximately 60–70% have autosomal dominant inheritance. They have moderate HS with mild-to-moderate anemia, splenomegaly, and intermittent jaundice. Hemoglobin is usually between 8% and 12 g/dL, reticulocytes usually >6%, and bilirubin >2 mg/dL.

Approximately, 20–30% of cases have mild phenotype and also have autosomal dominant inheritance. In such patients, bone marrow activity compensates for the persistent destruction of red cells, and they remain asymptomatic and are usually diagnosed later in life when they suffer from aplastic or hemolytic crises or through family screening. There is little or no splenomegaly. Lab studies show hemoglobin between 11 and 15 g/dL, reticulocytes between 3 and 6%, and bilirubin between 1 and 2 mg/dL.

Only 5% of all patients with HS have severe phenotype with recessive inheritance. Such patients require frequent red cell transfusions. Lab studies show hemoglobin in the range of 6–8 g/dL, reticulocytes usually >10%, and bilirubin >3 mg/dL [2, 4, 5].

7.2 Correlation of Results of Preliminary Investigations with Symptoms and Signs in Hereditary Spherocytosis

Q13. Correlate symptoms and signs with final diagnosis in this patient.

Answer: This child was becoming pale, irritable, lethargic, and has delayed developmental milestones. All these are symptoms of anemia. Pallor with jaundice and mild splenomegaly indicate possible hemolytic anemia. Young age of patient hints toward possible hereditary cause of disease.

Q14. How do CBC, blood film findings, and biochemical tests correlate with the diagnosis of HS in this patient? What was confirmatory test for HS?

Answer: This patient has anemia with MCV and MCH within normal limits, but MCHC is high. A normocytic normochromic anemia with high MCHC and evidence of hemolysis (reticulocytosis and NRBCs) indicate possible hemolytic anemia. Biochemical indicators of hemolysis (high Indirect bilirubin, high LDH, and low haptoglobin) further supported the possibility of hemolysis. Blood film showed spherocytes, which lead to suspicion of hereditary spherocytosis. Osmotic fragility test and SDS-PAGE confirmed the diagnosis of HS.

Q15. What laboratory tests may be required for excluding other conditions with hemolytic process?

Answer: Spherocytes can also be seen in autoimmune hemolytic anemia, G6PD deficiency, and following burns. For excluding hemolytic etiologies in this age group, direct Coombs test, G6PD estimation, HPLC, and rarely copper and lead level estimation are required. In a rare case of unconjugated hyperbilirubinemia where Gilbert's syndrome is a possibility, a liver biopsy may be required for confirmation of this syndrome.

7.3 Quick Information for Practicing Clinicians and Students

References [1–13]:

1. Typical symptoms of HS include anemia, jaundice, and splenomegaly.
2. Anemia in early childhood needs to be investigated keeping hereditary causes as priority.
3. A family history should be thoroughly investigated for hereditary cause.
4. Initial CBC result with anemia, high MCHC, and reticulocytosis are good indicators for suspecting HS.
5. Blood film examination is most important to exclude majority of causes of hemolysis.
6. Osmotic fragility test is the most commonly performed test for diagnosis and confirmation. However, DCT should be performed first if there is a suggestion of autoimmune hemolytic anemia. It is easy to perform as compared to OFT.
7. Current guidelines suggest flow cytometry for confirmation of HS.
8. SDS-PAGE analysis is optional and limited to institutions with facility to perform this test.
9. Few cases which require frequent blood transfusion should be evaluated for complete red cell phenotype, a hepatitis screen, folic acid levels, and human leukocyte antigen (HLA) typing.

10. Complications include aplastic crises, hemolytic crises, megaloblastic crises, gall bladder stone formation, etc.

To acquire further knowledge on the subject, following sources are advised:

1. BCSH guidelines
2. Br Jr. Hematology
3. ASH education book
4. Blood
5. NEJM
6. Int Jr. Lab Hematology

References

1. Ward PC. Investigation of nonpoikilocytic normochromic normocytic anemia. Postgrad Med. 1979;65(3):233–5. 238, 241–3
2. Bonnet JD. Normocytic normochromic anemia. Postgrad Med. 1977;61(6):139–42.
3. King MJ, Garçon L, Hoyer JD, et al. ICSH guidelines for the laboratory diagnosis of nonimmune hereditary red cell membrane disorders. Int J Lab Hematol. 2015;37(3):304–25.
4. Farias MG. Advances in laboratory diagnosis of hereditary spherocytosis. Clin Chem Lab Med. 2017;55(7):944–8.
5. Debaugnies F, Cotton F, Boutique C, Gulbis B. Erythrocyte membrane protein analysis by sodium dodecyl sulphate-capillary gel electrophoresis in the diagnosis of hereditary spherocytosis. Clin Chem Lab Med. 2011;49(3):485–92.
6. Yangyang W, Liao L, Lin F. The diagnostic protocol for hereditary spherocytosis-2021 update. J Clin Lab Anal. 2021;35(12):e24034. https://doi.org/10.1002/jcla.24034.
7. Bolton-Maggs PH, Stevens RF, Dodd NJ, Lamont G, Tittensor P, King MJ. Guidelines for the diagnosis and management of hereditary spherocytosis. Br J Haematol. 2004;126(4):455–74.
8. King MJ, Behrens J, Rogers C, et al. Rapid flow cytometric test for the diagnosis of membrane cytoskeleton-associated hemolytic anaemia. Br J Haematol. 2000;111:924–33.
9. Alexa J, Siddon AJ, Christopher AT. The chemical and laboratory investigation of hemolysis. Adv Clin Chem. 2019;89:215–58.
10. Da Costa L, Mohandas N, Sorette M, Grange MJ, Tchernia G, Cynober T. Temporal differences in membrane loss lead to distinct reticulocyte features in hereditary spherocytosis and in immune hemolytic anemia. Blood. 2001;98:2894–9.
11. Cynober T, Mohandas N, Tchernia G. Red cell abnormalities in hereditary spherocytosis: relevance to diagnosis and understanding of the variable expression of clinical severity. J Lab Clin Med. 1996;128:259–69.
12. Barcellini W, Bianchi P, Fermo E, Imperiali FG, Marcello AP, Vercellati C, et al. Hereditary red cell membrane defects: diagnostic and clinical aspects. Blood Transfus. 2011;9(3):274–7.
13. Chang L, Brenda JG. Red blood cell transfusion for hematologic disorders. Hematology Am Soc Hematol Educ Program. 2015;1:454–61.

Chapter 8
Hereditary Pyropoikilocytosis

A two -year-old child was referred to hematology OPD with a history of anemia since birth. The mother revealed a history of neonatal jaundice for which he was given phototherapy. The child had recurrent attacks of infection which were ascribed to poor immunity due to anemia since birth. Mild developmental delay was recorded by general pediatrician, who had also advised hematinics for some time, without any obvious beneficial outcome. The family had good socio-economic status. The mother and an elder brother of child had been diagnosed with hereditary elliptocytosis.

Examination revealed a pale-looking child with mild icterus. There was no lymphadenopathy or hepatomegaly. Tip of spleen was palpable. Table 8.1 shows CBC result done at presentation.

Table 8.1 CBC

CBC parameter	Patient's result	Reference range
WBC	5.3	3.7–10 × 10^9/L
RBC	3.9	4.5–5.4 × 10^{12}/L
HB	85	130–170 g/L
Hct	0.25	0.36–0.46 L/L
MCV	65	83–101 fL
MCH	23	27–32 pg
MCHC	319	315–345 g/L
RDW	40.2	11.6–14.6%
PLT	256	130–430 × 10^9/L
MPV	10	7–11 fL
Poly #	1.9	1.7–6 × 10^9/L
Lymp#	2.0	1–3 × 10^9/L
Mono#	0.9	0.2–1.0 × 10^9/L
EO#	0.5	0.02–0.5 × 10^9/L
Baso#	0	0.02–0.1 × 10^9/L
RETIC%	3.9	0.5–1.5%
ESR	29	0–20 mm 1st h Westergren

A. Gupta, *Decision Making Through Problem Based Learning in Hematology*, https://doi.org/10.1007/978-981-99-8933-1_8

8.1 Questions

Q1. Interpret the CBC result given above and suggest investigations for further evaluation in such case.

Answer: The CBC shows low values for red cell count, low hemoglobin, Hct, MCV, and MCH. RDW is high. Reticulocyte percentage is raised. ESR is slightly high. Thus, there is microcytic hypochromic anemia with very high RDW and mild reticulocytosis.

A combination of findings in this CBC (microcytic hypochromic anemia with very high RDW and reticulocytosis) suggests:

1. IDA (usually on treatment).
2. Combined deficiency of iron and B_{12}/folic acid.
3. Beta or alfa thalassemia (hemoglobin H disease).
4. Hereditary pyropoikilocytosis (HPP).
5. Congenital dyserythropoietic anemia (CDA).
6. Myelofibrosis.
7. Rarely, MDS can have marked anisopoikilocytosis.

For further evaluation, next best investigations should include examination of peripheral blood film, estimation of serum iron, ferritin, transferrin, transferrin saturation, serum B_{12}/folic acid levels, and analysis of hemoglobin by HPLC. Liver function tests and baseline biochemical tests for functions of kidney, thyroid, pancreas, and bone should be done. Routine examination of stools and urine should also be considered.

Q2. Given are images from blood film (Figs. 8.1 and 8.2), HPLC (Fig. 8.3), serum levels of iron, ferritin, transferrin, percentage of transferrin saturation, serum B_{12}/folic acid, and CRP (Table 8.2); results of liver, kidney, thyroid, pancreas, and bone profiles (Table 8.3); and urine + stool examination (Table 8.4). Interpret these results and suggest a provisional diagnosis.

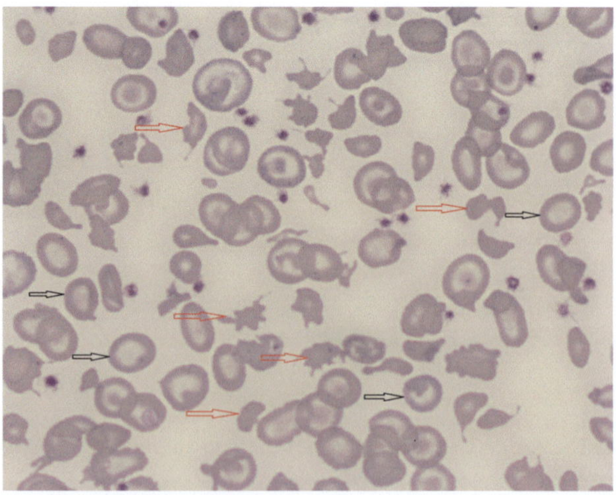

Fig. 8.1 PBF. Marked anisopoikilocytosis with microcytic hypochromic red cells (white arrows) and irregularly contracted cells (red arrows). Leishman stain ×100

Fig. 8.2 PBF. Marked anisopoikilocytosis, target cells (white arrows), budding (green arrows), and tear drop poikilocytes (red arrows). Leishman ×100

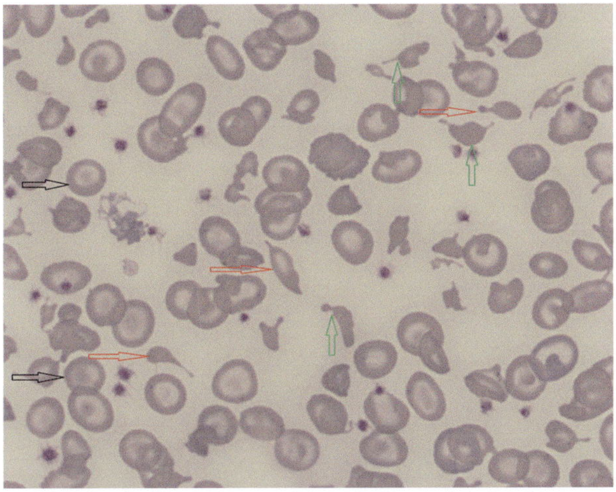

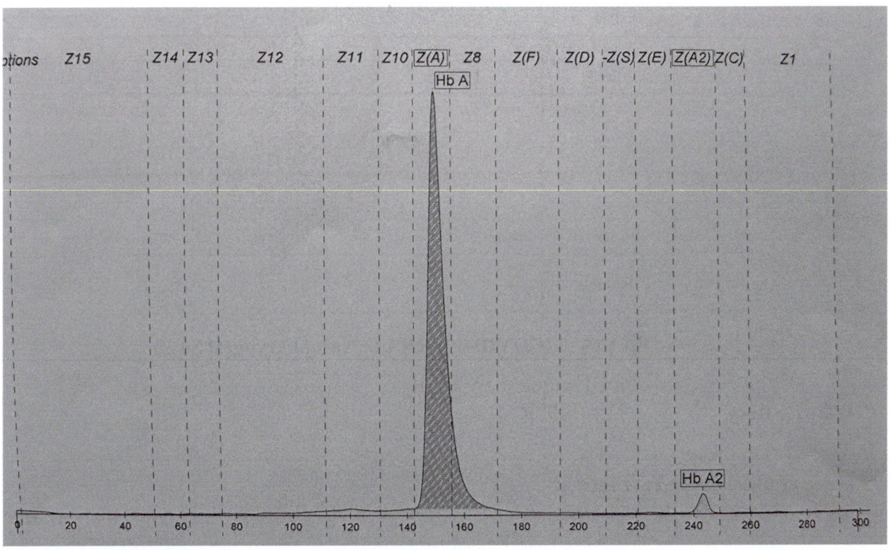

Fig. 8.3 Hemoglobin analysis (capillary electrophoresis) Hb A: 97.7% HbA2: 2.3%

Table 8.2 Serum iron profile, serum B_{12}, folic acid, red cell folate, and CRP

Test	Patient's result	Ref range
S. iron	31	11–31 umol/L
Transferrin	3.2	2.1–3.6 g/L
Trans. sat%	38	20–40%
Ferritin	400	11–307 ng/mL
S. B_{12}	565	150-700 pmol/L
S. folate	31.7	10–42 nmol/L
RBC folate	2554	1187–2854 nmol/L
CRP	8	0–10 mg/L

Table 8.3 Biochemical tests

Test	Patient's result	Ref range
Glu	5.0	3.9–6.1 mmol/L
Urea	2.8	2.5–6.6 mmol/L
Creat	90	60–120 μmol/L
Na+	139	136–146 mmol/L
Ca+	2.3	2.2–2.6 mmol/L
Mg+	1.0	0.08–1.1 mmol/L
T. Prot	68	63–80 mmol/L
Alb	39	35–47 mmol/L
Choles	2.5	1.5–5.2 mmol/L
TG	0.9	0.4–1.7 mmol/L
Urates	300	150–400 mmol/L
T Bil	35	3–20 μmol/L
Indirect Bil	30	5–20 μmol/L
D. Bil	5	0–5 μmol/L
Alk Ph	80	26–88 IU/L
ALT	55	10–60 IU/L
AST	32	10–42 IU/L
GGT	20	7–64 IU/L
LDH	250	90–180 IU/L
Hapto	0.2	0.2–2.0 g/L
T4	10.6	7.8–16 pmol/L
TSH	3.99	0.27–4.2 ulU/ml
Amylase	20	28-100 IU/L
Lipase	30	0–160 U/L
Direct antiglobulin test	Negative	Negative

Table 8.4 Urine and stool examination

Urine examination	Patient's result	Reference range
SG	1.020	1.005–1.030
Ph	6	5–7
Leu	Neg	Neg
Nit	Neg	Neg
Pro	Neg	Neg
Glu	Neg	Neg
Ket	Neg	Neg
Uro	Neg	Neg
Bil	Neg	Neg
Stool examination		
Occult blood	Neg	Neg
Ova/cysts	Neg	Neg

Answer: The blood film shows marked anisopoikilocytosis. Microcytic hypochromic red cells, tear drop poikilocytes, fragmented cells, irregularly contracted cells, and few target cells are noted. The result of HPLC is within normal range. Serum iron, transferrin, transferrin saturation, B_{12}, and folic acid are within normal limits. Serum ferritin is increased. The biochemical tests show mild indirect hyperbilirubinemia and mild increase in LDH. The haptoglobin level is at lower limits of normal. Urine and stool examination are unremarkable. A normal HPLC, normal iron levels, B_{12} and folic acid levels, and liver function tests exclude the diagnosis of thalassemia, iron +/− B12/folic acid deficiency, and liver disease. Also systemic pathologies resulting from kidney, bone, and thyroid organs are unlikely. The blood film findings of marked anisopoikilocytosis along with CBC changes (anemia, markedly high RDW, reticulocytosis) and evidence of hemolysis (red cell fragments, indirect hyperbilirubinemia, high LDH) suggest possibility of pyropoikilocytosis (HPP).

Q2. What other possible differential diagnoses should be considered at this stage of diagnosis?

Answer: Other possible diagnoses are CDA, myelofibrosis, and rare cases of MDS. A bone marrow examination is not indicated for HPP as it is nondiagnostic for this entity. However, it should be considered to exclude remote possibility of CDA and myelofibrosis. MDS is very rare in this age group. Also, there is no obvious morphological change in granulocytes and platelets in PBF. But a bone marrow examination can give better information of morphological changes for the evaluation of MDS [1].

Q3. Given are images from bone marrow trephine biopsy (Figs. 8.4 and 8.5). Interpret the findings and suggest final diagnosis.

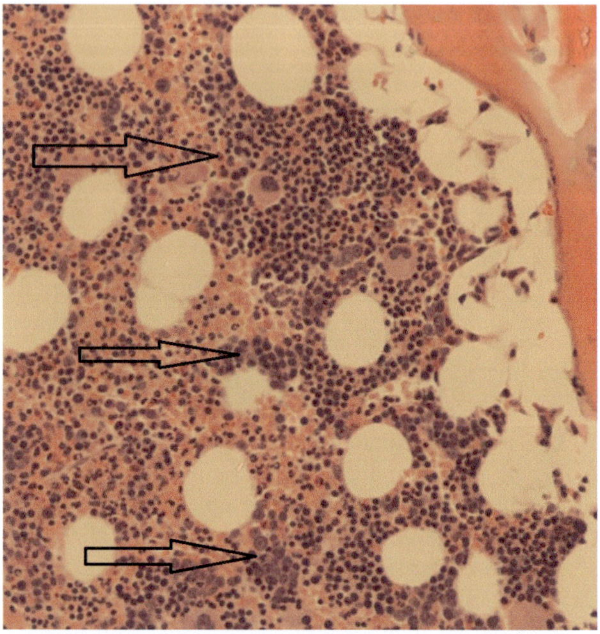

Fig. 8.4 BM trephine biopsy. Erythroid hyperplasia (arrows). H/E stain ×40

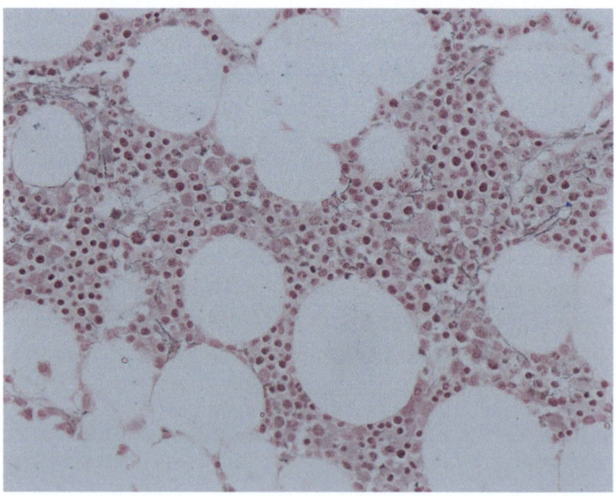

Fig. 8.5 BM trephine biopsy. Normal reticulin fibers. Reticulin stain ×40

Answer: The bone marrow biopsy shows marked erythroid hyperplasia, indicating increased response of bone marrow, secondary to hemolysis in peripheral blood. The aspirated smear did not show any dysplastic changes. The reticulin-stained slide shows normal tiny, scattered background twigs of reticulin fibers. Thus, CDA, MDS, and myelofibrosis are excluded, and the final diagnosis of pyropoikilocytosis (HPP) is confirmed.

Q4. What additional investigations can be considered in such patient which can help in exclusion of other close differential diagnosis of HPP?

Answer: Following test can give additional information on the diagnosis of HPP [2, 3]:

1. Osmotic fragility test: Hereditary pyropoikilocytosis can have normal or only mildly increased osmotic fragility.
2. Thermal sensitivity test: The test is performed by incubating the patient's blood sample for 10 min at 46 °C. Increased thermal denaturation with elongation and fragmentation of red cells is seen in HPP.
3. EMA-binding test: EMA-binding test often displays a very dim and sometimes dual peak pattern.
4. Molecular analysis of membrane protein genes will confirm diagnosis.
5. Osmotic gradient ektacytometry may be helpful.

Q5. What is the defect in HPP?

Answer: HPP is an autosomal-recessive disorder of the red blood cell membrane which results from mutations in the genes encoding for alfa-spectrin, β-spectrin, or protein 4.1R. The same molecular defect of spectrin is seen in HE. So HPP is considered a severe subtype of HE. There is partial deficiency as well as mutant spectrin protein. The lipid membrane of red cells is destabilized resulting in hemolytic anemia [4].

Q6. What is the usual clinical presentation of HPP?

Answer: HPP usually presents with severe hemolytic anemia at birth. The neonatal hyperbilirubinemia requires phototherapy or exchange transfusion. Chronic hemolytic state of HPP may lead to the formation of bile stones and subsequent cholecystitis. The family history typically includes nonhemolytic hereditary elliptocytosis in a parent and the other parent may or may not have a history of a previously undiagnosed spectrin deficiency [2, 4].

Q7. Correlate signs and symptoms with the clinical diagnosis of this patient.

Answer: This child has anemia since birth and neonatal jaundice. He had a history of recurrent infections most likely secondary to anemia. Delayed developmental milestones were recorded that probably suggests effect of chronic anemia on growth and development.

Q8. How do CBC parameters correlate with diagnosis in this patient?

Answer: Anemia is microcytic hyperchromic with very high RDW, which indicates a lot of variation in cell shape and size. There is mild reticulocytosis suggesting bone marrow response to anemia. Low MCV with high RDW indicates conditions which come in differential diagnosis of HPP as discussed above. Diagnosis is usually confirmed on morphology, and additional tests are optional as they require a dedicated setup for further investigations. A family screening will be more helpful to correlate the presence of disease entity in the index patient.

Q9. Which other conditions have high RDW?

Answer: The red cell distribution width (RDW) refers to variation of red cell morphology. Possible conditions with high RDW as correlated with MCV are presented in Table 8.5. A high RDW may indicate red cell fragmentation or agglutination [5, 6].

Table 8.5 Differential diagnosis of high RDW

	MCV high	MCV normal	MCV low
RDW high	1. B_{12}/folate deficiency 2. Chronic liver disease 3. Immune hemolysis	1. Early iron/B_{12}/folic acid deficiency 2. MDS 3. Chronic liver disease	1. Iron deficiency 2. Sickle cell-β-thalassemia 3. HPP

Q9. What are typical changes in blood film in HPP?

Answer: Marked anisopoikilocytosis is observed. Microcytes, ovalocytes, tear drop cells, fragmented cells, irregularly contracted cells, and microspherocytes are also noted. The poikilocytes in HPP are due to greater amount of spectrin dimer content in red cell membranes [7].

Q10. What are indicators of hemolytic anemia in this patient?

Answer: Red cell fragments, reticulocytosis, high indirect bilirubin, and high LDH are indicators of hemolysis. The bone marrow response (erythroid hyperplasia) substantiates it.

Q11. What suggests that anemia is chronic in this patient?

Answer: History of developmental delay, recurrent attacks of infection, no improvement in spite of oral hematinics, and presence of high ferritin are indicators which suggest that this child could have long-standing (chronic) anemia. A family history of hereditary elliptocytosis (mother and brother) also suggests a possibility of inherited anemia, possibly chronic.

Q12. What are other hereditary defects of cell membrane proteins which can also result in hemolysis?

Answer: Hereditary defects such as spherocytosis (HS), hereditary elliptocytosis (HE), South East Asian ovalocytosis (SAO), stomatocytosis, and xerocytosis also have red cell membrane defects.

(a) HS: defect in spectrin, ankyrin, band 3, or protein 4.2.
(b) HE: defects in spectrin, adducin, protein 4.1, and glycophorin C can be seen.
(c) SAO: defect in band 3.
(d) Stomatocytosis: defect in a component of band 3 complex.
(e) Xerocytosis: defect in cation permeability [8].

Q13 How is HPP related to hereditary elliptocytosis?

Answer: HPP is considered a severe form of HE and may result from compound heterozygosity for two HE alleles or homozygosity for HE.

HE results from mutation in gene for protein 4.1, which impairs binding of spectrin to ankyrin. It has also been seen as a result of defect in gene for spectrin, ankyrin, adducin, and glycophorin C.

When morphology is uniformly elliptical, it is called HE. Hemolytic anemia is associated with more distorted forms which are also heat labile. Both HE and HPP are considered a group of hemolytic anemia with heterogeneous clinical presentations.

Frequently, HE is diagnosed by chance on blood film examination and may have marginally raised bilirubin only, indicating compensated anemia. Confirmation and identification of protein defect may be done by SDS-PAGE analysis as is done in HS. Those phenotypes with mild hemolysis may get more anemic during pregnancy, infections, or folate deficiency [1, 9].

Given are images of blood film from a patient of hereditary elliptocytosis (Figs. 8.6 and 8.7).

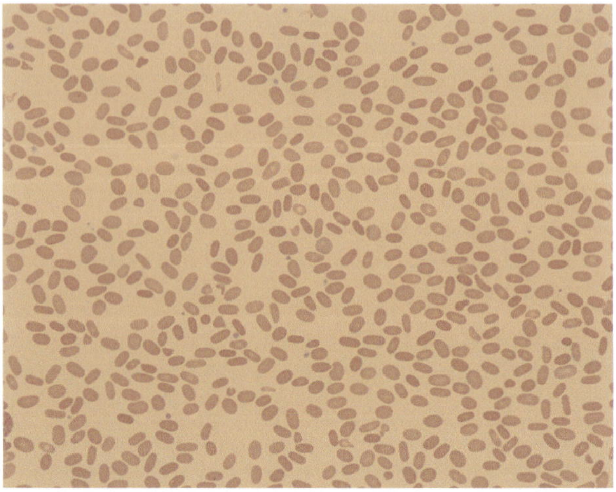

Fig. 8.6 PBF. Elliptocytes. Leishman ×40

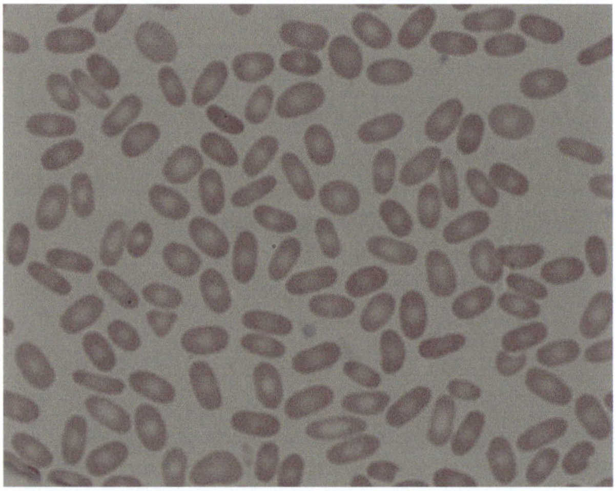

Fig 8.7 PBF. Elliptocytosis. Leishman ×100

Q14. In which other conditions elliptocytes can be seen?

Answer: Blood films of patients with deficiency of iron, folate, vitamin B_{12}, microangiopathic hemolytic anemia, thalassemia intermedia, and CDA can also show variable number of elliptical red cells.

Q15. How is HPP related to South East Asian ovalocytosis (SAO) and hereditary stomatocytosis?

Answer: In SAO, defect in band 3 results in tighter binding of band 3 to ankyrin, resulting in increased red cell rigidity. The red cell morphology is oval rather than elliptical. Most patients have no hemolysis, but a few may present with mild anemia. Ovalocytes (Fig. 8.8) are rigid and have reduced expression of many red cell antigens. They are resistant to invasion by *Plasmodium falciparum* [10, 11].

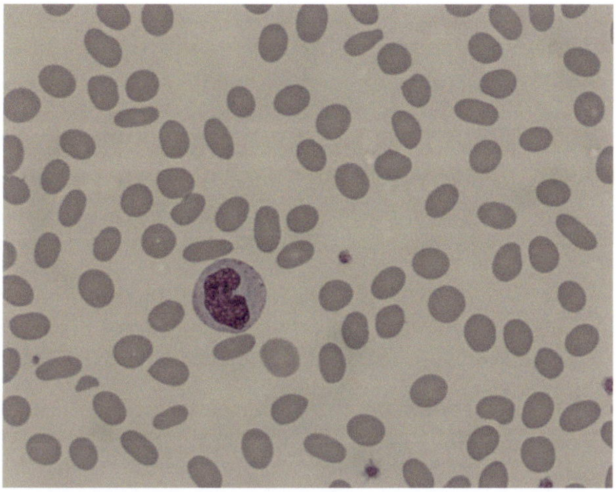

Fig. 8.8 PBF. Ovalocytes. Leishman stain ×40

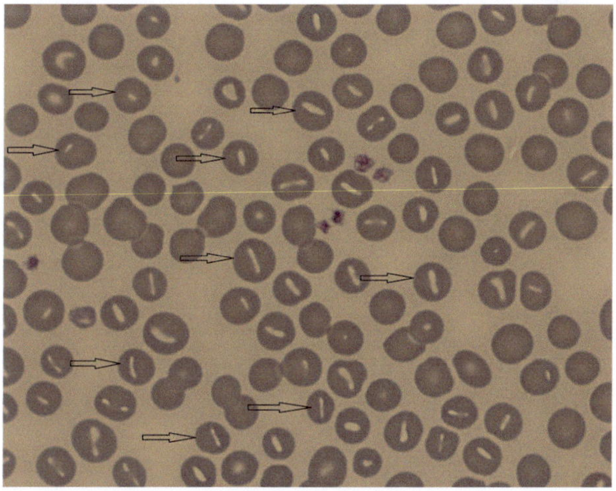

Fig. 8.9 PBF. Stomatocytes. Leishman stain ×40

In hereditary stomatocytosis (Fig. 8.9), fish-mouth like stoma are seen in red cells. This appearance is produced during preparation through folding of red cell membrane. The condition is inherited in autosomal dominant fashion and produces mild hemolytic anemia. Stomatocytes are leaky to potassium, which comes out rapidly from the cells at room temperature, and pseudohyperkalemia can occur. Lab investigations are done to test for hemolysis.

There are two variants—one is overhydrated stomatocytosis, in which MCHC is low, and a dehydrated stomatocytosis, in which MCHC is high. The condition is most often asymptomatic, but signs of mild hemolysis such as intermittent jaundice and gallstones have been reported. Blood film examination reveals stomatocytes and suggests the diagnosis. The confirmation of the condition can be done by genetic assays to confirm mutation of the SLC4A1 gene [10–12].

Q15. Which abnormalities of metabolism can affect red cell structure?

Answer: Acanthocytosis, abetalipoproteinemia, and McLeod phenotype are some of the conditions in which red cell structure is affected by lipids.

Acanthocytosis (Fig. 8.10) is also called spur cell anemia. The red cells show projections on the surface. They are formed when additional lipids get deposited on outer lipid layer of red cell membrane. The condition occurs usually with severe liver disease with abnormal plasma lipid level. Confirmation may require scanning electron microscopy.

In, abetalipoproteinemia, beta-apolipoprotein is absent. There is increased amount of sphingomyelin and reduced cholesterol. The sphingomyelin enters the cell membrane and produces acanthocytes [13].

In McLeod phenotype, there is decreased expression of Kell antigen. Patients may present with few acanthocytes and mild anemia [14].

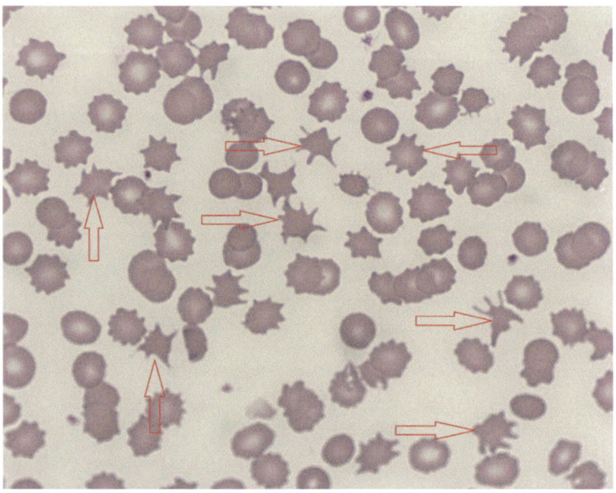

Fig. 8.10 PBF. Acanthocytes. Leishman stain ×40

8.2 Correlation of Results of Preliminary Investigations with symptoms and Signs in Hereditary Pyropoikilocytosis

Q16. Corelate symptoms and signs with final diagnosis of HPP in this patient.

Answer: This child had history of anemia since birth. The mother revealed a history of neonatal jaundice and recurrent attacks of infection possibly reduced immunity due to anemia. Mild developmental delay and pale appearance with mild icterus was present. All these symptoms and signs corelate with current diagnosis in this child. Young age of patient hints toward possible hereditary cause of disease. An important clue is presence of hereditary elliptocytosis in mother and brother.

Q17. How do CBC, blood film findings, and biochemical tests correlate with the diagnosis of HPP in this patient?

Answer: The CBC shows low values for red cell count, low hemoglobin, Hct, MCV, and MCH. RDW is high. Reticulocyte percentage is raised. The biochemical tests show mild indirect hyperbilirubinemia and mild increase in LDH indicating hemolytic process The blood film findings of marked anisopoikilocytosis, microcytic hypochromic red cells, tear drop poikilocytes, fragmented cells, irregularly contracted cells, and few target cells along with CBC changes (anemia, markedly high RDW, reticulocytosis) and evidence of hemolysis (red cell fragments, indirect hyperbilirubinemia, high LDH) corelate well with possibility of Pyropoikilocytosis (HPP).

8.3 Quick Information for Practicing Clinicians and Students

References [1–14]:

1. The most common form of HPP is diagnosed in infants who present with neonatal jaundice and frequently with transfusion-dependent anemia.
2. Anemia with low MCV, reticulocytosis, and distinct red cell morphology is quite helpful for the diagnosis of HPP.
3. In HPP, auto-hemolysis test shows increased RBC hemolysis, and heat sensitivity test is abnormal (hemolysis and fragmentation occurs at 46 °C).
4. Molecular analysis of membrane protein genes may be required in suspected cases with de novo mutation. However, it may not be required if there is a family history of HPP.
5. HPP is considered a severe form of HE.
6. HE patients are usually asymptomatic with minimal or no hemolysis. They may present with neonatal jaundice or come to attention when they undergo an episode of hemolysis following infections.

7. In HE, the hemoglobin is usually normal with borderline reticulocytosis. It is diagnosed by chance on blood film examination and may have marginally raised bilirubin only, indicating compensated anemia.
8. In ovalocytosis, most patients have no hemolysis, but a few may present with mild anemia.
9. Stomatocytes are leaky to potassium, which leaks rapidly from the cells at room temperature. It can result in pseudohyperkalemia.
10. In abetalipoproteinemia, acanthocytes are noted. The condition occurs usually with severe liver disease with abnormal plasma lipid level.
11. In all these conditions, genetic analysis of red cell membrane proteins can confirm the diagnosis.

To acquire further knowledge on the subject, following sources are advised:

1. BCSH guidelines
2. Br Jr. Hematology
3. ASH education book
4. Blood
5. NEJM
6. Int Jr. Lab Hematology

References

1. Mohandas N. Inherited hemolytic anemia: a possessive beginner's guide. Hematology Am Soc Hematol Educ Program. 2018;1:377–81. https://doi.org/10.1182/asheducation-2018.1.377.
2. King MJ, Garçon L, Hoyer JD, Iolascon A, Picard V, Stewart G, et al. ICSH guidelines for the laboratory diagnosis of nonimmune hereditary red cell membrane disorders. Int J Lab Hematol. 2015;37(3):304–25.
3. Da Costa L, Suner L, Galimand J, Bonnel A, Pascreau T, Couque N, et al. Diagnostic tool for red blood cell membrane disorders: assessment of a new generation ektacytometer. Blood Cells Mol Dis. 2016;56:9–22.
4. Niss O, Chonat S, Dagaonkar N, Almansoori MO, Kerr K, Rogers ZR, et al. Genotype-phenotype correlations in hereditary elliptocytosis and hereditary pyropoikilocytosis. Blood Cells Mol Dis. 2016;61:4–90.
5. Sultana GS, Haque SA, Sultana T, Ahmed AN. Value of red cell distribution width (RDW) and RBC indices in the detection of iron deficiency anemia. Mymensingh Med J. 2013;22(2):370–6.
6. Tekce H, Kin Tekce B, Aktas G, Tanrisev M, Sit M. The evaluation of red cell distribution width in chronic hemodialysis patients. Int J Nephrol. 2014;2014:754370.
7. King MJ, Zanella A. Hereditary red cell membrane disorders and laboratory diagnostic testing. Int J Lab Hematol. 2013;35(3):237–43.
8. Theodosia AK. Diagnosis and clinical management of red cell membrane disorders. Hematology Am Soc Hematol Educ Program. 2021;2021(1):331–40.
9. Lux SE. Disorders of the red cell membrane. In: Orkin SH, Fisher DE, Ginsburg D, et al., editors. Nathan and Oski's hematology and oncology of infancy and childhood. Saunders Elsevier; 2015. p. 515–79.
10. Amanda AL, Ruzzieatul AR, Munirah AR, et al. Homozygous Southeast Asian ovalocytosis in five live-born neonates. Haematologica. 2021;106(6):1758–61. https://doi.org/10.3324/haematol.2020.268581.

11. Rosanas-Urgell A, Lin E, Manning L. Reduced risk of Plasmodium vivax malaria in Papua New Guinean children with Southeast Asian Ovalocytosis in two cohorts and a case-control study. PLoS Med. 2012;9(9):e1001305. https://doi.org/10.1371/journal.pmed.1001305.
12. Joanna FF, Lesley JB. The hereditary stomatocytosis. Haematologica. 2009;94:1039–41.
13. Lee J, Hegele RA. Abetalipoproteinemia and homozygous hypobetalipoproteinemia: a framework for diagnosis and management. J Inherit Metab Dis. 2014;37:333–9.
14. Frey BM, Gassner C, Jung HH. Neurodegeneration in the elderly – when the blood type matters: an overview of the McLeod syndrome with focus on hematological features. Transfus Apher Sci. 2015;52(3):277–84.

Chapter 9
G6PD Deficiency

A 12-year-old boy was referred to OPD with a 5-day history of weakness and fatigue. The mother informed that child had mild fever one week back. He was diagnosed with upper respiratory infection, for which he took antipyretics and was given antibiotics by a local practitioner. The fever had resolved, but the weakness and symptoms of being tired were persisting. Also, the child observed passage of high-colored (tea-colored) urine for the last 4 days, the color of which has gradually cleared to become light yellow now.

A review of his past history revealed that this child had reported to her mother about passing high-colored urine a number times in the last few months. His father was diagnosed with G6PD deficiency. It was detected as he used to suffer from attacks of extreme weakness following ingestion of fava beans. He had been advised to avoid specific medications and foods.

Examination revealed skin and mucous membrane pallor and mild jaundice. Tiny, less than 1 cm, cervical lymph nodes were palpable. There was no hepatosplenomegaly. Result of CBC done at presentation is given (Table 9.1).

A. Gupta, *Decision Making Through Problem Based Learning in Hematology*, https://doi.org/10.1007/978-981-99-8933-1_9

Table 9.1 CBC

CBC parameter	Patient's result	Reference range
WBC	11.0	3.7–10 × 10^9/L
RBC	3.5	4.5–5.4 × 10^{12}/L
HB	80	130–160 g/L
Hct	0.24	0.33–0.43 L/L
MCV	84	83–101 fL
MCH	30	27–32 pg
MCHC	320	315–345 g/L
RDW	14	11.6–14.6%
PLT	260	130–430 × 10^9/L
MPV	10	7–11 fL
Poly #	8	1.7–6 × 10^9/L
Lymp#	1.5.0	1–3 × 10^9/L
Mono#	0.6	0.2–1.0 × 10^9/L
EO#	0.4	0.02–0.5 × 10^9/L
Baso#	0	0.02–0.1 × 10^9/L
RETIC%	6%	0.5–1.5%
ESR	34	0–20 mm 1st h Westergren

9.1 Questions

Q1. Interpret the CBC result given above and suggest investigations for further evaluation in this case.

Answer: The CBC shows low values for red cell count, Hb, and Hct. Other red cell indices are normal. The differential count shows mild neutrophilia. Reticulocyte % is high, and ESR is also little raised. So, there is normocytic normochromic anemia with high reticulocyte count.

Normocytic normochromic anemia can be seen in the following conditions [1, 2]:

(a) *Decreased production from marrow (will have low reticulocyte count)*: Chronic pathological conditions (such as chronic inflammations, neoplastic pathologies, and infections), chronic renal failure, chronic liver disease, endocrinopathies, marrow infiltration, and hypoplastic anemias.

(b) *Increased destruction (will have increased reticulocytes with normal marrow):*

1. Red cell defects: Defects of red cell membrane (HS HE), hemoglobin (structural hemoglobinopathies), or enzyme deficiency (G6PD, pyruvate kinase, nicotinamide adenine dinucleotide phosphate [NADPH], glutathione).
2. Without any defect of red cells (defects lies outside red cells): Autoimmune hemolytic anemia, micro-angiopathic hemolytic anemia (DIC/TTP/HUS).
3. PNH.

(c) *Sequestration: splenomegaly.*
(d) *Hemorrhage.*

Next best investigation will be to examine a blood film and tests for renal functions and liver functions. As there is reticulocytosis indicating either bone marrow response or hemolysis, hemolytic parameters (LDH and haptoglobin) and test of urine for hemoglobin, urobilinogen and hemosiderin should also be considered.

Q2. Given are images from blood film (Figs. 9.1 and 9.2), results of kidney functions, liver functions with hemolytic parameters (Table 9.2), and examination of urine (Table 9.3). Interpret these results and suggest a differential diagnosis. What further investigations should be done to exclude various possibilities?

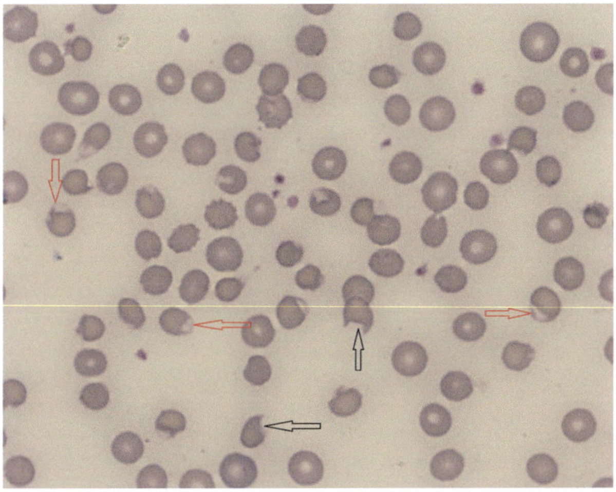

Fig. 9.1 Blood film. Blister cells (red cells), Bite cells (white arrows). Leishman stain ×100

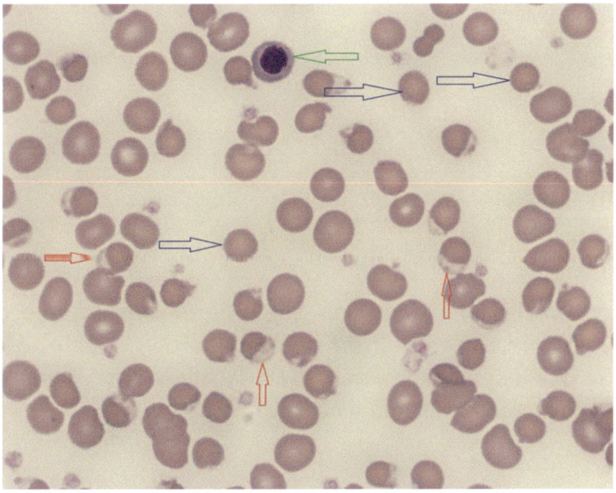

Fig. 9.2 Blood film. spherocytes (blue arrows), blister cells (red arrows), nucleated red cells (green arrow). Leishman stain ×100

Table 9.2 Biochemical tests

Test	Patient's result	Ref range
Glu	5.1	3.9–6.1 mmol/L
Urea	4.1	2.5–6.6 mmol/L
Creat	88	60–120 μmol/L
Na^+	141	136–146 mmol/L
K^+	4.2	3.7–5.0 mmol/L
Ca^+	2.0	2.2–2.6 mmol/L
Mg^+	1.0	0.08–1.1 mmol/L
T. Prot	73	63–80 mmol/L
Alb	40	35–47 mmol/L
Choles	3.4	1.5–5.2 mmol/L
TG	0.7	0.4–1.7 mmol/L
Urates	332	150–400 mmol/L
T Bil	**48**	3–20 μmol/L
D. Bil	9	0–5 μmol/L
I Bil	**39**	5–15 μmol/L
Alk Ph	60	26–88 IU/L
ALT	55	10–60 IU/L
AST	36	10–42 IU/L
GGT	10	7–64 IU/L
LDH	**280**	90–180 IU/L
Hapto	**0.17**	0.2–2.0 g/L

Table 9.3 Urine examination

Urine examination	Patient's result	Reference range
SG	1.022	1.005–1.030
Ph	6.2	5–7
Leu	Neg	Neg
Nit	Neg	Neg
Pro	Neg	Neg
Glu	Neg	Neg
Ket	Neg	Neg
Uro	Traces	0.1–1.8 μmol/L
Bil	Neg	Neg
Hemoglobin	Positive	Neg
Hemosiderin	Positive	Negative

Answer: The blood films show normocytic normochromic red cells, bite cells (white arrows), blister cells (red arrows), nucleated red cell (green arrow), and spherocyte (blue arrow). These finding are highly suggestive of enzyme deficiency (G6PD deficiency).

The biochemical tests show indirect hyperbilirubinemia (raised total and indirect bilirubin), raised LDH, and low haptoglobin. Urine examination shows hemoglobinuria and hemosiderinuria. These findings are consistent with hemolytic anemia (intravascular) with a high possibility of enzyme deficiency state.

Based on these results (bite cells, blister cells, and evidence of hemolysis), possible diagnoses are enzyme deficiencies like G6PD deficiency, pyruvate kinase deficiency (PKD), NADPH deficiency, glutathione deficiency, immune-mediated hemolysis, micro-angiopathic hemolytic anemia (MAHA), and unstable hemoglobin. The blood film examination, however, excludes the possibility of MAHA.

Further investigations required in this case will be to test for Heinz bodies, G6PD screening (fluorescent spot test), estimation of G6PD enzyme level, and detection of unstable hemoglobin. Direct Coombs test and screening for immunological causes (ANA) may also be considered. OFT is optional and should be done at a later stage as only a few spherocytes were also noted on blood films.

NADPH and glutathione are part of hexose monophosphate shunt pathway (HMP pathway), where G6PD plays its role, and their deficiencies are extremely rare. Determination of a specific enzyme activity using a spectrophotometric assay is required for exact identification.

Q3. Given are results of test for Heinz bodies (Fig. 9.3), G6PD screening (Fig. 9.4), and result of G6PD assay, isopropanol precipitation test, heat denaturation test, OFT, antinuclear antibodies (ANA), and direct Coombs test (DAT; Table 9.4). Interpret these tests and suggest a final diagnosis. What are other specialized tests which may be considered in this patient to exclude rare possibilities?

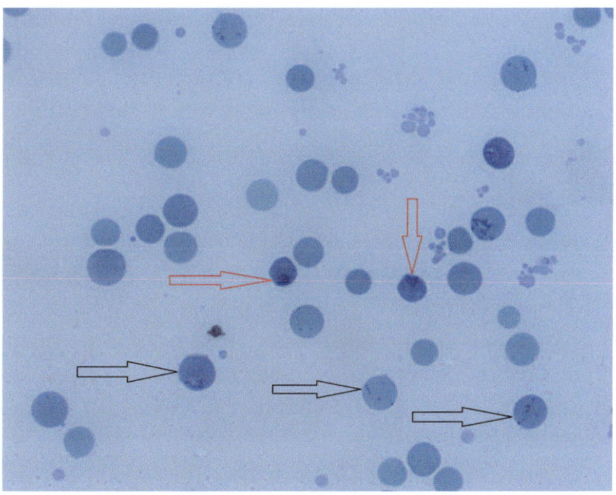

Fig. 9.3 PBF. Heinz bodies (red arrows) and normal reticulocytes (black arrows). New methylene blue stain ×100

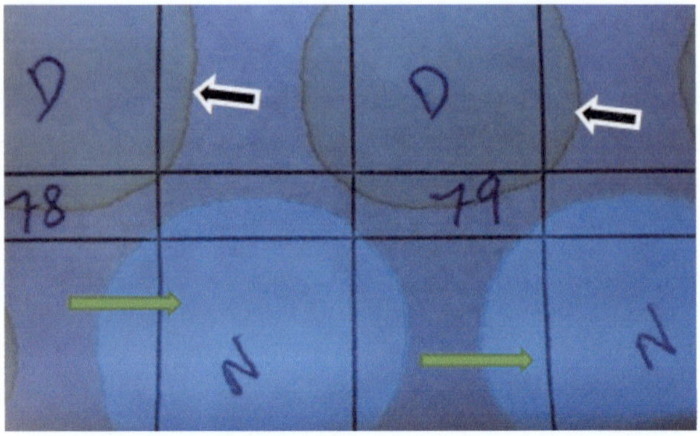

Fig. 9.4 G6PD fluorescent screening test (FST). Normal G6PD (green arrows). G6PD deficient (white arrows)

Table 9.4 Specialized tests

Test	Patient's result	Ref range
G6PD enzyme assay	**3**	**5–20 units/gm Hb**
Isopropanol precipitation test	Negative	Negative
Heat denaturation test	Negative	Negative
Direct antiglobulin test	Negative	Negative
ANA screen	Negative	Negative
Osmotic fragility test (OFT)	Negative	Negative

Answer: Blood film with supravital stain (new methylene blue) shows Heinz bodies and normal reticulocytes. The G6PD screening test (FST) shows no fluorescence (black arrow compared to normal for green arrows) for patient, suggesting G6PD enzyme-deficient state. The G6PD enzyme assay shows the level of enzyme far below the normal value, confirming a diagnosis of G6PD deficiency in this patient. Rest of the tests for unstable hemoglobin, immune causes of hemolysis, and hereditary spherocytosis are negative. Thus a final diagnosis of G6PD deficiency resulting in hemolytic anemia in this patient is confirmed.

Once G6PD enzyme deficiency is confirmed by enzyme assay, no further investigations are required in routine clinical practice. However, some patients, especially females, may require genetic testing for the confirmation of deficiency state (see below). Deficiencies of NADPH and glutathione are extremely rare, and their enzyme activity is estimated using a spectrophotometric assay.

OFT is recommended only if a number of spherocytes are significantly high, the patient has splenomegaly, and there is a family history suggestive of spherocytosis. HPLC is, sometimes, done to evaluate such cases as a part of hereditary nonspherocytic hemolytic anemia (HNSHA). In this patient, both OFT and HPLC were normal.

Q4. What laboratory investigations will help to exclude pyruvate kinase deficiency?

Answer: Pyruvate kinase deficiency (PKD) is an autosomal-recessive disease with a defect in *PKLR* gene located on chromosome 1. Because of rarity of condition and wide clinical presentations, many patients remain undiagnosed.

PK deficiency is diagnosed under appropriate clinical symptoms and signs of hemolytic anemia, splenomegaly, jaundice, and a history of gallstones, and supported by laboratory markers of hemolysis, including reticulocytosis and indirect hyperbilirubinemia [3].

Investigations for PKD deficiency should be done after other causes of hemolysis are ruled out. Peripheral blood film shows anisocytosis, poikilocytosis, and contracted red blood cells (Fig. 9.5) along with occasional blister cells. Spherocytes are absent. G6PD enzyme activity is normal; direct antiglobulin test and hemoglobin electrophoresis are normal. The incubated osmotic fragility test may be abnormal with hemolysis, which can be corrected by ATP but not by glucose. Confirmation will require quantitative estimation of enzyme. Genetic study for PKLR mutational analysis is diagnostic.

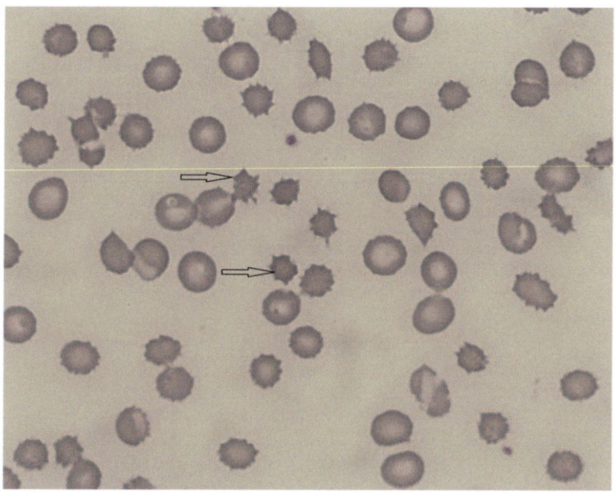

Fig. 9.5 Pyruvate kinase deficiency. Leishman stain ×100

Q5. Which patients require genetic testing and why?

Answer: The G6PD gene is located on X chromosome and is an X-linked recessive disorder. Males have only one X allele (XY), and females have two X alleles (XX). Males with a single X chromosome will have either a normal working G6PD gene (allele) or a defective G6PD gene (allele). So they will be either normal or deficient [4].

But females have two alleles (XX). So if one is a defective allele, still the other allele will produce sufficient enzyme to keep the enzyme level between 30 and 80%. This is a heterozygous state with one normal and one abnormal G6PD allele. They have two populations of red cells—one with normal enzyme and the other with deficient enzyme activity. If the G6PD activity is less than 30% in female, she is considered as G6PD deficient. She is considered as homozygous for G6PD-deficient alleles. So such females who are heterozygous or homozygous for deficiency may require genetic analysis for exact categorization. Any female whose red cell G6PD activity is 80% or more is considered as normal for G6PD. There are approximately 230 G6PD variants with known mutations (Table 9.5) [5].

Table 9.5 Genotype–phenotype correlation in G6PD patients

	Genotype	Phenotype	Enzyme activity
Male	$X^N Y^N$	Normal	Above 80%
	$X^0 Y^N$	Deficient	Below 30%
Female	$X^N X^N$	Normal	Above 80%
	$X^O X^N$	Intermediate	30–80%
	$X^0 X^0$	Deficient	Below 30%

X^N normal; Y^N normal; X^0 deficient.

Q6. What tests are normally required for establishing a diagnosis of G6PD in clinical setting?

Answer:

1. The Heinz body test.
2. Fluorescent spot test.
3. Methemoglobin reduction test.
4. G6PD assay.
5. Genetic analysis in select cases.

Screening procedures are not suitable for diagnosis in female heterozygotes and in patients with relatively milder forms of G6PD deficiency. The correct diagnosis of patients who have recently undergone hemolysis may be obscured by the large proportion of young cells (reticulocytes) in the circulation. In female heterozygotes, blood contains varying proportions of normal and deficient cells. There is no biochemical method that is entirely reliable in the detection of heterozygotes. Only DNA analysis is helpful in definite diagnosis [5].

Q7. In which other conditions Heinz bodies are seen?

Answer: Heinz bodies can also be seen in thalassemia, methemoglobinemia, and unstable hemoglobin, e.g., HB Koln. They may also be due to the effect of drugs, plants, or chemicals with oxidative properties [6].

Q8. What is pathogenesis of G6PD deficiency?

Answer: G6PD enzyme has a role in hexose monophosphate shunt pathway. When oxygen enters red cells, it combines with hemoglobin to form oxyhemoglobin. Subsequently methemoglobin (Fe^{3+}) and superoxide radicals are produced, both of which need to be reduced. The methemoglobin (Fe^{3+}) is rapidly reduced back to Hb (Fe^{2+}) by methemoglobin reductase, and superoxide radicals are converted to hydrogen peroxide (H_2O_2), which is a powerful oxidizing agent.

Also, oxidized glutathione needs to be reduced back to reduced glutathione; the latter is capable of neutralizing reactive oxygen species. All these reactions require NADPH, which is a powerful reducing agent. NADPH is formed from NADP by G6PD enzyme. In the absence of G6PD, NADPH will not be formed. In such circumstances, H_2O_2 persists, and oxidative damage of red cells occurs [7].

Q9. What are trigger factors for hemolysis in G6PD deficiency?

Answer: Fava beans, drugs, and infections are three most common triggers for hemolysis.

1. Fava beans: Divicine and isouramil present in fava beans can generate oxygen free radicals.
2. Drugs: Antimalarial drugs and antibiotics like ciprofloxacin, moxifloxacin, nalidixic acid, norfloxacin, niridazole, nitrofurantoin, ofloxacin, phenazopyridine, rasburicase, sulfamethoxazole, sulfadiazine, sulfasalazine, and sulfonylurea are some of the important drugs implicated in formation of oxygen free radicals. Aspirin also has dose-dependent effect.

3. Infections: *Streptococcus*, *Staphylococcus*, *Brucella*, *Rickettsia*, *Clostridium difficile*, and viral infections like hepatitis and CMV. During inflammation and infections, free radicals are produced, which diffuse into the red cells [8].

Q10. Why G6PD-deficient patients are considered to be protected against malaria?
Answer: The oxidative stress in G6PD-deficient red cells seems to be detrimental to the survival of parasites, and also possibly, G6PD-deficient cells are phagocytosed early. The explanations are debatable [8].

Q11. How is G6PD deficiency classified?
Class I—associated with chronic non-spherocytic hemolytic anemia (CNSHA).
Class II—severely deficient: less than 10% residual activity.
Class III—moderately deficient: 10–60% residual activity.
Class IV—normal activity: 60–150%.
Class V—increased activity [9].

Q12. What are the factors which affect G6PD activity?
Answer: Factors that can affect G6PD activity are:

1. G6PD variant.
2. Age of RBCs.
3. Anemia.
4. Associated hemoglobinopathies.
5. Reticulocytes with high G6PD levels (resistance to oxidative stress).

Q13. What is the ideal time for conducting G6PD assay in patients with a history of G6PD deficiency?
Answer: The G6PD levels are falsely high at the time of hemolysis. This is due to the presence of reticulocytes, which are high in G6PD content. Ideally, this assay should be done after 3–4 weeks of recovery from hemolytic attack.

9.2 Correlation of Results of Preliminary Investigations with Symptoms and Signs in G6PD Deficiency

Q14. How do symptoms and signs in this patients correlate with diagnosis.
Answer: This child has symptoms of anemia following respiratory tract infection treated with antibiotics. Presence of jaundice and passage of tea-colored urine indicate intravascular hemolysis, and a family history of G6PD deficiency correlates well with a diagnosis of G6PD deficiency in this child.

Q15. How do CBC, blood film, and biochemical tests guide in the evaluation of this case?
The CBC shows normocytic normochromic anemia with reticulocytosis. The blood film shows bite cells, blister cells, and occasional spherocytes. The biochemical tests show evidence of hemolysis in the form of raised unconjugated bilirubin,

high LDH, and reduced amount of haptoglobin indicating intravascular hemolysis. All these findings guide us to a possibility of G6PD deficiency in which normocytic normochromic anemia, intravascular hemolysis, and typical red cell abnormalities are observed.

Q16. What is the mechanism of formation of bite cells (keratocyte), blister cells (helmet cell), and few spherocytes in this case?

Answer: The denatured hemoglobin gets accumulated as small inclusions on one side of the red cell and appears as Heinz bodies. The Heinz bodies are selectively removed by macrophages in spleen, and the removed part appears as a bite on red cell membrane. Following bite, the cell membrane is reformed through fibrin strands, and a vacuole or blister like appearance is imparted to the cells. Some of the cells regenerate their membrane, and these cells look like a spherocyte.

Q17. What were confirmatory tests in this case, and why G6PD level is not markedly suppressed?

Answer: Markedly reduced G6PD enzyme level was confirmatory in this patient. This patient has a G6PD enzyme level of 3, which is most likely due to the presence of reticulocytes which are high in G6PD content. Ideally, this test should be repeated 3–4 weeks after recovery from hemolytic episode to check the exact level of enzyme. If the patient is female with an enzyme level of 30–80% (heterozygous or homozygous for deficiency), she may require genetic analysis for exact categorization [10].

Q18. What is the principle of fluorescent spot test (FST), methemoglobin reduction test, and enzyme assays?

Answer: The FST is the most widely used qualitative screening test that has a sensitivity and specificity of around 94–95%. The results are of limited value when enzyme levels are less than 15–20%. The test is based on the principle that it measures G6PD enzyme activity by detecting the conversion of coenzyme nicotinamide adenine dinucleotide phosphate (NADP) into its reduced form (NADPH). The reduced form (NADPH) is observed directly using fluorescent light (due to its property of autofluorescence) [11].

In methemoglobin reduction test, oxyhemoglobin is first converted to methemoglobin, and then the rate of methemoglobin reduction is observed in the presence of methylene blue and glucose [12].

The enzyme assay is a quantitative test that requires spectrophotometry, which estimates G6PD by measuring the formation of NADPH from NADP by G6PD enzyme present in red cells. The rate of reduction of NADP to NADPH is measured as an increase in absorbance at 340 nm produced in the reaction catalyzed by the enzyme which is proportional to the G6PD activity in the sample [13].

Q19. How should the patients of G6PD be followed up?

Answer: Such patients are required to avoid fava beans and certain drugs (antibiotics, antimalarials, and analgesics). Repeat enzyme levels should be done when a patient is in remission (non-hemolytic condition). Management mainly consists of preventing hemolysis by avoiding triggers.

9.3 Quick Information for Practicing Clinicians and Students

References [1–12]:

1. G6PD deficiency is the commonest red cell enzyme defect. It is inherited as X-linked recessive disease.
2. Male are either normal or deficient. Females can be normal, deficient, or have intermediate levels of enzymes.
3. Triggers for hemolysis include ingestion of fava beans, certain drugs, and some infections.
4. Avoidance of trigger factors is key to prevent hemolysis.
5. Always ask for the family history of G6PD deficiency.
6. Massive intravascular hemolysis produces tea-colored urine.
7. Anemia is normocytic normochromic with reticulocytosis.
8. Always ask for biochemical tests which help to establish hemolytic anemia.
9. Confirmation of diagnosis is done by fluorescent spot test and estimation of G6PD enzyme level.
10. Avoid test for G6PD assay during an acute episode of hemolysis when reticulocytosis is present. This test should be ideally done at least 2–3 weeks after recovery from hemolytic episode.

To acquire further knowledge on the subject, following sources are advised:

1. BCSH guidelines
2. Br Jr. Hematology
3. ASH education book
4. Blood
5. NEJM
6. Int Jr. Lab Hematology

References

1. Ward PC. Investigation of nonpoikilocytic normochromic normocytic anemia. Postgrad Med. 1979;65(3):233–5, 238, 241-3
2. Ford J. Red blood cell morphology. Int J Lab Hematol. 2013;35:351–7. https://doi.org/10.1111/ijlh.12082.
3. Bianchi P, Elisa Fermo E, Glader B, et al. Addressing the diagnostic gaps in pyruvate kinase (PK) deficiency: consensus recommendations on the diagnosis of PK deficiency. Am J Hematol. 2019;94(1):149–61.
4. Lauden SM, Chongwain S, Achidi A, Helm E, Cusick SE, Krug A, Slusher TM, Lund TC. Prevalence of glucose-6-phosphate dehydrogenase deficiency in Cameroonian blood donors. BMC Res Notes. 2019;12(1):195.
5. Luzzatto L, Nannelli C, Notaro R. Glucose-6-phosphate dehydrogenase deficiency. Hematol Oncol Clin North Am. 2016;30(2):373–93.

6. Rodak BF, Carr JH. Inclusions in erythrocytes. In: Clinical hematology atlas. 5th ed. St. Louis: Elsevier Inc.; 2017. p. 107–14.
7. Ong KIC, Iwagami M, Araki H, Khattignavong P, Soundala P, Keomalaphet S, Prasayasith P, Lorpachan L, Xangsayalath P, Pongvongsa T, Hongvanthong B, Brey PT, Kano S, Jimba M. Prevalence of G6PD Viangchan variant in malaria endemic areas in Lao PDR: an implication for malaria elimination by 2030. Malar J. 2019;18(1):75.
8. Allison AC. Malaria and glucose-6-phosphate dehydrogenase deficiency. Nature. 1963;197:609–609.
9. Caterina N, Andrea B, Jane C, Pierre-Antoine D, Luzzatto L. Genetic variants causing G6PD deficiency: clinical and biochemical data support new WHO classification. Br J Haematol. 2023;202:1–9.
10. David R, Mark L, David R, et al. Laboratory diagnosis of G6PD deficiency. A British Society rheumatology guideline. Br J Haematol. 2020;189:24–38.
11. Betke K, Brewer GJ, Kirkman HN, Luzzatto L, Motulsky AG, Ramot B, Siniscalco M. Standardization of procedure for the study of glucose-6-phosphate dehydrogenase: report of a WHO Scientific Group. World Health Org Techn Rep Ser. 1979;366:1–53.
12. Minucci A, Giardina B, Zuppi C, Capoluongo E. Glucose-6-phosphate dehydrogenase laboratory assay: how, when, and why? IUBMB Life. 2009;61(1):27–34.
13. Beutler E. Red cell metabolism: a manual of biochemical methods. 3rd ed. New York: Grune & Strattan; 1984.

Chapter 10
Autoimmune Hemolytic Anemia

A 70-year-old male reports to hematology OPD with a history of gradually progressive weakness for the last 3 months. He was diagnosed with CLL 6 months back and was kept on followup without any specific medications. Currently, he is experiencing low-grade fever, exertional dyspnea, lethargy, and weight loss. Physical examination showed pallor and mild tinge of jaundice. Examination revealed tiny, 1–2 cm, cervical, axillary, and inguinal lymph nodes. There was no hepatomegaly. Only the tip of the spleen was palpable. Result of CBC done at presentation is given (Table 10.1):

Table 10.1 CBC

CBC parameter	Patient's result	Reference range
WBC	75	3.7–10 × 10^9/L
RBC	3.6	4.5–5.4 × 10^{12}/L
HB	8.5	130–160 g/L
Hct	0.26	0.33–0.43 L/L
MCV	105	83–101 fL
MCH	27	27–32 pg
MCHC	360	315–345 g/L
RDW	14	11.6–14.6%
PLT	150	130–430 × 10^9/L
MPV	10	7–11 fL
Poly #	1.4	1.7–6 × 10^9/L
Lymp#	33	1–3 × 10^9/L
Mono#	0.4	0.2–1.0 × 10^9/L
EO#	0.2	0.02–0.5 × 10^9/L
BASO#	0	0.02–0.1 × 10^9/L
RETIC%	3.9	0.5–1.5%
ESR	57	0–20 mm 1st h Westergren

A. Gupta, *Decision Making Through Problem Based Learning in Hematology*, https://doi.org/10.1007/978-981-99-8933-1_10

10.1 Questions

Q1. Interpret the CBC result given above and suggest investigations for further evaluation in such case.

Answer: The CBC result shows high total leukocytic count, low number of RBCs, decreased hemoglobin level and hematocrit, and high MCV and MCHC. There is absolute lymphocytosis. Reticulocyte count is increased. ESR value is also high.

So there is leukocytosis with lymphocytosis. Anemia is macrocytic with high MCHC. Reticulocytosis indicates a bone marrow response to anemia.

Causes of macrocytic anemia in this age group include:

1. Megaloblastic anemia: Deficiency or impaired utilization of B_{12}/folic acid.
2. Non-megaloblastic etiologies: Myelodysplasia, liver disease, hypothyroidism, aplastic anemia, erythroleukemia, reticulocytosis, alcoholism, and certain drugs.
3. In addition pseudo-macrocytosis (falsely high MCV) also needs to be excluded.

In the presence of high reticulocyte %, the possible cause of anemia is either peripheral destruction or bleeding.

Next best investigation in this case will be examination of blood film. Also estimation of serum levels of vitamin B_{12} and folic acid, and serum chemistry for functions of liver, kidney, and thyroid are indicated for evaluation. Routine urine and stool examination (for occult blood) are also suggested.

Q2. Given are images from blood film (Figs. 10.1 and 10.2), results of serum levels of vitamin B_{12} and folic acid (Table 10.2), liver, kidney, thyroid functions (Table 10.3), and examination of urine and stools (Table 10.4). Interpret these results and suggest a differential diagnosis. What further investigations should be done to exclude various possibilities?

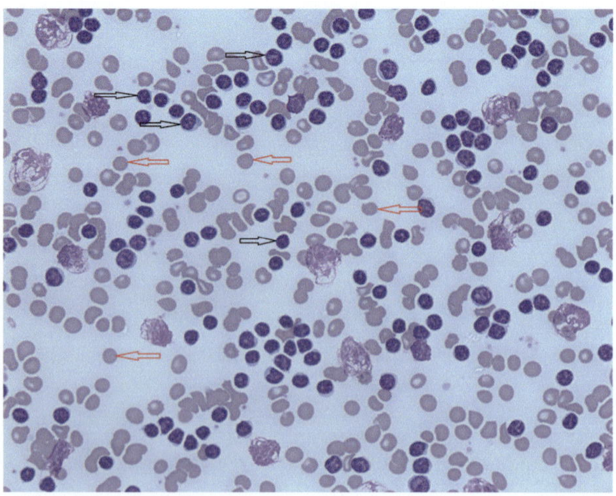

Fig. 10.1 PBF. Lymphocytes (black arrows) and spherocytes (red arrows). Leishman stain ×40

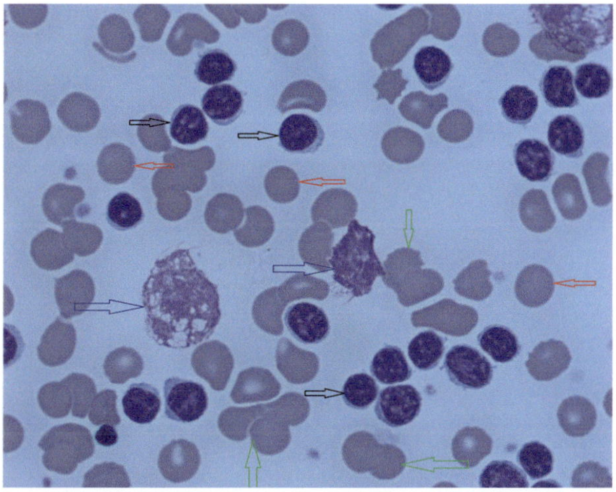

Fig. 10.2 PBF. Spherocytes (red arrows) and mature lymphocytes (black arrows), red cell clumps (green arrows), smudge cells (blue arrows). Leishman stain ×100

Table 10.2 Serum B_{12}, folic acid, and CRP

Test	Patient's result	Ref range
S. B_{12}	665	150–700 pmol/L
S. folate	31.7	10–42 nmol/L
RBC folate	2554	1187–2854 nmol/L
CRP	3	0–10 mg/L

Table 10.3 Biochemical tests

Test	Patient's result	Ref range
Glu	5.5	3.9–6.1 mmol/L
Urea	5.9	2.5–6.6 mmol/L
Creat	99	60–120 μmol/L
Na^+	142	136–146 mmol/L
K^+	4.9	3.7–5.0 mmol/L
Ca^+	2.3	2.2–2.6 mmol/L
Mg^+	1.0	0.08–1.1 mmol/L
T. Prot	78	63–80 mmol/L
Alb	44	35–47 mmol/L
Choles	3.5	1.5–5.2 mmol/L
TG	0.9	0.4–1.7 mmol/L
Urates	398	150–400 mmol/L
T Bil	42	3–20 μmol/L
D. Bil	5	0–5 μmol/L
I Bil	37	5–15 μmol/L
Alk Ph	60	26–88 IU/L
ALT	54	10–60 IU/L
AST	33	10–42 IU/L
GGT	55	7–64 IU/L
LDH	280	90–180 IU/L
Hapto	0.1	0.2–2.0 g/L
T4	10.6	7.8–16 pmol/L
TSH	3.99	0.27–4.2 μlU/ml
Amylase	20	28–100 IU/L
Lipase	30	0–160 U/L

Table 10.4 Urine and stool examination

Urine examination	Patient's result	Reference range
SG	1.021	1.005–1.030
Ph	6.1	5–7
Leu	Neg	Neg
Nit	Neg	Neg
Pro	Neg	Neg
Glu	Neg	Neg
Ket	Neg	Neg
Uro	Neg	Neg
Bil	Neg	Neg
Hemosiderin	Positive	Neg
Stool examination		
Occult blood	Neg	Neg
Ova/cysts	Neg	Neg

Answer: The blood film confirms Leukocytosis. All are mature-looking lymphocytes. Smudge cells are also seen. No immature cells are seen. Many spherocytes are noted. In addition, a few tiny clumps of two to three red cells are also observed. The biochemical tests show indirect hyperbilirubinemia, high levels of LDH, and reduced level of haptoglobin, which suggest a hemolytic process.. The serum levels of vitamin B_{12} and folic acid are within normal limits. The urine examination shows hemosiderinuria, suggestive of chronic intravascular hemolysis. The high WBC count with mature lymphocytes suggests chronic lymphocytic leukemia. All these results combined together indicate CLL with hemolytic anemia.

Possible causes of anemia in CLL include the following:

1. Marrow infiltration by abnormal lymphocytes resulting in the replacement of marrow erythroid precursors.
2. Bleeding.
3. Vitamin deficiencies.
4. Renal disease.
5. Autoimmune hemolytic anemia (AIHA).

However, except for AIHA, none of them causes hemolysis. For further evaluation and confirmation of AIHA, antiglobulin test (AGT) with IgG and C3d are required. For confirmation of CLL, immunophenotyping and cytogenetic analysis are helpful. Bone marrow biopsy is usually necessary to document the extent of CLL infiltration and to rule out other causes [1].

Q3. Given are the results of direct antiglobulin test (DAT), immunological tests (Table 10.5), bone marrow biopsy (Fig. 10.3), and flow cytometry and cytogenetics analysis on bone marrow–aspirated sample (Table 10.6). Analyze these results and suggest final diagnosis in this patient.

Table 10.5 DAT and immunology screen

Test	Patient's result	Ref range
Direct antiglobulin test	Positive (2+) – IgG	Negative
Anti ds-DNA antibody	Negative	0–20 Iu/mL
ANA screen	Negative	Negative
AnA pattern	Negative	Negative
ANA titer	Negative	Negative
Sm B	Negative	Negative
RNP A and C	Negative	Negative
SS-A	Negative	Negative
SS-B	Negative	Negative
Scl-70	Negative	Negative
Jo-1	Negative	Negative
Ribosomal P	Negative	Negative
Histone	Negative	Negative
MPO Ab	Negative	Negative
Proteinase Ab	Negative	Negative

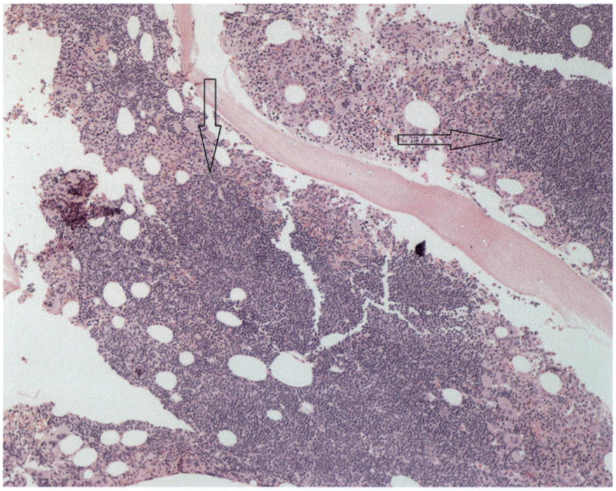

Fig. 10.3 BM trephine biopsy. Infiltration of mature lymphocytes. H/E stain ×40

Table 10.6 Flow cytometry and cytogenetic analysis

CD marker	CD5	CD10	CD19	CD20	CD23	CD79b	FMC-7	CD25	CD11c	CD103
% positivity	80	1	70	68 (weak)	75	5	1	10	8	1
Cytogenetic analysis: Normal male karyotype (46XY)										

Answer: The DAT is positive for IgG. The immunological screen tests are negative. The bone marrow biopsy shows mature lymphoid cells infiltrating all marrow spaces. These lymphoid cells are mostly distributed in aggregates as well as interspersed in interstitial spaces. There is no fibrosis. The erythroid precursors are also present. The flow cytometry for CD markers on aspirated sample shows these cells to be positive for CD5, CD23, CD22 (weak), CD19, and are negative for FMC-7. Cytogenetics shows normal male karyotype. All these findings confirm a final diagnosis of warm autoimmune hemolytic anemia secondary to CLL.

Q4. What are the causes of warm autoimmune hemolytic anemia?

Answer: The autoimmune hemolytic anemia is either warm antibody or cold antibody induced. The warm antibody hemolytic anemia can be idiopathic (primary) or secondary to autoimmune diseases like SLE and RA, lymphoproliferative disorders such as chronic lymphocytic leukemia, lymphoma, ovarian tumors, and also some infections, e.g., babesiosis. Few medicines like methyldopa and penicillin can also induce warm antibody immune hemolytic anemia. The cold antibody autoimmune hemolytic anemia can also be idiopathic (primary) and is mostly induced by infections such as mycoplasma, infectious mononucleosis, and CMV infection. Chronic lymphoproliferative diseases can also produce cold antibody autoimmune hemolytic anemia [2].

Q5. What are diagnostic laboratory findings in warm antibody AIHA?

Answer: A diagnosis of warm AIHA is made mostly if Hb is less than 110 G/L with the presence of hemolytic markers (unconjugated hyperbilirubinemia, high lactate dehydrogenase, reduced haptoglobin, reticulocytosis) and positive AGT (IgG alone or IgG + C3d) [3].

Presence of spherocytes and red cell clumps are initial pointers to immune process. Other causes such as drug-induced immune hemolytic anemia, allo-immune-mediated hemolysis, glucose-6-phosphate deficiency(G6PD), burns, and transfusion of old blood can also show some spherocytes on blood film [4].

Q6. What is the pathogenesis of warm-type immune hemolytic anemia in CLL patients?

Answer: CLL lymphocytes are responsible of a number of pathogenic mechanisms, including aberrant antigen presentation and cytokine production. The pathogenic B-cell lymphocytes may induce the emergence of autoreactive B-cells producing anti-red blood cells and antiplatelet autoantibodies.

1. IgG autoantibodies coat erythrocytes, platelets, and neutrophils with consequent antibody-dependent cellular cytotoxicity and complement-mediated destruction in the reticuloendothelial system (spleen and liver) or in the blood stream.
2. Anti-erythroblast and megakaryocyte autoantibodies can impair bone marrow compensatory response.
3. Autoreactive T cells produce inflammatory cytokines and further inhibit myelopoiesis [5].

Autoimmune hemolytic anemia (AIHA) is caused by the destruction of red blood cells (RBCs) by anti-RBC autoantibodies. IgG antibodies are directed mainly against epitopes of the Rh system. It can happen with or without complement activation.

RBC destruction may occur by a direct lysis through complement activation (MAC) or by antibody-dependent cell-mediated cytotoxicity (ADCC). Direct complement-mediated lysis takes place mainly in the circulation resulting in intravascular hemolysis. ADCC and phagocytosis occur in the spleen and lymphoid organs producing extravascular hemolysis [6].

CD4+ CD25+ regulatory T cells (Tregs) are now recognized as key players in immunologic tolerance. Tregs produce IL-10 and transforming growth factor β (TGF-β), which may play an essential role in AIHA [7].

(Note: Tregs are a specialized subpopulation of T cells that act to suppress immune response, thereby maintaining homeostasis and self-tolerance.)

10.2 Correlation of Results of Preliminary Investigations with Symptoms and Signs in Auto immune Hemolytic Anemia

Q7. Correlate signs and symptoms with the clinical diagnosis of this patient.

Answer: Gradually progressive weakness, exertional dyspnea, and lethargy are all symptoms of anemia. Pallor is due to anemia and jaundice is due to the presence of bilirubin following hemolysis. These correlate with the diagnosis of a hemolytic anemia. Presence of lymphadenopathy is part of CLL.

Q8 How do CBC, blood film, and biochemical tests guide in the evaluation of this case?

Answer: CBC shows anemia with high MCV and MCHC. Examination of blood film does not show macrocytes, but high MCV is due to tiny two to three red cell clumps (pseudo-macrocytosis), which are detected by autoanalyzer as cells with high MCV. High MCHC is due to the presence of spherocytes. Reticulocytosis suggests good bone marrow response and excludes inhibitory effect of disease on erythroblastic production and maturation. A high indirect bilirubin, high LDH, and low haptoglobin are pointers toward intravascular hemolytic process which along with the presence of spherocytes, reticulocytosis, and a positive DAT test confirm the diagnosis of AIHA. Mature lymphocytes and smudge cells are part of CLL.

Q9. What are other causes of pseudo-macrocytosis?

Answer: Clumping of red cells is more prominent in cold agglutinin disease and may also occur due to inflammatory or neoplastic conditions. Severe leukocytosis or hyperglycemia may also result in overestimation of MCV by autoanalyzers [8].

Q9. In which other conditions DAT positivity is seen, and what are the causes of false negative DAT?

Answer: DAT can be positive in patients without AIHA following transfusion of intravenous immunoglobulin, increased serum immunoglobulin, spontaneous red cell agglutination, elevated blood urea nitrogen levels, and if there is improper sample collection(clotted sample) or over centrifugation. Between 2% and 10% of all AIHA patients are DAT negative. DAT can be falsely negative if there is improper cell washing, delay in adding antiglobulin reagent after the washing step, or if antiglobulin reagent is ineffective [9].

Q10. What are pathophysiological differences between different types of autoimmune hemolytic anemias?

Answer: AIHA is warm, cold, or mixed types.

1. In warm AIHA: DAT is positive for IgG or IgG + C3d. The IgG antibody is directed mainly against epitopes of the Rh system.
2. Cold AIHA is further categorized into:
   (a) Cold agglutinin disease (CAD): DAT is positive for C3d. IgM antibody is directed against the I/i system.
   (b) Paroxysmal cold hemoglobinuria (PCH): Donath-Landsteiner antibodies are seen. These are biphasic IgG antibodies directed against the red cell P antigen. It binds to RBCs at cold temperatures and causes complement-mediated lysis when warmed to 37 °C.
3. Mixed AIHA: DAT is positive for both IgG and C3d. There is coexistence of warm IgG autoantibodies and high-titer IgM cold agglutinins [2, 10].

10.3 Quick Information for Practicing Clinicians and Students

References [1–10]:

1. Anemia with high MCV, MCHC, and reticulocytosis should be investigated for possible autoimmune pathology.
2. Hemolytic markers—reticulocytosis, indirect hyper bilirubinemia, and reduced haptoglobin indicate intravascular hemolysis, and if blood film shows spherocytes with red cell clumps, it is highly suggestive of autoimmune hemolytic anemia.
3. Direct antiglobulin test (DAT) with IgG and C3d should be done to confirm autoimmune process.
4. Viral infections, autoimmune diseases, and malignancies are most commonly associated diseases.
5. A detailed history especially of drug intake and thorough clinical examination is quite helpful in narrowing the differential diagnosis.

6. Autoanalyzers will show high MCV in the presence of red cell clumps seen in autoimmune diseases. So examination of blood film is important to exclude false positive high MCV (pseudo-macrocytosis).
7. High MCHC is due to the presence of spherocytes in blood.
8. DAT can be falsely negative due to technical reasons, i.e., improper cell washing, delay in adding antiglobulin reagent after the washing step, or if antiglobulin reagent is ineffective.
9. Up to 10% of AIHA can have negative DAT due to low titer of antibodies which may not be detected by DAT.
10. An immunology profile should be done in all cases to exclude more than one pathology producing AIHA.

To acquire further knowledge on the subject, following sources are advised:

1. BCSH guidelines
2. Br Jr. Hematology
3. ASH education book
4. Blood
5. NEJM
6. Int Jr. Lab Hematology

References

1. Visco C, Barcellini W, Maura F, Neri A, Cortelezzi A, Rodeghiero F. Autoimmune cytopenias in chronic lymphocytic leukemia. Am J Hematol. 2014;89:1055–62. https://doi.org/10.1002/ajh.23785.
2. Hill QA, Hill A, Berentsen S. Defining autoimmune hemolytic anemia: a systematic review of the terminology used for diagnosis and treatment. Blood Adv. 2019;3:1897–906. https://doi.org/10.1182/bloodadvances.2019000036.
3. Tsang M, Parikh SA. A concise review of autoimmune cytopenias in chronic lymphocytic leukemia. Curr Hematol Malig Rep. 2017;12:29–38. https://doi.org/10.1007/s11899-017-0366-1.
4. Bessis M. Red cell shapes. An illustrated classification and its rationale. Nouv Rev Fr Hematol. 1972;12:721–46.
5. Hamblin TJ, Oscier DG, Young BJ. Autoimmunity in chronic lymphocytic leukaemia. J Clin Pathol. 1986;39:713–6. https://doi.org/10.1136/jcp.39.7.713.
6. Gehrs BC, Friedberg RC. Autoimmune hemolytic anemia. Am J Hematol. 2002;69:258–71.
7. Abbas AK, Lichtman AH, Pillai S. Cellular and molecular immunology. Philadelphia: Saunders; 2012.
8. van Duijnhoven HL, Treskes M. Marked interference of hyperglycemia in measurements of mean (red) cell volume by Technicon H analyzers. Clin Chem. 1996;42:76–80.
9. Boven LA, de Haar-Holleman A, Folman CC, Kraaijenhagen RJ, Fijnheer R. Diagnostic and therapeutic challenges of severe Rh e-specific IgA-mediated autoimmune hemolytic anemia. Ann Hematol. 2012;91:641–2.
10. Brodsky RA. Warm autoimmune hemolytic anemia. N Engl J Med. 2019;381:647–54.

Chapter 11
Cold Agglutinin Disease (CAD)

A 62-year-old lady reports to hematology OPD with 5 days history of weakness, fatigue, dyspnea, and palpitations on walking. She also has mild fever and has observed pallor and blanching of her fingers and toes when exposed to cold. During the previous winter months, she had felt dusky color of nose, ears, and lips on exposure to cold.

A review of her past history revealed that she had been diagnosed to have low grade non-Hodgkins lymphoma 2 years back based on biopsy of axially lymph node, for which she was being followed up by oncologist. There is no history of recent treatment.

Examination revealed pallor of skin and mucous membrane, mild jaundice, pale digits, and few patches of bluish network of discoloration of skin on both lower legs. Tiny, less than 2 cm, cervical and axillary lymph nodes were palpable. There was no hepatosplenomegaly. Result of CBC is presented in Table 11.1.

A. Gupta, *Decision Making Through Problem Based Learning in Hematology*,
https://doi.org/10.1007/978-981-99-8933-1_11

Table 11.1 CBC

CBC parameter	Patient's result	Reference range
WBC	9.0	3.7–10 × 10^9/L
RBC	3.6	4.5–5.4 × 10^{12}/L
HB	8.9	130–160 g/L
Hct	0.20	0.33–0.43 L/L
MCV	110	83–101 fL
MCH	39	27–32 pg
MCHC	360	315–345 g/L
RDW	24	11.6–14.6%
PLT	160	130–430 × 10^9/L
MPV	10	7–11 fL
Poly#	5.4	1.7–6 × 10^9/L
Lymp#	3.0	1–3 × 10^9/L
Mono#	0.4	0.2–1.0 × 10^9/L
EO#	0.2	0.02–0.5 × 10^9/L
BASO#	0	0.02–0.1 × 10^9/L
RETIC%	12%	0.5–1.5%
ESR	90	0–20 mm 1st h Westergren

11.1 Questions

Q1. Interpret the CBC result given above and suggest investigations for further evaluation in such case.

Answer: The CBC result shows low number of RBCs, decreased hemoglobin level and hematocrit. The MCV, MCH, and MCHC values are high. Reticulocyte count is increased. ESR value is also high. Hb and hematocrit values do not correlate with each other.

So there is macrocytic anemia with reticulocytosis. In the presence of high reticulocyte %, the possible cause of anemia is either peripheral destruction or bleeding.

Causes of macrocytic anemia are as follows:

1. Megaloblastic anemia: Deficiency or impaired utilization of B12/folic acid.
2. Non-megaloblastic pathologies: Myelodysplasia, liver disease, hypothyroidism, aplastic anemia, congenital dyserythropoietic anemia (CDA-I and III), erythroleukemia, reticulocytosis, alcoholism, certain drugs, and some inherited disorders of DNA synthesis (e.g., inherited orotic aciduria, Lesch-Nyhan syndrome).
3. Pseudo macrocytosis (falsely high MCV) also needs to be excluded [1–3].

Next best investigation in this case will be examination of blood film and estimation of serum levels of vitamin12 and folic acid. Serum chemistry for functions of liver, kidney, thyroid, and hemolytic parameters is also indicated for evaluation. Routine urine and stool examination (occult blood) are also suggested.

Q2. Given are images from blood film (Figs. 11.1 and 11.2), result of serum levels of vitamin B12 and folic acid (Table 11.2), liver, kidney, thyroid functions (Table 11.3), and examination of urine and stools (Table 11.4). Interpret these findings and suggest a differential diagnosis? what further investigations should be done to arrive at a final diagnosis?

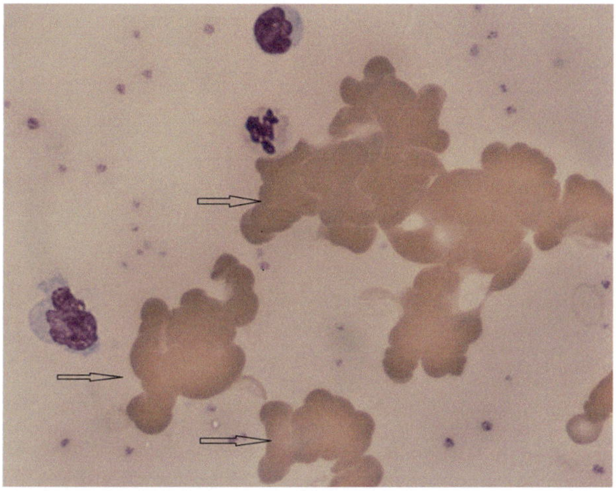

Fig. 11.1 PBF. Red cell clumps. Leishman stain ×100

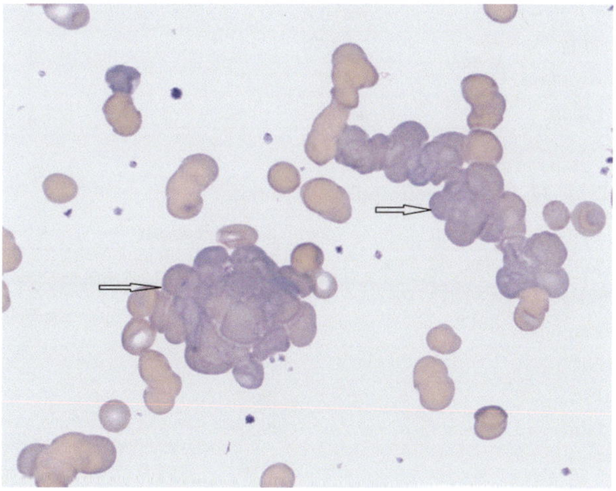

Fig. 11.2 PBF. Red cell clumps and polychromatic cells. Leishman stain ×100

Table 11.2 Serum levels of vitamin B12, folate, and CRP

Test	Patient's result	Ref range
S. B12	522	150–700 pmol/L
S. Folate	20.7	10–42 nmol/L
RBC folate	2253	1187–2854 nmol/L
CRP	6	0–10 mg/L

Table 11.3 Biochemical tests

Test	Patient's result	Ref range
Glu	5.5	3.9–6.1 mmol/L
Urea	5.9	2.5–6.6 mmol/L
Creat	99	60–120 μmol/L
Na^+	142	136–146 mmol/L
K^+	4.9	3.7–5.0 mmol/L
Ca^+	2.3	2.2–2.6 mmol/L
Mg^+	1.0	0.08–1.1 mmol/L
T. Prot	78	63–80 mmol/L
Alb	44	35–47 mmol/L
Choles	3.5	1.5–5.2 mmol/L
TG	0.9	0.4–1.7 mmol/L
Urates	398	150–400 mmol/L
T Bil	62	3–20 μmol/L
D. Bil	5	0–5 μmol/L
I Bil	57	5–15 μmol/L
Alk Ph	60	26–88 IU/L
ALT	54	10–60 IU/L
AST	33	10–42 IU/L
GGT	55	7–64 IU/L
LDH	280	90–180 IU/L
Hapto	0.02	0.2–2.0 g/L
T4	10.6	7.8–16 pmol/L
TSH	3.99	0.27–4.2 μlU/ml
Amylase	20	28–100 IU/L
Lipase	30	0–160 U/L

Table 11.4 Urine and stool examination

Urine examination	Patient's result	Reference range
SG	1.021	1.005–1.030
Ph	6.1	5–7
Leu	Neg	Neg
Nit	Neg	Neg
Pro	Neg	Neg
Glu	Neg	Neg
Ket	Neg	Neg
Uro	Neg	Neg
Bil	Neg	Neg
Hemosiderin	Neg	Neg
Hemoglobin	Pos	Neg
Stool examination		
Occult blood	Neg	Neg
Ova/cysts	Neg	Neg

Answer: The blood films show clumps of red cells of variable sizes. Many clumps show polychromatic cells. The leukocytes and platelets appear unremarkable. No immature cells were seen. The biochemical tests show indirect hyperbilirubinemia, high levels of LDH, and reduced value for haptoglobin. The serum levels of vitamin B 12 and folic acid are within normal limits. The urine shows hemoglobinuria while stool examination is normal. All these findings suggest hemolytic anemia.

This patient is known to have non-Hodgkins lymphoma. Possible causes of anemia in NHL include:

1. Anemia of chronic diseases (ACD).
2. Marrow infiltration by abnormal lymphocytes resulting in bone marrow failure.
3. Iron or vitamin deficiencies.
4. Autoimmune hemolytic anemia (AIHA).

However, except for AIHA, none of them causes hemolysis [4]. Our patient has evidence of hemolysis (reticulocytosis, polychromatic cells on blood film, high indirect bilirubin, high LDH, and low haptoglobin).

For further evaluation of hemolysis, examination of blood film after rewarming blood sample and a direct antiglobulin test (DAT) with IgG and C3d are required. Also based on these results, immunology profile will be required. Bone marrow biopsy is usually necessary to document relapse of NHL and to assess extent of infiltration.

Q3. Blood film image after rewarming blood is presented (Fig. 11.3). Also results of direct antiglobulin test (DAT), antibody titers, immunological tests (Table 11.5), and bone marrow biopsy (Fig. 11.4) are given. Interpret the results and suggest final diagnosis.

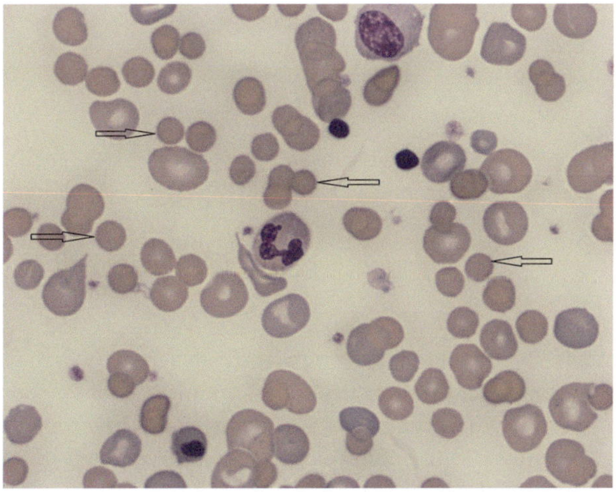

Fig. 11.3 PBF: Blood film after rewarming blood to 37 °C. Shows Spherocytes (arrows). The red cell clumps which were seen in Figs. 11.2 and 11.2 have disappeared. Leishman stain ×100

Table 11.5 DAT and immunological tests

Test	Patient's result	Ref Range
Direct antiglobulin test	Monospecific DAT -positive for C3d; cold antibody titers 1: 1024 at 4 deg. C; negative for IgG	Negative
Anti ds-DNA antibody	Negative	0–20 Iu/mL
ANA screen	Negative	Negative
AnA pattern	Negative	Negative
ANA titer	Negative	Negative
Sm B	Negative	Negative
RNP A and C	Negative	Negative
SS-A	Negative	Negative
SS-B	Negative	Negative
Scl-70	Negative	Negative
Jo-1	Negative	Negative
Ribosomal P	Negative	Negative
Histone	Negative	Negative
MPO Ab	Negative	Negative
Proteinase Ab	Negative	Negative
C3	0.537 g/L	0.83–1.77 g/L
C4	0.116 g/L	0.2–0.8 g/L

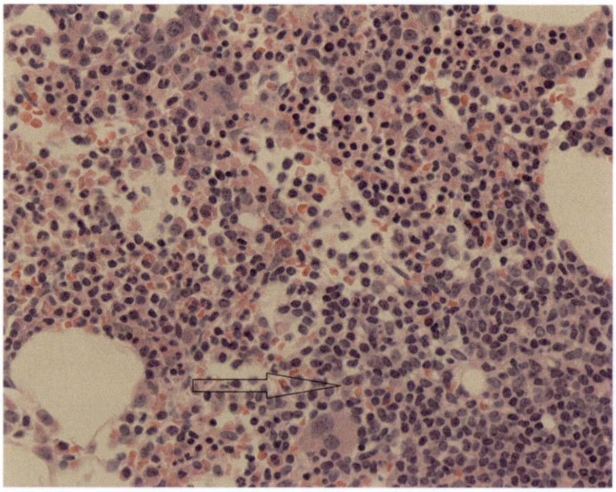

Fig. 11.4 BM Trephine biopsy. Lymphoid infiltration. H/E ×40

Answer: The blood film prepared from sample which was rewarmed to 37 °C shows disappearance of red cell agglutination. Many spherocytes are noted along with normocytic normochromic red cells. No macrocytes are seen. Thus, this patient has false high value for MCV due to red cell clumping. This is called pseudo macrocytosis.

The DAT is positive with anti-C3d and negative with anti-IgG. Cold antibody titer is 1:1024 at 4 °C. The immunological screen tests show reduced levels of C3 and C4. Other test results are normal. The bone marrow biopsy shows predominantly normocellular marrow with only an occasional tiny aggregate and few scattered-interstitial lymphoid cells. Differential cell count on bone marrow aspirate had shown less than 20% lymphoid cells. The erythroid precursors and megakaryocytes are sufficiently represented. Immunohistochemical stain with CD20 had shown scattered B- lymphoid cells. There is no fibrosis.

These findings along with CBC indices, blood film changes, hemolytic parameters, and DAT positivity with anti-C3d confirm a diagnosis of cold agglutinin (antibody) disease (CAD) most likely secondary to NHL.

Q4. What are other diagnostic possibilities in patients of CAD with this presentation?

Answer: In patients with this clinical presentation and evidence of hemolysis, the differential diagnosis includes paroxysmal cold hemoglobinuria, cryoglobulinemia, paroxysmal nocturnal hemoglobinuria, connective tissue diseases, antiphospholipid syndrome, monoclonal gammopathy of undetermined significance (MGUS), Waldenstrom's macroglobulinemia, and drug-induced immune hemolytic anemia [5].

(a) When hemolysis is episodic in nature, possibilities can be paroxysmal cold hemoglobinuria, march hemoglobinuria, and PNH.
(b) When cold induced peripheral vaso-occlusive symptoms are present, the possibility of cryoglobulinemia and Raynaud's phenomena should be considered.
(c) In presence of lymph node enlargement with or without fever, infectious mononucleosis, mycoplasma pneumonia, and lymphoma should be kept in mind under appropriate clinical setting.

Q5. what additional tests (other than done so far in this case) may be required in a case of CAD?

Answer: Following tests may be required for further analysis of such case to evaluate differential diagnosis [5, 6].

1. Quantification of IgG, IgA, IgM, serum protein electrophoresis (SPEP), and immune fixation to check for monoclonality of immunoglobulins.
2. Donath Landsteiner test (D-L antibody screening), if patient has hemoglobinuria with episodic hemolysis.
3. Cryoglobulin levels are tested if patient has vascular purpura or history of hepatitis.
4. Tests for viruses as EBV, influenza, mycoplasma, and CMV if patient has fever and clinical suspicion of CAD.
5. Immunological tests for SLE, RA, scleroderma, etc. in appropriate clinical setting.

Q6. What is etiopathogenesis of CAD?

Answer: Classic cold agglutinin diseases is idiopathic. It can occur secondary to infections like mycoplasma pneumonia and infectious mononucleosis, influenza, HIV, CMV, and rubella. Persistent CAD is seen in lymphoproliferative disorders including lymphoma, CLL, and Waldenstrom's macroglobulinemia. Autoimmune disorders are also responsible for cold agglutinin production [5, 6].

In CAD, the antibody is IgM which is usually monoclonal with Kappa or Lambda light chains. The antibody is directed against I/i antigen on red cell membrane. This antibody attaches to red cells and produces agglutination at temperature below 37 °C. Maximum agglutination is seen at around 4 °C deg. [5–7].

The agglutination usually occurs when circulating blood goes to cooler exposed parts of body especially digits, nose, and ears. When blood returns to warmer parts of body (higher temperature), C3 component of complement fixes to the red cell agglutinins. IgM antibodies dissociate from RBC at warmer core temperatures but complement components remain on RBC surface. These C3 complement coated cells are phagocytosed by macrophage in liver (Kupffer's cells) that have specific complement receptors (while in warm AIHA, macrophage Fc_ receptors on splenic macrophages recognize IgG on RBC surface). If the complement cascade progresses on surface of red cells with formation of membrane attack complex, intravascular hemolysis takes place, resulting in hemoglobinuria. So both intra- and extra- vascular hemolysis can occur in CAD. If this disease becomes chronic, the complement tends to be depleted due to consumption (decreased serum levels of C3 and C4). Monoclonal cold IgM antibodies found in patients with lymphoma are product of abnormal clone of lymphoid cells [5–7].

Q7. How is CAD different from warm AIHA and PCH?

Answer: Table 11.6 shows some of the differences seen in these three conditions [8].

Table 11.6 Differences between warm AIHA, CAD, and PCH

Disease	Warm -AIHA	CAD	PCH
Ig class involved	IgG mainly	IgM mainly	D-L biphasic antibody (IgG)
Common Etiology	LPD, autoimmune diseases	Mycoplasma, HIV, infectious mononucleosis, LPD	Infectious mononucleosis
	DAT + with IgG+/− C3	DAT + with C3	DAT + with C3
Blood film	Spherocytes	Agglutinins	Hemolysis
Blood group system involved	Rh system	I/i system	P system

In CAD: Antibodies are agglutinins-IgM.
In PCH: Antibodies are hemolysins- DL antibodies which are biphasic.
In both, DAT is positive with anti-complement antibodies.

Q8. What are common clinical presentations of CAD?
Answer: CAD presents with symptoms of anemia associated with clinical manifestations of cold induced circulatory symptoms such as livedo reticularis, Raynaud phenomena, acrocyanosis and, rarely, cutaneous necrosis.
In livedo reticularis, there is mottled discoloration of the skin with reticular (net-like, lace-like) appearance. Cyanotic discoloration surrounds pale central skin.
In Raynaud's disease, there is episodic reduction in the blood supply to the fingers, toes, or nipple occurring when exposed to cold (vasospastic disease) [9].

Q9. How should the samples be handled for suspected case of CAD?
Answer: For CBC, EDTA blood should be collected in tubes which are prewarmed at 37 °C. Similarly, for cold agglutinin titer, estimation of Ig levels, serum protein electrophoresis, and immunofixation, blood is drawn into prewarmed vacuum tubes and kept at this temperature until serum/plasma has been removed. After that samples can be handled at room temperature. For flowcytometry on bone marrow aspirate samples, samples are collected in EDTA or heparinized tube and pre-warming before analysis is sufficient.

11.2 Correlation of Results of Preliminary Investigations with Symptoms and signs in Cold Agglutinin Disease

Q10. How do symptoms and signs in this patients corelate with diagnosis of CAD?
Answer: Patient has symptoms of anemia (weakness, fatigue, dyspnea, and palpitations on walking). She has jaundice which corelate with possible hemolytic anemia. She has history of blanching of her fingers and toes when exposed to cold. During the previous winter months, she had felt dusky color of nose, ears, and lips on exposure to cold. Pale digits and few patches of bluish network of discoloration of skin on both lower legs are present. All these are symptoms and signs of cold induced vaso-occlusive disease which corelate with diagnosis of CAD.

Q11. How do CBC, blood film, and biochemical tests guide and corelate in evaluation of this case?
Answer: Patient has anemia with high MCV, MCH, and MCHC and reticulocytosis. There is mismatch between values for Hb and hematocrit, which indicates possibility of agglutinins and subsequently blood film shows red cell agglutination which disappeared on rewarming the sample at 37°°C. The biochemical tests confirm hemolytic anemia (indirect hyper bilirubinemia, high LDH, and low haptoglobin). Low C3 and C4 levels suggest consumption of complement. Rest of the immunological tests are normal, thus excluding immunological diseases. Hemoglobinuria indicates intravascular hemolysis. All these findings corelate well with diagnosis of CAD.

The MCV, MCH, and MCHC values are high because of red cell agglutination. If the samples are not collected in prewarmed tubes, agglutination will start from the time sample of blood put in CBC tube. The auto analyzer will read tiny clumps of red cells together and will interpret it as having high red cell parameters. False high values will be produced. Thus pseudo macrocytosis is observed. High MCHC is due to the presence of spherocytes. Similar analytical error produces miscorrelation between hemoglobin values and hematocrit.

Q12. What were confirmatory tests in this case?
Answer: Monospecific DAT positive for C3d, cold antibody titers 1: 1024 at 4 °C, negativity for IgG and presence of low complement C3 and C4 confirmed CAD. The history of previously diagnosed lymphoma suggests that the most likely cause of CAD in this case is non-Hodgkins lymphoma.

Q13. What is diagnostic criteria for CAD?
Answer: (1) Chronic hemolysis, (2) positive polyspecific DAT, (3) strongly positive monospecific C3d DAT, (4) cold agglutinin titer =/> 1:64 at 4 °C [10].

11.3 Quick Information for Practicing Clinicians and Students

References [1–10]:

1. Anemia with high MCV, MCH, MCHC and reticulocytosis in presence of mismatch between hemoglobin and hematocrit should raise suspicion of cold agglutinin disease.
2. Blood film with red cell clumps which disappear when blood film is re-examined after warming sample to 37 °C strongly suggests cold immune pathology. Hemolytic markers- reticulocytosis, indirect hyper bilirubinemia and reduced haptoglobin complement the diagnostic possibility of hemolytic anemia.
3. Direct antiglobulin test (DAT) positive with C3d and negative with IgG confirms CAD.
4. Viral infections, auto immune diseases and malignancies are the most commonly associated diseases.
5. A detailed history and thorough clinical examination is quite helpful in narrowing the differential diagnosis.
6. Auto analyzers will show high MCV in presence of red cell clumps seen in auto immune diseases. So examination of blood film is important to exclude false positive high MCV (pseudo macrocytosis).
7. High MCHC is due to presence of spherocytes in blood.
8. DAT can be falsely negative due to technical reasons, i.e., improper cell washing, delay in adding antiglobulin reagent after the washing step or if antiglobulin reagent is ineffective.

9. Up to 10% of AIHA can have negative DAT due to low titer of antibodies which may not be detected by DAT.
10. An immunology profile should be done in all cases to exclude more than one pathology producing AIHA.
11. Patients with mild anemia or compensated hemolysis and no clinical symptoms have not been shown to benefit from treatment.
12. Always ask about the history of drug intake.

To acquire further knowledge on the subject, following sources are advised:

1. BCSH guidelines
2. Br Jr. Hematology
3. ASH education book
4. Blood
5. NEJM
6. Int Jr. Lab Hematology

References

1. Savage DG, Ogundipe A, Allen RH, Stabler SP, Lindenbaum J. Etiology and diagnostic evaluation of macrocytosis. Am J Med Sci. 2000;319(6):343–52.
2. Aslinia F, Mazza JJ, Yale SH. Megaloblastic anemia and other causes of macrocytosis. Clin Med Res. 2006;4(3):236–41.
3. Dali-Youcef N, Andres E. An update on cobalamin deficiency in adults. QJM. 2009;102(1):17–28.
4. Hill QA, Hill A, Berentsen S. Defining autoimmune hemolytic anemia: a systematic review of the terminology used for diagnosis and treatment. Blood Adv. 2019;3:1897–906. https://doi.org/10.1182/bloodadvances.2019000036.
5. Swiecicki PL, Hegerova LT, Gertz MA. Cold agglutinin disease. Blood. 2013;122:1114–21. https://doi.org/10.1182/blood-2013-02-474437.
6. Gehrs BC, Friedberg RC. Autoimmune hemolytic anemia. Am J Hematol. 2002;69:258–71.
7. Petz LD. Cold antibody autoimmune hemolytic anemias. Blood Rev. 2008;22:1–15. https://doi.org/10.1016/j.blre.2007.08.002.
8. Win N, Stamps R, Knight R. Paroxysmal cold haemoglobinuria/Donath-Landsteiner test. Transfus Med. 2005;15(3):254.
9. Berentsen S, Ulvestad E, Langholm R, et al. Primary chronic cold agglutinin disease: a population based clinical study of 86 patients. Haematologica. 2006;91(4):460–6.
10. Berentsen S, Tjønnfjord GE. Diagnosis and treatment of cold agglutinin mediated autoimmune hemolytic anemia. Blood Rev. 2012;26:107–15. https://doi.org/10.1016/j.blre.2012.01.002.

Chapter 12
Cryoglobulinemia

A 30-year-old lady presented with history of pruritic rash involving buttocks, thighs, and legs for the previous 5 days. There was no history of cold sensitivity and allergy to food or drugs. She gave history of arthralgias affecting the proximal interphalangeal and metacarpophalangeal joints of the hands and pain in ankles. Recently, she had been feeling tired and easily fatigued with frequent nonspecific myalgias. She also gave past history of being tested positive for hepatitis C, which was detected during her previous pregnancy one year back.

Physical examination revealed mild pallor without jaundice. No organomegaly was detected. A palpable macular rash involving both thighs and legs was observed. Result of CBC done is presented in Table 12.1:

Table 12.1 CBC

CBC parameter	Patient's result	Reference range
WBC	18	3.7–10 × 10^9/L
RBC	3.9	4.5–5.4 × 10^{12}/L
HB	110	130–160 g/L
Hct	0.29	0.33–0.43 L/L
MCV	99	83–101 fL
MCH	31	27–32 pg
MCHC	340	315–345 g/L
RDW	21	11.6–14.6%
PLT	1200	130–430 × 10^9/L
MPV	12	7–11 fL
Poly#	4.8	1.7–6 × 10^9/L
Lymp#	12	1 3 × 10^9/L
Mono#	1.0	0.2–1.0 × 10^9/L
EO#	0.3	0.02–0.5 × 10^9/L
BASO#	0	0.02–0.1 × 10^9/L
RETIC%	3.0	0.5–1.5%
ESR	79	0–20 mm 1st h Westergren

A. Gupta, *Decision Making Through Problem Based Learning in Hematology*,
https://doi.org/10.1007/978-981-99-8933-1_12

12.1 Questions

Q1. Interpret the CBC result given above and suggest investigations for further evaluation in such case

Answer: The CBC result shows leukocytosis with lymphocytosis, low number of RBCs, decreased hemoglobin level and hematocrit level, and high value for RDW. The red cell indices are within normal range. Platelet count and ESR are high. There is mild reticulocytosis.

So, there is normocytic normochromic anemia with mild reticulocytosis.

Causes of normocytic normochromic anemia include [1, 2]:

(a) *Decreased production from marrow (will have low reticulocyte count)*: Chronic pathological conditions (such as chronic inflammations, neoplastic pathologies, and infections), chronic renal failure, chronic liver disease, endocrinopathies, marrow infiltration, and hypoplastic anemias.

(b) *Increased destruction (will have increased reticulocytes with normal marrow)*:

1. Red cell defects: Defects of red cell membrane, enzymes, or hemoglobin.
2. Without any defect of red cells (defects lies outside red cells): Autoimmune hemolytic anemia, micro-angiopathic hemolytic anemia (DIC/TTP/HUS), cryoglobulinemia, PNH, warm AIHA.

(c) *Sequestration: splenomegaly.*

A high total leukocytic and platelet count needs to be investigated. Next best investigation will be examination of blood film.

Q2. Given are images from blood film (Figs. 12.1 and 12.2). Interpret the findings and suggest further workup.

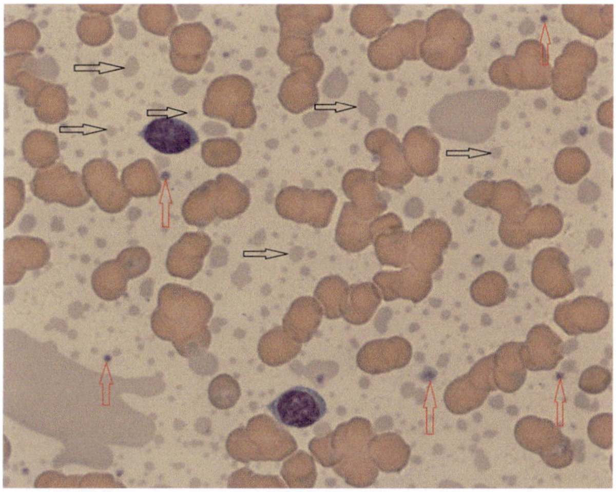

Fig. 12.1 PBF: Cryoglobulins (black arrows) Platelets (red arrows). Leishman ×100

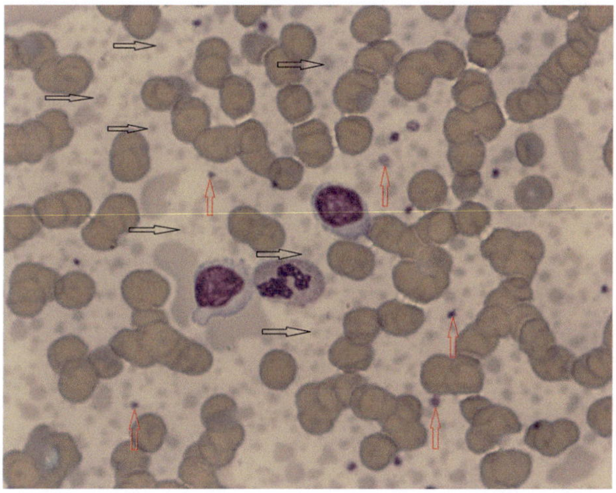

Fig. 12.2 PBF Cryoglobulins (black arrows) Platelets (red arrows). Leishman ×100

Answer: The blood film shows normocytic normochromic red cells with plenty of rouleaux formation. In addition, small irregular grayish-blue extracellular precipitates and large number of tiny variable sized granules of same color are seen in the background. These are possibly cryoglobulins but require confirmation. The leukocytes appear normal except for some activated lymphocytes. The platelets number also appears normal on smear. No abnormal cells are seen.

So when correlated with CBC, the number of leukocytes and platelets appear normal on smear (this is referred as pseudo leukocytosis and pseudo thrombocytosis). To evaluate further, a CBC done after collection of blood at 37 °C is required. Also, immunoglobulin levels, DAT, immunological profile, and viral serology will aid in evaluating etiology. Tests for cryoglobulinemia should also be considered.

Q3. Given are results of CBC done after warming sample to 37 °C (Table 12.2), DAT, immunoglobulin levels, and immunology profile (Table 12.3), biochemical tests (Table 12.4) and viral screen (Table 12.5). Interpret the results and suggest differential diagnosis.

Table 12.2 CBC result after collection of blood at 37 °C

CBC parameter	Patient's result	Reference range
WBC	7.5	3.7–10 × 10^9/L
RBC	4.0	4.5–5.4 × 10^{12}/L
HB	114	130–160 g/L
Hct	0.34	0.33–0.43 L/L
MCV	98	83–101 fL
MCH	30	27–32 pg
MCHC	331	315–345 g/L
RDW	12	11.6–14.6%
PLT	208	130–430 × 10^9/L
MPV	10	7–11 fL
Poly#	3.0	1.7–6 × 10^9/L
Lymp#	3.3	1–3 × 10^9/L
Mono#	1.0	0.2–1.0 × 10^9/L
EO#	0.2	0.02–0.5 × 10^9/L
BASO#	0	0.02–0.1 × 10^9/L
RETIC%	3.0	0.5–1.5%
ESR	70	0–20 mm 1st h Westergren

Table 12.3 DAT and immunology profile

Test	Patient's result	Ref range
Direct antiglobulin test (DAT)	Positive with IgG	Negative
Anti ds-DNA antibody	Negative	Negative
ANA	Negative	Negative
ANCA	Negative	Negative
Anti LKM antibodies	Neg	
Anti mitochondrial antibodies	Neg	
Anti CCP antibodies	Neg	
Rh-factor	Positive	Negative
Rh titer	1460	0–20 IU/mL
C3	0.832 g/L	0.83–1.77 g/L
C4	0.116 g/L	0.2–0.8 g/L
IgG	64	6–16 g/L
IgM	12	0.5–2.0 g/L
IgA	3	0.8–4.0 g/L
CRP	18	0–10 mg/L

Table 12.4 Biochemical tests

Test	Patient's result	Ref Range
Glu	5.6	3.9–6.1 mmol/L
Urea	5.5	2.5–6.6 mmol/L
Creat	101	60–120 μmol/L
Na+	142	136–146 mmol/L
K^+	4.5	3.7–5.0 mmol/L
Ca^+	2.3	2.2–2.6 mmol/L
Mg^+	1.0	0.08–1.1 mmol/L
T. Prot	70	63–80 mmol/L
Alb	32	35–47 mmol/L
Choles	3.5	1.5–5.2 mmol/L
TG	0.9	0.4–1.7 mmol/L
Urates	395	150–400 mmol/L
T Bil	35	3–20 μmol/L
D. Bil	5	0–5 μmol/L
I Bil	30	5–15 μmol/L
Alk Ph	60	26–88 IU/L
ALT	66	10–60 IU/L
AST	40	10–42 IU/L
GGT	55	7–64 IU/L
LDH	280	90–180 IU/L
Hapto	0.6	0.2–2.0 g/L
T4	10.6	7.8–16 pmol/L
TSH	3.99	0.27–4.2 μlU/mL
Amylase	20	28-100 IU/L
Lipase	30	0–160 U/L

Table 12.5 Viral serology

Test name	Result	Ref range
CMV-DNA	Not detected by real-time PCR	
CMV-IgG	Reactive	
CMV-IgM	Non-reactive	
EBV-DNA	Not detected by real-time PCR	
EBV-IgG	Reactive	
EBV- IgM	Non-reactive	
HBs Ag	Non-reactive	
HCV-Ab	Reactive	
HCV-Ag	Not detected	
HIV Ag/Ab	Non-reactive	

Answer: The CBC done after warming blood sample shows almost similar comparable values for hemoglobin and red cell indices. However, the leukocyte count and platelet number are calculated within reference range (so there was pseudoleukocytosis and pseudothrombocytosis which have disappeared). There is, however, mild reticulocytosis and high ESR.

The immunological tests show positive DAT with IgG, a positive rheumatoid factor (1460 IU/mL), mildly reduced complement component C4, and increased IgG and IgM levels. CRP is also high.

The biochemical tests show mild hypo-albuminemia, mild hyper-indirect hyperbilirubinemia, high LDH, and borderline increase in ALT.

The viral screen indicates past infection with CMV, EBV, and HCV with no evidence of recent/active infection.

These findings suggest a diagnosis of rheumatoid arthritis with possible presence of cryoglobulins/agglutinins with hyperglobulinemia and mild hemolysis. High CRP indicates mild active inflammation, and elevated ESR is due to presence of high globulins.

The differential diagnosis includes cryoglobulinemia (precipitates), cold agglutinin disease (rouleaux formation and red cell agglutination), multiple myeloma (high IgG), and Waldenstrom's macroglobulinemia (high IgM). For final diagnosis, test for cryoglobulins, DAT with C3d, serum protein electrophoresis, and immunofixation should be done.

Q4. Given are results of DAT with C3d, test for cryoglobulins (Table 12.6), serum protein electrophoresis (Fig. 12.3), and immunofixation (Fig. 12.4). Interpret the results and suggest final diagnosis in this case.

Table 12.6 Result of DAT and cryoglobulins

DAT IgG+	Positive
DAT C3d	Negative
Cryoglobulins	Positive
Cryocrit level: 20%	N: Less than 0.5%

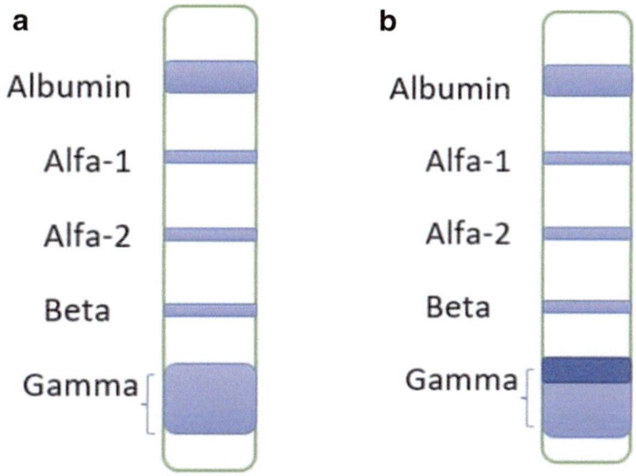

Fig. 12.3 Serum protein electrophoresis. Normal bands (left). Dense band in gamma region (right)

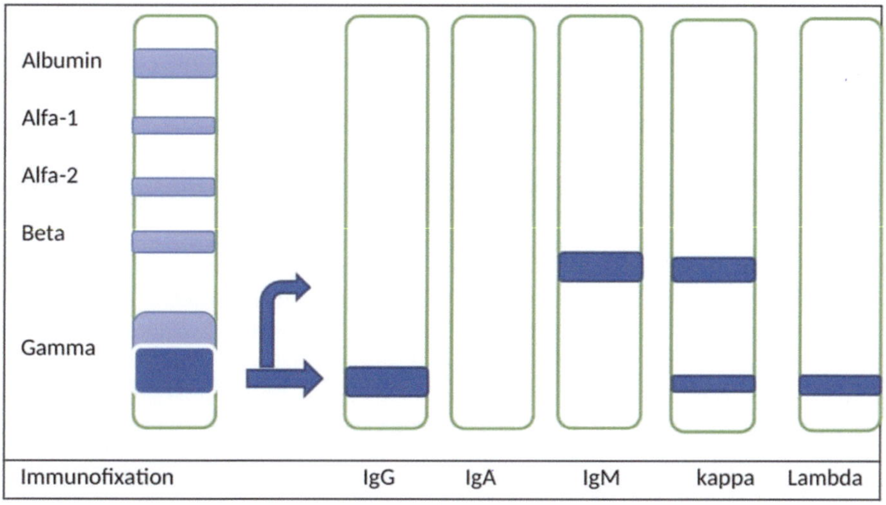

Fig. 12.4 Immunofixation. Both IgG and IgM are present. IgG is polyclonal with both kappa and lambda chains. IgM is monoclonal with only kappa chains

Answer: The DCT is positive with IgG and negative with C3d, excluding presence of CAD. The serum protein electrophoresis shows a dense band in gamma region. Further analysis by immuno-electrophoresis shows both IgG and IgM. However there is only lambda band associated with IgM (monoclonal), while IgG shows presence of both Kappa and lambda light chains, making it polyclonal. The test for cryoglobulins is positive with cryocrit of 20% concentration. Thus a final diagnosis of cryoglobulinemia Type II – secondary to rheumatoid arthritis is established.

Q5. What additional tests (other than done so far) may be required in this case.

Answer: Skin biopsy which may show leukocytoclastic vasculitis. U/S, CT scan or a kidney biopsy may be considered under appropriate clinical situation. In rare cases, bone marrow examination may be required to exclude other conditions related to monoclonal proteins.

Q6. What is etiopathogenesis of cryoglobulinemia?

Answer: Cryoglobulins are single or complexes of immunoglobulins. These have property of undergoing precipitation at temp less than 37 °C which is reversed at higher temperatures [3] Deposition of these cryoglobulins (immune complexes) on walls of blood vessels restricts blood flow to various organs. Inflammatory response and damage to the blood vessels follows, resulting in a clinical syndrome of systemic inflammation, mostly affecting the kidneys and skin. Cryoglobulinemia may be classified based on cryoglobulin composition. Three types are described [4]:

Type I: Composed of a single monoclonal immunoglobulin, IgM, mostly. It is seen in plasma cell disorders. Very rare it is IgA or IgG.

Types II and III: Composed of both IgG and IgM components These are classified as mixed cryoglobulinemia. In these cases, abnormal immune complex formation occurs. Both types contain an IgM rheumatoid factor, which is an autoantibody that complexes with IgG. The IgM is monoclonal in Type II and polyclonal in Type III. Types II and III cryoglobulinemia comprise approximately 80% of all cases of cryoglobulinemia.

Mixed cryoglobulinemia (containing more than one type of immunoglobulin) is a multifactorial disease resulting from interaction of environmental factors like chronic infection with the hepatitis C virus, immunological disorders such as RA, systemic lupus erythematosus, and human immunodeficiency virus (HIV). Rare cases of lymphoma also develop mixed cryoglobulinemia (MC). When no cause of MC is identified, it is referred to as essential mixed cryoglobulinemia [5].

Q7. What are the causes of spurious cell counts with automated analyzers?

Answer: False elevation of Hb measurement by automated methods is related to high levels of immunoglobulins that interact with reagents of the lysis solution. Hb is overestimated, and MCHC usually exceeds 36 g/dL. In order to obtain accurate results, determine plasma Hb after centrifugation of the sample. Other situations where spurious results can be obtained are [6]:

High hemoglobin: in presence of lipids, high WBC counts, immunoglobulins, and cryoglobulins.

High MCV: in presence of cold agglutinins, warm agglutinins, high WBC counts, hyperglycemia.

High MCH: in presence of cold agglutinins, warm agglutinins, lipids, immunoglobulins.

High WBC: in presence of cryoglobulin, cryofibrinogen, immunoglobulins, lipids, and platelet aggregates.
Platelets: in presence of fragmented erythrocytes, fragments of nucleated cells, bacteria, fungi, lipids, and cryoglobulins.

Q8. How should samples be processed to estimate cryocrit in such cases?
Answer: A fasting blood sample should be collected and transported at 37 °C in preheated tubes. These should be immediately transported and kept at this temperature for at least 1 h till clotting is complete. Centrifugation is also done at 37 °C. For detecting cryoglobulins, incubate serum at 4 °C for 7 days and observe for precipitate. This precipitate is separated and quantified to calculate % cryocrit. (percentage of precipitate in relation to total plasma used) [7].

Q9. In which cases cryoglobulins be tested or suspected?
Answer: Patients presenting with arthralgia, purpura, skin ulcers, glomerulonephritis, and peripheral neuropathy should be assessed and investigated for cryoglobulinemia [8].

Q10. What is clinical triad of mixed cryoglobulinemia?
Answer: Mixed cryoglobulinemia is characterized by the clinical triad of palpable purpura, arthralgia, and weakness.
Meltzer triad (i.e., purpura, arthralgia, and weakness) was first described in 1966 by Meltzer and Franklin in cases of essential mixed cryoglobulinemia. This triad is generally seen with types II and III cryoglobulinemia in up to 25–30% of patients [9].

12.2 Correlation of Results of Preliminary Investigations with Symptoms and signs in Cryoglobulinemia

Q11. How do symptoms and signs in this patients correlate with diagnosis?
Answer: This patient has classical history suggestive of cryoglobulinemia. She has purpura, arthralgia, and weakness—the triad is highly suggestive of this condition.

Q12 How do CBC, blood film, and biochemical tests guide in evaluation of this case?
Answer: The CBC shows typical findings of anemia, pseudoleukocytosis, and pseudothrombocytosis which occur due to presence of cryoglobulins. Blood film shows background precipitates of cryoglobulins, thus guiding for further evaluation and confirmation.

Q13. What were confirmatory tests in this case.
Answer: DAT positive in presence of high rheumatoid factor, positive testing for cryoglobulins, high immunoglobulins-polyclonal IgG, and monoclonal IgM and low C4 levels are confirmatory for diagnosis of cryoglobulinemia.

12.3 Quick Information for Practicing Clinicians and Students

References [1–10]:

1. Patients presenting with arthralgia, purpura, skin ulcers, glomerulonephritis, levido reticularis, and peripheral neuropathy should be assessed and investigated for cryoglobulinemia.
2. Meltzer triad (i.e., purpura, arthralgia, and weakness) is generally seen with types II and III cryoglobulinemia in up to 25–30% of patients.
3. The target organs are the skin, nerves, kidney, liver, and joints. More than 80% of patients have evidence of hepatitis C infection.
4. Blood film should be examined in all cases with high WBC and platelets for confirmation of values and exclude pseudoleukocytosis and pseudothrombocytosis.
5. A CBC and blood film re-examined after collecting blood at 37 °C is highly recommended.
6. Blood film findings of gray blue granular deposits are highly indicative of cryoglobulins.
7. Confirmation of diagnosis and typing of cryoglobulin class require cryoglobulins levels, DAT with C3d, serum protein electrophoresis, and immunofixation.
8. Patients suspected to have kidney involvement require urine examination and kidney biopsy for evaluation.
9. Fasting blood samples are advised for analysis of cryoglobulins that are collected and transported at 37 °C in preheated tubes.
10. A combination of cryoglobulin measurement along with a low C4 complement level is typical of cryoglobulinemia syndromes [10]

To acquire further knowledge on the subject, following sources are advised:

1. BCSH guidelines
2. Br Jr. Hematology
3. ASH education book
4. Blood
5. NEJM
6. Int Jr. Lab Hematology

References

1. Ward PC. Investigation of nonpoikilocytic normochromic normocytic anemia. Postgrad Med. 1979;65(3):233–5, 238, 241–3
2. Bonnet JD. Normocytic normochromic anemia. Postgrad Med. 1977;61(6):139–42.
3. Ramos-Casals M, Stone JH, Cid MC, Bosch X. The cryoglobulinaemias. Lancet. 2012;379:348–60.

4. Gulli F, Basile U, Gragnani L, Napodano C, Pocino K, Miele L, et al. IgG cryoglobulinemia. Eur Rev Med Pharmacol Sci. 2018 Sep;22(18):6057–62.
5. Brouet JC, Clauvel JP, Danon F, Klein M, Seligmann M. Biologic and clinical significance of cryoglobulins. A report of 86 cases. Am J Med. 1974;57(5):775–88.
6. Cornbleet J. Spurious results from automated hematology cell counters. Lab Med. 1983;14:509–14. https://doi.org/10.1093/labmed/14.8.509.
7. Sargur R, White P, Egner W. Cryoglobulin evaluation: best practice? Ann Clin Biochem. 2010;47(Pt 1):8–16. https://doi.org/10.1258/acb.2009.009180.
8. Della Rossa A, Trevisani G, Bombardieri S. Cryoglobulins and cryoglobulinemia. Diagnostic and therapeutic considerations. Clin Rev Allergy Immunol. 1998;16(3):249–64.
9. Meltzer M, Franklin EC, Elias K, McCluskey RT, Cooper N. Cryoglobulinemia–a clinical and laboratory study. II. Cryoglobulins with rheumatoid factor activity. Am J Med. 1966;40(6):837–56.
10. Gorevic PD, Kassab HJ, Levo Y, Kohn R, Meltzer M, Prose P, Franklin EC. Mixed cryoglobulinemia: clinical aspects and long-term follow-up of 40 patients. Am J Med. 1980;69(2):287–308.

Chapter 13
Paroxysmal Cold Hemoglobinuria

A 5-year-old boy is brought to OPD with history of fever for 7 days which had developed following exposure to a cold night. He also had sore throat, dry cough, myalgias, intermittent pain abdomen, nausea, and headache. He had vomited once the previous night. Four days back, his urine color was dark red which had gradually cleared over next 24 h.

Examination revealed pallor and mild tinge of jaundice. Tiny bilateral cervical lymph nodes and tip of spleen were palpable. Result of CBC (Table 13.1) done at presentation is given below:

Table 13.1 CBC

CBC parameter	Patient's result	Reference range
WBC	12	3.7–10 × 10^9/L
RBC	3.5	4.5–5.4 × 10^{12}/L
HB	105	130–160 g/L
Hct	0.32	0.33–0.43 L/L
MCV	100	83–101 fL
MCH	31	27–32 pg
MCHC	330	315–345 g/L
RDW	14	11.6–14.6%
PLT	150	130–430 × 10^9/L
MPV	10	7–11 fL
Poly#	2.3	1.7–6 × 10^9/L
Lymp#	7.5	1–3 × 10^9/L
Mono#	2.0	0.2–1.0 × 10^9/L
EO#	0.2	0.02–0.5 × 10^9/L
BASO#	0	0.02–0.1 × 10^9/L
RETIC%	3.9	0.5–1.5%
ESR	49	0–20 mm 1st h Westergren

A. Gupta, *Decision Making Through Problem Based Learning in Hematology*, https://doi.org/10.1007/978-981-99-8933-1_13

13.1 Questions

Q1. Interpret the CBC result given above and suggest investigations for further evaluation in such case

Answer: The CBC result shows that low number of RBCs and decreased hemoglobin level and hematocrit. MCV, MCH, and MCHC are within normal limits. Reticulocyte count is increased. ESR value is also high. So, there is normocytic normochromic anemia.

Causes of normocytic normochromic anemia include: [1, 2]

(a) *Decreased production from marrow (will have low reticulocyte count)*: Chronic pathological conditions (such as chronic inflammations, neoplastic pathologies, and infections), chronic renal failure, chronic liver disease, endocrinopathies, marrow infiltration, and hypoplastic anemias.

(b) *Increased destruction (will have increased reticulocytes with normal marrow)*:

1. Red cell defects: Defects of red cell membrane, enzymes, or hemoglobin.
2. Without any defect of red cells (defects lies outside red cells): Autoimmune hemolytic anemia, PNH, PCH, CAD, and micro-angiopathic hemolytic anemia (DIC/TTP/HUS).

(c) *Sequestration: splenomegaly.*

As there is reticulocytosis, a possibility of peripheral destruction, consumption, or bleeding should be kept in mind. Next best investigation in this case will be examination of blood film and investigate with serum chemistry for evaluation of liver and kidney functions along with hemolytic markers. Routine urine and stool examination are also suggested.

Q2. Given are images from blood film (Figs. 13.1 and 13.2), results of liver and kidney functions along with hemolytic markers (Table 13.2) and examination of urine and stools (Table 13.3). Interpret these findings and suggest a differential diagnosis? what further investigations should be done to exclude various differential diagnoses?

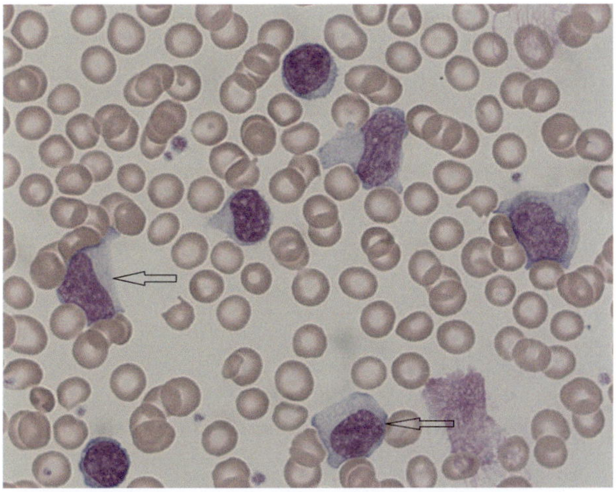

Fig. 13.1 PBF. Activated and transformed lymphocytes (arrows). Leishman stain ×100

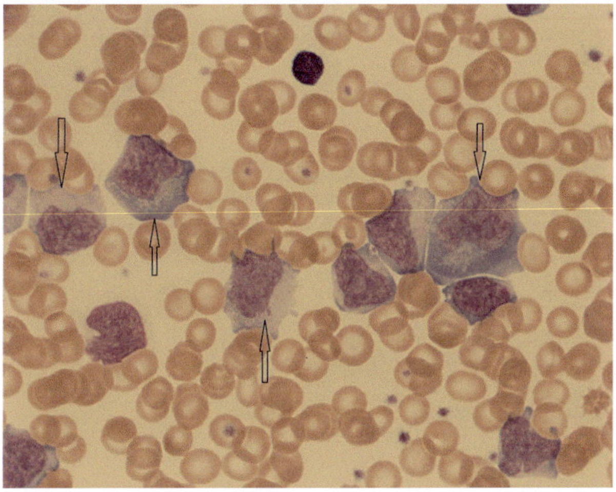

Fig. 13.2 PBF. Atypical lymphocytes with skirting of cytoplasm (arrow). Leishman stain ×100

Table 13.2 Biochemical tests

Test	Patient's result	Ref range
Glu	5.0	3.9–6.1 mmol/L
Urea	4.0	2.5–6.6 mmol/L
Creat	99	60–120 μmol/L
Na^+	142	136–146 mmol/L
K^+	4.7	3.7–5.0 mmol/L
Ca^+	2.5	2.2–2.6 mmol/L
Mg^+	1.0	0.08–1.1 mmol/L
T. Prot	75	63–80 mmol/L
Alb	44	35–47 mmol/L
Choles	3.5	1.5–5.2 mmol/L
TG	0.9	0.4–1.7 mmol/L
Urates	330	150–400 mmol/L
T Bil	43	3–20 μmol/L
D. Bil	5	0–5 μmol/L
I Bil	38	5–15 μmol/L
Alk Ph	60	26–88 IU/L
ALT	54	10–60 IU/L
AST	33	10–42 IU/L
GGT	55	7–64 IU/L
LDH	266	90–180 IU/L
Hapto	0.16	0.2–2.0 g/L
T4	10.6	7.8–16 pmol/L
TSH	3.91	0.27–4.2 μlU/ml
Amylase	20	28–100 IU/L
Lipase	30	0–160 U/L

Table 13.3 Urine and stool examination

Urine examination	Patient's result	Reference range
SG	1.023	1.005–1.030
Ph	6.3	5–7
Leu	Neg	Neg
Nit	Neg	Neg
Pro	Neg	Neg
Glu	Neg	Neg
Ket	Neg	Neg
Uro	Neg	Neg
Bil	Neg	Neg
Hemosiderin	Neg	Neg
Hemoglobin	Pos	Neg
Stool examination		
Occult blood	Neg	Neg
Ova/cysts	Neg	Neg

Answer: The blood films show many activated, transformed and atypical lymphocytes. These are larger than normal lymphocytes and have big nucleus with clumped chromatin, moderate cytoplasm, and cytoplasmic projections. The cytoplasm tends to be invaginated by adjacent red cells giving appearance of "Skirting." Some of them show monocytic appearance with large cytoplasm and cytoplasmic vacuolations. The red cells show mild rouleaux formation. No immature cells are seen.

The biochemical tests show indirect hyperbilirubinemia, high LDH, and reduced level of haptoglobin. The urine shows hemoglobinuria while stool examination is normal. All these findings suggest possibility of hemolytic anemia. The appearance of lymphocytic cells suggests a viral infection, most likely infectious mononucleosis due to EBV infection.

For further evaluation of hemolytic anemia, antiglobulin test (DAT) with IgG and C3d is required. To assess cause of signs and symptoms, test for heterophile antibody and screening for viruses especially Epstein–Barr virus are advised.

Q3. Given are result of direct antiglobulin test (DAT), Donath-Landsteiner test, heterophile antibody test, and viral serology (Table 13.4). Interpret the results and suggest final diagnosis.

Table 13.4 Serology and immunological tests

Test	Patient's result
Direct antiglobulin test	Monospecific DAT -positive for C3d; negative for IgG
Donath-Landsteiner ab test	Positive
Heterophile antibody test	Positive
Epstein–Barr virus-specific antibodies	Anti-VCA IgM and anti-VCA IgG Positive
Adenovirus DNA	Not detected by PCR
Coronavirus-E229RNA	Not detected by PCR
CMV-DNA	Not detected
Enterovirus RNA	Not detected
HSV-DNA	Not detected
Metapneumovirus RNA	Not detected
Influenza A virus RNA	Not detected
Influenza B virus RNA	Not detected
Mycoplasma pneumoniae DNA	Not detected
Parainfluenza virus 1,2,3,4 RNA	Not detected
RSV A/B RNA	Not detected
Rhinovirus RNA	Not detected

Answer: The DAT is positive with C3d, and D–L antibody is detected. This confirms the diagnosis of paroxysmal cold hemoglobinuria (PCH). Further, the heterophile antibody test and EBV-specific antibodies (anti-VCA IgM and anti-VCA IgG) are positive which confirms the signs and symptoms due to EBV-infectious mononucleosis. Other viruses are not detected by PCR. So the final diagnosis will be Paroxysmal cold hemoglobinuria (PCH) secondary to infectious mononucleosis.

Q4. What additional tests (other than done so far in this case) may be required in a case of PCH?

Answer: In situations where initial test result (heterophile antibody test) is negative and tests for EBV-specific antibodies (viral capsid antigen: VCA IgG, VCA IgM) are also negative, tests for early antigen (EA) may be done. Anti-EA IgG appears in the acute phase of illness. Usually, detection of antibody to EA is a sign of active infection. Antibody to EBV nuclear antigen (EBNA) is not seen in the acute phase of EBV infection. It appears 2 to 4 months after onset of symptoms and persists for the rest of life [3].

In addition to this, immunological profile, complement levels, and flowcytometry to exclude PNH and test for cryoglobulins may be considered in evaluation.

Q5. What is etiopathogenesis of PCH?

Answer: Donath-Landsteiner antibodies have specificity for the human P blood group antigen and are produced mostly following a viral infection. Hemolytic anemia occurs as a single post-viral episode in children. Pathogenetic organisms identified are measles, mumps, influenza, varicella-zoster virus (VZV), cytomegalovirus (CMV), Epstein–Barr virus (EBV), adenovirus, parvovirus B19, hemophilus influenzae, mycoplasma pneumoniae, and Klebsiella pneumoniae [4].

During severe cold, blood is exposed to low temperatures in peripheral circulation. The Donath-Landsteiner antibody and early-acting complement components bind to RBC at this lowered temperature. On return of these red cells to 37 °C in central circulation, they are lysed by activation of complement pathway. The Donath-Landsteiner antibody itself dissociates from the RBC at 37 °C (98.6 °F). However, prior to dissociation, it initiates the classical pathway of complement [5, 6].

Q6. What are classic clinical symptoms in PCH?

Answer: Following exposure to cold, the patient develops myalgia, arthralgia, headache, pain in the back or legs, and sometimes abdominal cramps. It is usually followed by fever. The first urine passed after onset of symptoms typically contains hemoglobin and jaundice may follow [6].

Q7. How should the blood samples be handled for suspected case of PCH?

Answer: For CBC, EDTA blood should be collected in tubes which are prewarmed at 37 °C. For flowcytometry, samples are collected in EDTA or heparinized tube and prewarming before analysis is sufficient.

13.2 Correlation of Results of Preliminary Investigations with Symptoms and Signs of Paroxysmal Cold Hemoglobinuria

Q8. How do symptoms and signs in this patients corelate with diagnosis?

Answer: This child had history of fever which had developed following exposure to a cold night, sore throat, dry cough, myalgias, nausea, and headache, all of which indicate an infectious process and observation of jaundice and change in change in urine color to dark red (possible hemoglobinuria) suggest hemolytic episode during this infection. Lymphadenopathy and palpable spleen were noticed which are part of infectious process. These symptoms and signs correlate well with diagnosis of PCH.

Q9 How do CBC, blood film, and biochemical tests guide in evaluation of this case?

Answer: The CBC shows anemia with reticulocytosis. Blood film shows atypical lymphocytes and mild red cell agglutination- rouleaux formation. Biochemical tests show evidence of hemolysis (indirect hyperbilirubinemia, high LDH, and low haptoglobin). There is lymphocytosis with many atypical and reactive lymphocytes in peripheral blood, suggesting viral infection. So evidence of hemolysis in a patient with atypical lymphocytes (seen in viral infections) and red cell agglutination guide for further evaluation in this case.

Q10. What were confirmatory tests in this case?

Answer: The DAT is positive with C3d (negative with IgG), and D–L antibody is detected. This suggests the diagnosis of paroxysmal cold hemoglobinuria (PCH) as a cause of hemolysis. Further, the heterophile antibody test and EBV-specific antibodies (Anti-VCA IgM and anti-VCA IgG) are positive which confirms the diagnosis of EBV- infectious mononucleosis. Other viruses are not detected by PCR. So all these results correlate with the final diagnosis of PCH secondary to Infectious mononucleosis.

Q11. How to differentiate between hemoglobinuria, myoglobinuria, and hematuria?

Answer: Urine dipstick gives positive result with all. Centrifuge the urine sample. If the sediment is red and supernatant is clear, it is hematuria. If there is uniform reddish color of urine, it is hemoglobinuria or myoglobinuria. To differentiate these two conditions, plasma will be required. Centrifuge the blood. If color of plasma is pink to red, it is hemoglobinuria but if it is clear, it is myoglobinuria.

Q12. What are the causes of hemoglobinuria?

Answer: In addition to PCH, common conditions where hemoglobinuria can be seen include PNH, hemolytic uremic syndrome, G6PD deficiency, blood transfusion reactions, crush injury and burns, etc.

Q13. What is Donath-Landsteiner test?

Answer: In this test, the patient's serum is incubated with group O, P antigen positive red cells in ice water and fresh normal serum. The mixture is warmed to 37 °C. The test is positive if red cells hemolyze on rewarming [8].

13.3 Quick Information for Practicing Clinicians and Students

References [1–12]:

1. PCH is a disease seen exclusively in children and accounts for approximately 1–5% of all childhood autoimmune hemolytic anemia.
2. Paroxysmal cold hemoglobinuria frequently occurs shortly after upper respiratory or gastrointestinal infections.
3. Typical presentation is myalgia, arthralgia, headache, pain in the back or legs, and sometimes abdominal cramps following exposure to cold. Fever develops shortly.
4. In infectious mononucleosis, blood film reveals lymphocytosis mostly more than 50% of total leukocytic count, of which over 10% are atypical in morphology.
5. Presence of RBC engulfment by neutrophils within the peripheral blood has a stronger association with paroxysmal cold hemoglobinuria and should raise suspicion for this entity.
6. The diagnosis of infectious mononucleosis should be confirmed with a heterophile antibody test or through EBV-specific antibodies. The monospot (or heterophile antibody) test is almost 100% specific and 85% sensitive for infectious mononucleosis.
7. Donath-Landsteiner test is used for diagnosis of PCH. If this test is negative, but there is strong suspicion of cold reacting antibodies, cold agglutinin titer should be done to exclude cold autobody autoimmune hemolytic anemia.
8. Transfuse warmed, packed red blood cells (RBCs) which are p-antigen negative.

To acquire further knowledge on the subject, following sources are advised:

1. BCSH guidelines
2. Br Jr. Hematology
3. ASH education book
4. Blood
5. NEJM
6. Int Jr. Lab Hematology

References

1. Ward PC. Investigation of nonpoikilocytic normochromic normocytic anemia. Postgrad Med. 1979;65(3):233–5, 238, 241-3
2. Bonnet JD. Normocytic normochromic anemia. Postgrad Med. 1977;61(6):139–42.
3. Ref Hislop AD, Taylor GS, Sauce D, Rickinson AB. Cellular responses to viral infection in humans: lessons from Epstein-Barr virus. Annu Rev Immunol. 2007;25:587–617.
4. Ref Sokol RJ, Hewitt S, Stamps BK, Hitchen PA. Autoimmune haemolysis in childhood and adolescence. Acta Haematol. 1984;72(4):245–57.
5. Taylor CJ, Neilson JR, Chandra D, Ibrahim Z. Recurrent paroxysmal cold haemoglobinuria in a 3-year-old child: a case report. Transfus Med. 2003;13(5):319–21.
6. Bell CA, Zwicker H, Rosenbaum DL. Paroxysmal cold hemoglobinuria (P.C.H.) following mycoplasma infection: anti-I specificity of the biphasic hemolysin. Transfusion. 1973;13(3):138–41.
7. Win N, Stamps R, Knight R. Paroxysmal cold haemoglobinuria/Donath-Landsteiner test. Transfus Med. 2005;15(3):254.
8. Eder AF. Review: acute Donath-Landsteiner hemolytic anemia. Immunohematology. 2005;21(2):56–62.
9. Ref BS. Role of complement in autoimmune Hemolytic Anemia. Transfus Med Hemother. 2015;42(5):303–10.
10. Garratty G. Erythrophagocytosis on the peripheral blood smear and paroxysmal cold hemoglobinuria. Transfusion. 2001;41(8):1073–4.
11. Ref Koester TM, Meece JK, Fritsche TR, Frost HM. Infectious mononucleosis and Lyme disease as confounding diagnoses: a report of 2 cases. Clin Med Res. 2018;16(3–4):66–8.
12. Roy-Burman A, Glader BE. Resolution of severe Donath-Landsteiner autoimmune hemolytic anemia temporally associated with institution of plasmapheresis. Crit Care Med. 2002;30(4):931.

Chapter 14
Paroxysmal Nocturnal Hemoglobinuria

A 50-year-old lady was admitted to hospital with pain abdomen and lower back of 5 days duration. There was no vomiting or diarrhea. For the last 1 week, she had been observing high colored urine early in morning which used to clear off with time during the day. She also had been feeling weak and lethargic for the past 2 weeks. There was no history of fever or drug intake. Similar observation of dark urine in morning with color lightening with time had been observed three times in the past 6 months. Examination revealed pallor and mild tinge of jaundice. There was no organomegaly. Initial CBC result is provided in Table 14.1.

A. Gupta, *Decision Making Through Problem Based Learning in Hematology*,
https://doi.org/10.1007/978-981-99-8933-1_14

Table 14.1 CBC

CBC parameter	Patient's result	Reference range
WBC	2.5	3.7–10 × 10^9/L
RBC	4.0	4.5–5.4 × 10^{12}/L
HB	100	130–160 g/L
Hct	0.30	0.33–0.43 L/L
MCV	88	83–101 fL
MCH	29	27–32 pg
MCHC	325	315–345 g/L
RDW	12	11.6–14.6%
PLT	60	130–430 × 10^9/L
MPV	10	7–11 fL
Poly#	1.5	1.7–6 × 10^9/L
Lymp#	0.5	1–3 × 10^9/L
Mono#	0.9	0.2–1.0 × 10^9/L
EO#	0.1	0.02–0.5 × 10^9/L
BASO#	0	0.02–0.1 × 10^9/L
RETIC%	7	0.5–1.5%
ESR	28	0–20 mm 1st h Westergren

14.1 Questions

Q1. Interpret the CBC result given above and suggest investigations for further evaluation in such case

Answer: The CBC shows low values for WBC, red cell count, and platelet count. The Hb is low with normal red cell indices. The differential white cell count shows neutropenia and lymphocytopenia. Reticulocyte % is high, and ESR is also raised.

So there is pancytopenia with high reticulocyte count. Such alterations can be seen in:

1. Infections
2. Hypersplenism
3. Bleeding
4. Nutritional deficiencies (such as B12/ iron) on treatment
5. Autoimmune disorders
6. PNH, some cases of MDS, neoplastic conditions, etc.

Next best test will be to examine a blood film and also estimate level of serum B12 and folic acid, CRP, urine and stools for blood loss, immunology profile as well as baseline tests for liver, kidney, and pancreatic functions. There is no history of fever. So the possibility of infection is unlikely. Also, there is no organomegaly or history of neoplastic pathology.

Q2. Given is image from blood film (Fig. 14.1). Results of liver, kidney, pancreatic functions (Table 14.2); serum B12, folic acid levels, CRP (Table 14.3), immunology profile (Table 14.4); and examination of urine and stools (Table 14.5) are also provided. Interpret these results and suggest a differential diagnosis? what further investigations should be done to exclude various possibilities?

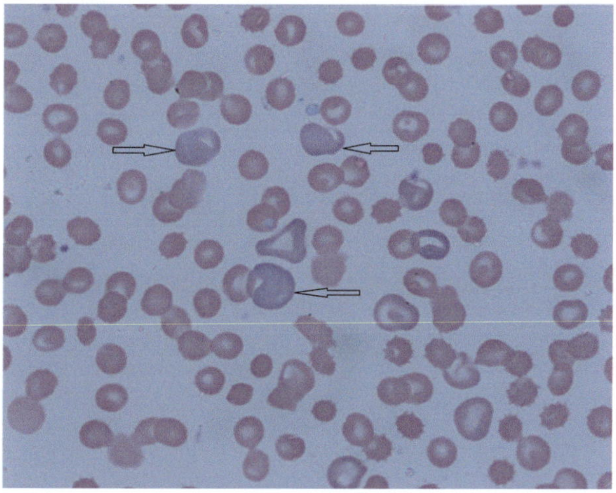

Fig. 14.1 PBF: Normocytic normochromic red cells and polychromatic cells (black arrows). Leishman stain × 100

Table 14.2 Biochemical tests

Test	Patient's result	Ref range
Glu	5.0	3.9–6.1 mmol/L
Urea	4.0	2.5–6.6 mmol/L
Creat	99	60–120 μmol/L
Na+	142	136–146 mmol/L
K^+	4.7	3.7–5.0 mmol/L
Ca+	2.5	2.2–2.6 mmol/L
Mg+	1.0	0.08–1.1 mmol/L
T. Prot	75	63–80 mmol/L
Alb	44	35–47 mmol/L
Choles	3.5	1.5–5.2 mmol/L
TG	0.9	0.4–1.7 mmol/L
Urates	330	150–400 mmol/L
T Bil	49	3–20 μmol/L
D. Bil	7	0–5 μmol/L
I Bil	42	5–15 μmol/L
Alk Ph	60	26–88 IU/L
ALT	54	10–60 IU/L
AST	33	10–42 IU/L
GGT	55	7–64 IU/L
LDH	286	90–180 IU/L
Hapto	0.26	0.2–2.0 g/L
T4	10.6	7.8–16 pmol/L
TSH	3.91	0.27–4.2 μlU/ml
Amylase	40	28–100 IU/L
Lipase	50	0–160 U/L

Table 14.3 Serum B12, folic acid and CRP

Test	Patient's result	Ref range
S. B12	522	150–700 pmol/L
S. folate	20.7	10–42 nmol/L
RBC folate	2253	1187–2854 nmol/L
CRP	6	0–10 mg/L

Table 14.4 DAT and immunology tests

Test	Patient's result	Ref range
Direct antiglobulin test	Negative	Negative
Anti ds-DNA antibody	Negative	0–20 Iu/mL
ANA screen	Negative	Negative
AnA pattern	Negative	Negative
ANA titer	Negative	Negative
Sm B	Negative	Negative
RNP A and C	Negative	Negative
SS-A	Negative	Negative
SS-B	Negative	Negative
Scl-70	Negative	Negative
Jo-1	Negative	Negative
Ribosomal P	Negative	Negative
Histone	Negative	Negative
MPO ab	Negative	Negative
Proteinase ab	Negative	Negative
C3	0.537 g/L	0.83–1.77 g/L
C4	0.116 g/L	0.2–0.8 g/L

Table 14.5 Urine and stool examination

Urine examination	Patient's result	Reference range
SG	1.022	1.005–1.030
Ph	6.2	5–7
Leu	Neg	Neg
Nit	Neg	Neg
Pro	Neg	Neg
Glu	Neg	Neg
Ket	Neg	Neg
Uro	Neg	Neg
Bil	Neg	Neg
Hemoglobin	Positive	Neg
Prussian blue stain on urine sediment	Positive for hemosiderin	Neg
Stool examination		
Occult blood	Neg	Neg
Ova/cysts	Neg	Neg

Answer: The blood film shows mainly normocytic normochromic red cells. Polychromatic cells are also seen (arrows). No abnormal leukocytes are seen. The biochemical tests show indirect hyper-bilirubinemia and high LDH and low normal levels of haptoglobin. Serum B12, folic acid, and red cell folate levels are within normal limits. Immunology profile is normal except for mildly reduced C3 and C4 levels. The urine shows hemoglobinuria and hemosiderinuria. These findings suggest intravascular hemolysis with mildly reduced complement levels. There is no evidence of hematological malignancy. Autoimmune disorders are excluded.

The possible causes of intravascular hemolysis are as follows:

1. Prosthetic cardiac valves.
2. Glucose-6-phosphate dehydrogenase (G6PD) deficiency.
3. Thrombotic thrombocytopenic purpura (TTP).
4. Disseminated intravascular coagulation (DIC).
5. Transfusion of ABO incompatible blood.
6. Paroxysmal nocturnal hemoglobinuria (PNH).

There is no history of prosthetic heart valve. No red cell fragments are seen on blood film excluding DIC and TTP. Also there is no history of recent blood transfusion or history of G6PD deficiency.

None of these conditions are associated with decreased complement levels except PNH. The cause of pain abdomen needs further investigations. An ultrasound examination/ CT abdomen is required to assess cause of pain abdomen and a bone marrow examination to assess any specific cause of pancytopenia. For exclusion of PNH, flowcytometric analysis (FLAER based) of peripheral blood for CD55 and CD59 is advised.

Q3. Given are images from bone marrow biopsy (Fig. 14.2), flow cytometry on peripheral blood (Table 14.6), and result of Ultrasound abdomen (Fig. 14.3). Interpret the results and suggest final diagnosis.

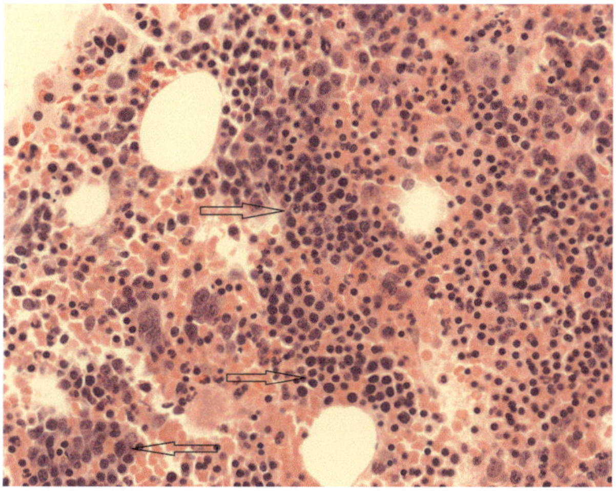

Fig. 14.2 BM Trephine biopsy. Erythroid hyperplasia H/E × 40

Table 14.6 Flowcytometric analysis of peripheral blood. Deficiency of CD55 and CD59 (red cells), CD24 (neutrophils), and CD14 (monocytes) is recorded

Cell type	Anchoring protein	Deficiency%
Red cells	CD55 and CD59	40% deficient
Neutrophils	CD24	80% deficient
Monocytes	CD 14	60% deficient

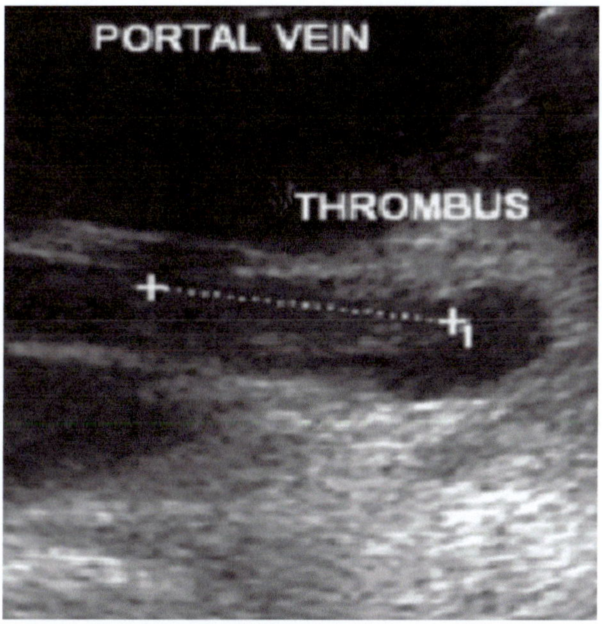

Fig. 14.3 Ultrasound of abdomen showing thrombus in portal vein

Answer: The bone marrow biopsy is mildly hypercellular for age and shows increase in erythroid precursors which are seen as aggregates as well as interstitially distributed cells. The granulocytic precursors and megakaryocytes are unremarkable. The ultrasound abdomen shows portal vein thrombosis which is most likely cause of pain abdomen. The flow cytometric result of peripheral blood for PNH screening shows deficiency of CD55 and CD59 on red cells and deficiency of CD24 and CD 14 on neutrophils and monocytes, respectively.

These findings confirm a final diagnosis of paroxysmal nocturnal hemoglobinuria (PNH) with portal vein thrombosis.

Q4. What additional tests (other than done so far) may be considered in this case?

Answer: Analysis of *PIGA* gene can be used to confirm a diagnosis of PNH but its availability is limited to specialized centers. Red cell acetylcholine esterase or neutrophil alkaline phosphatase assays can also support diagnosis of PNH.

Q5. What is etiopathogenesis of PNH?

Answer: PNH is an acquired hemolytic anemia due to defect in hematopoietic stem cell resulting from mutation in PIGA gene linked to X-chromosome.

Normally PIGA gene is responsible for formation of anchor proteins-glycosylphosphatidylinositol (GPI) which holds CD55 and CD59 on red cell membrane. In PNH, due to somatic mutation in this gene, synthesis of these anchors is impaired. The stem cells lacking CD55 and CD59 anchor proteins, clonally expand into red blood cells (RBCs) and white blood cells (WBCs) that are susceptible to lysis by complement, resulting in intravascular hemolysis and cytopenias.

Complement system is an important first-line defense in our body. It consists of many precursor proteins that are synthesized by the liver. Three biochemical pathways activate the complement system, namely the classical pathway, the alternative pathway, and the lectin pathway. The hemolysis of PNH is caused by abnormal regulation of the alternative pathway.

When complement pathway is activated, it results in a series of reactions. Of all intermediary reaction steps, reactions involving C3 convertase and C5 convertase are important. C5 convertase cleaves C5 into C5a and C5b. C5b initiates formation of membrane attack complex (MAC) which are combinations of C5b-C6-C7-C8- C9. These MACs insert into the lipid bilayer of the cell and results in osmotic lysis with resultant intravascular hemolysis. Red cells are normally protected from such attacks due to presence of CD55 (DAF) which blocks the formation C3 and C5 convertases and CD59 (MIRL) which blocks the formation of the MAC. In absence of CD55 and CD59, cells are unprotected and undergo lysis [1, 2].

Q6. Which diseases are associated with PNH?

Answer: PNH is a clonal hematopoietic stem cell disorder that manifests with hemolytic anemia, bone marrow failure, and thrombosis. Patients with aplastic anemia and myelodysplasia can develop PNH clone subsequently [3].

Q7. What is the cause of thrombosis in PNH?

Answer: Thrombophilia in PNH is multifactorial. Exact mechanism is not known. However, possibilities offered are as follows: [4–7]

1. Depletion of nitric oxide which may result in activation of platelet.
2. Complement activation contributes to the prothrombotic tendency.
3. Lack of urokinase receptor and tissue factor pathway inhibitor (TFPI), which are also part of anchor proteins. There is defective fibrinolysis that contribute to the thrombophilic state.

Q8. What is the cause of pancytopenia in PNH?.

Answer: As PNH is clonal hematopoietic stem cell disorder, all cell lines are effected by lack of anchor proteins. There is bone marrow failure and defective blood cell production.

Approximately, 30–45% of PNH patients have some kind of bone marrow failure syndromes such as aplastic anemia, myelodysplastic syndrome, refractory anemia, and unexplained cytopenia(s) [8].

Q9. Which cells are best suited for analysis of PNH?

Answer: Ideally, at least two GPI-linked markers from two different lineages should be tested, i.e., red cells and granulocytes/monocytes. However, in some situations where the number of red cells is less due to severe hemolysis, granulocytes are preferred cells for analysis. A FLAER based flowcytometric assessment is recommended [9].

Q10. How is PNH classified clinically?

Answer: As proposed by the International PNH Interest Group, PNH is classified into 3 categories: [3].

1. Classical PNH: It includes patients with hemolytic anemia and thrombosis.
2. PNH associated with other primary bone marrow disorders: Aplastic anemia and myelodysplastic syndrome.
3. Subclinical PNH: Patients have small PNH clones but no clinical or laboratory evidence of hemolysis or thrombosis.

Q11. What are the other diagnostic possibilities in patients with Coombs negative hemolytic anemia?

Answer: In patients with anemia only, other possibilities with intravascular hemolysis include prosthetic cardiac valves, glucose-6-phosphate dehydrogenase deficiency, thrombotic thrombocytopenic purpura, disseminated intravascular coagulation, and transfusion of ABO incompatible blood. In patients presenting with pancytopenia, aplastic/hypoplastic anemia and MDS are also considered in differential diagnosis.

Q12. How is PNH different from warm AIHA, CAD, and PCH?

Answer: Following are some of the main points which help in differentiating these conditions: (Table 14.7) [3, 5, 10].

Table 14.7 Differences between Warm AIHA, CAD, PCH and PNH

Disease	Warm AIHA	CAD	PCH	PNH
Ig class involved	IgG mainly	IgM mainly	D-L biphasic antibody (IgG)	No Ig involved
Common etiology	LPD, autoimmune diseases	Mycoplasma, HIV, infectious mononucleosis	Infectious mononucleosis	Mutation in PIGA gene
	DAT + with IgG +/− C3	DAT + with C3	DAT + with C3	DAT negative
Blood film	Spherocytes	Agglutinins	Hemolysis	Hemolysis
Blood group system involved	Rh system	I/i system	P system	No blood group involved

Q13. What are the common clinical presentations of PNH?

Answer: The most common presentation is anemia with passage of dark colored urine. Also thrombosis at unusual sites like hepatic, abdominal, cerebral, and subdermal veins is seen in many patients. Erectile dysfunction and esophageal spasms also occur [11, 12].

Q14. What is the cause of dark colored urine in early morning samples?

Answer: The hemolysis is triggered by acidosis during sleep which activates complement resulting in hemolysis of abnormal red cells. However, it has been shown that hemolysis occurs throughout the day and is not actually paroxysmal.

Q15. What is the cause of symptoms like fatigue, erectile dysfunctions, and esophageal spasms?

Answer: Following intra vascular hemolysis, the released hemoglobin scavenges nitric oxide. Under normal conditions, nitric oxide maintains the vascular tone and prevents platelet activation. When it is depleted, muscle spasms occur manifesting as fatigue, dysphagia, and abdominal pain and erectile dysfunction occur [13].

14.2 Correlation of Results of Preliminary Investigations with Symptoms and Signs in PNH

Q16. How do symptoms and signs in this patients correlate with diagnosis?

Answer: The patient was feeling weak and lethargic which are the symptoms of anemia. A high colored urine in early morning samples is typical of PNH due to intravascular hemolysis. Pain abdomen is explained by presence of portal vein thrombosis.

Q17. How do CBC, blood film, and biochemical tests guide in evaluation of this case?

Answer: Anemia with reticulocytosis, indirect hyperbilirubinemia and raised LDH suggest intravascular hemolysis. Reticulocytosis indicates response of bone marrow. Presence of hemoglobin and hemosiderin in urine are indicators of intravascular hemolysis with recent as well as recurrent episodes in recent past. A decrease in complement C3 and C4 suggests their consumption, indirectly pointing to activation of complement pathway.

Q18. What were the confirmatory tests in this case?

Answer: The flowcytometry on blood cells which revealed deficiency of 2 GPI-linked molecules–red blood cells and granulocytes confirmed the diagnosis of PNH.

Q19. How should the patients be followed up?

Answer: Patients with PNH should be assessed annually for clone size if they remain stable clinically. More frequent assessment is required in patients with fluctuating clinical parameters.

Q20. Which patients should be investigated for PNH?

Answer: Patients presenting with hemoglobinuria, unexplained hemolysis with suspicion of thrombosis at unusual sites, unexplained cytopenias, DCT negative hemolytic anemia or if there is evidence of bone marrow failure syndrome especially with granulocytopenia or thrombocytopenia (hypoplastic/aplastic anemia and MDS) should be investigated for PNH.

Unexplained thrombosis (such as stroke, myocardial infarction, pulmonary emboli, and deep vein thrombosis) or thrombosis at unusual sites (such as hepatic vein thrombosis, portal or mesenteric vein thrombosis, cerebral sinus thrombosis, and dermal vein thrombosis) should raise suspicion of PNH.

Any thrombotic episode seen in association with hemolysis or unexplained cytopenia should undergo investigations for PNH [14, 15].

Q21. What is the diagnostic triad of PNH? What is the minimal criteria for diagnosing PNH?

Answer: Hemolytic anemia, pancytopenia, and thrombosis are considered a diagnostic triad of PNH. Minimum criteria for diagnosis require evidence of deficiency of GPI anchor proteins on red cells, white cells, or preferably both by FLAER-based flow cytometry [3].

Q21. Which test methods are recommended for confirmation of PNH?

Answer: Flow cytometry is the preferred technique. Best specimen is peripheral blood, and estimation of both WBC and RBC clone size is recommended. Specific GPI-linked monoclonal antibodies are used. GPI-linked proteins that can be assayed include CD59 and CD55, as well as the CD14, CD15, CD16, CD24, CD45, and CD64. Analysis using fluorescent labeled aerolysin (FLAER) is now considered GOLD STANDARD test for diagnosis of PNH. Aerolysin is a bacterial protein that binds directly to the GPI anchor proteins. When this is combined with CD157, CD15, and CD64, the accuracy of test is very high. FLAER is more sensitive than monoclonal antibodies like CD59 when granulocytic population is less. It can detect PNH cells as low as 0.5%. Ham test is now obsolete [14–17].

14.3 Quick Information for Practicing Clinicians and Students

References [1–20]:

1. Coombs negative hemolytic anemia, pancytopenia, and thrombosis are considered a diagnostic triad of PNH.
2. Patients presenting with hemoglobinuria, unexplained hemolysis with suspicion of thrombosis at unusual sites, unexplained cytopenias, DCT negative hemolytic anemia or if there is evidence of bone marrow failure syndrome especially with granulocytopenia or thrombocytopenia should be investigated for PNH.
3. PNH is a clinical diagnosis that needs confirmation with peripheral blood flow cytometry to detect deficiency of GPI-APs on 2 lineages.
4. The "Gold standard" test for diagnosis is flow cytometry with FLAER-based testing.
5. Absence of CD59 is most responsible for the clinical manifestations in PNH.
6. The hemolysis is chronic but paroxysms may result from increase in complement activation due to infection, surgery, strenuous activity, and excessive alcohol intake.
7. Unexplained thrombosis (such as stroke, myocardial infarction, pulmonary emboli, and deep vein thrombosis) or thrombosis at unusual sites (such as hepatic vein thrombosis, portal or mesenteric vein thrombosis, cerebral sinus thrombosis, and dermal vein thrombosis) should raise suspicion of PNH.
8. Thrombosis is the leading cause of mortality. The PNH clone size of >50% in granulocytes correlates highly with thrombotic risk.
9. The bone marrow is normocellular to hypercellular with erythroid hyperplasia. The reticulocyte count is increased with high LDH. Hemoglobinuria, smooth muscle dystonias (e.g., esophageal spasm and erectile dysfunction), severe fatigue, and thrombosis are common.
10. Hemosiderin is nearly always present in the urine sediment.
11. Depending on the complement sensitivity to lysis, PNH cells are categorized into type I (normal sensitivity), type II (3–5 times more sensitive), and type III cells (15–25 times more sensitive to lysis).

To acquire further knowledge on the subject, following sources are advised:

1. BCSH guidelines
2. Br Jr. Hematology
3. ASH education book
4. Blood
5. NEJM
6. Int Jr. Lab Hematology

References

1. Robert AB. Paroxysmal nocturnal hemoglobinuria. Blood. 2014;124(18):2804–11. https://doi.org/10.1182/blood-2014-02-522128.
2. Risitano AM, Notaro R, Marando L, et al. Complement fraction 3 binding on erythrocytes as additional mechanism of disease in paroxysmal nocturnal hemoglobinuria patients treated by eculizumab. Blood. 2009;113:4094–100.
3. Parker C, Omine M, Richards S, et al. Diagnosis and management of paroxysmal nocturnal hemoglobinuria. Blood. 2005;106(12):3699–709. https://doi.org/10.1182/blood-2005-04-1717.
4. Neal SY, Janis LA, Luzzatto L. New insights into the pathophysiology of acquired cytopenias. Hematology Am Soc Hematol Educ Program. 2000;1:18–38. https://doi.org/10.1182/asheducation-2000.1.18.
5. Brodsky RA. New insights into paroxysmal nocturnal hemoglobinuria. Hematology Am Soc Hematol Educ Program. 2006;1:24–28.
6. Bessler M, Hiken J. The pathophysiology of disease in patients with paroxysmal nocturnal hemoglobinuria. Hematology Am Soc Hematol Educ Program. 2008;1:104–108.
7. Rønne E, Pappot H, Grøndahl-Hansen J, et al. The receptor for urokinase plasminogen activator is present in plasma from healthy donors and elevated in patients with paroxysmal nocturnal haemoglobinuria. Br J Haematol. 1995;89:576–81.
8. Schrezenmeier H, Muus P, Socie G, et al. Baseline characteristics and disease burden in patients in the international paroxysmal nocturnal Hemoglobinuria registry. Haematologica. 2014;99:922–9. https://doi.org/10.3324/haematol.2013.093161.
9. Hernandez-Campo PM, Almeida J, Sanchez ML, Malvezzi M, Orfao A. Normal patterns of expression of glycosylphosphatidylinositol-anchored proteins on different subsets of peripheral blood cells: a frame of reference for the diagnosis of paroxysmal nocturnal hemoglobinuria. Cytometry B Clin Cytom. 2006;70:71–81.
10. Win N, Stamps R, Knight R. Paroxysmal cold haemoglobinuria/Donath-Landsteiner test. Transfus Med. 2005;15(3):254.
11. Brodsky RA. How I treat paroxysmal nocturnal hemoglobinuria. Blood. 2009;113(26):6522–7.
12. Mukhina GL, Buckley JT, Barber JP, Jones RJ, Brodsky RA. Multilineage glycosylphosphatidylinositol anchor-deficient haematopoiesis in untreated aplastic anaemia. Br J Haematol. 2001;115:476–82.
13. Rother RP, Bell L, Hillmen P, Gladwin MT. The clinical sequelae of intravascular hemolysis and extracellular plasma hemoglobin: a novel mechanism of human disease. JAMA. 2005;293:1653–62.
14. Borowitz MJ, Craig FE, JA DG, On behalf of the Clinical Cytometry Society, et al. Guidelines for the diagnosis and monitoring of paroxysmal nocturnal hemoglobinuria and related disorders by flow cytometry. Cytom B Clin Cytom. 2010;78:211–30.
15. Sharma VR. Paroxysmal nocturnal hemoglobinuria: pathogenesis, testing and diagnosis. Clin Adv Hematol Oncol. 2013;11:2–8.
16. Brodsky RA, Mukhina GL, Li S, Nelson KL, et al. Improved detection and characterization of paroxysmal nocturnal hemoglobinuria using fluorescent aerolysin. Am J Clin Pathol. 2000;114:459–66.
17. Parker CJ. Update on the diagnosis and management of paroxysmal nocturnal hemoglobinuria. Hematology Am Soc Hematol Educ Program. 2016;2016(1):208 16.
18. Hall SE, Rosse WF. The use of monoclonal antibodies and flow cytometry in the diagnosis of paroxysmal nocturnal hemoglobinuria. Blood. 1996;87:5332–40.
19. Sutherland DR, Kuek N, Davidson J, et al. Diagnosing PNH with FLAER and multiparameter flow cytometry. Cytom B Clin Cytom. 2007;72:167–77. https://doi.org/10.1002/cyto.b.20151.
20. Latour RP, Mary JY, Salanoubat C, et al. Paroxysmal nocturnal hemoglobinuria: natural history of disease subcategories. Blood. 2008;112:3099–106. https://doi.org/10.1182/blood-2008-01-133918.

Chapter 15
Microangiopathic Hemolytic Anemia

A 45-year-old female patient reports with history of sudden development of confusion, giddiness, and headache. She was also experiencing low-grade fever and had history of exertional dyspnea and lethargy for the past 1 week. One day before presentation, she had observed few petechial spots on chest, abdomen, and upper arms. There is no history of bleeding from any site other than skin. There is no past or current history of hypertension, migraine, problem with eyesight, ear, nose, or throat. Physical examination showed pallor and mild tinge of jaundice. There was no organomegaly. Result of CBC is presented in Table 15.1.

Table 15.1 CBC

CBC parameter	Patient's result	Reference range
WBC	8	3.7–10 × 10^9/L
RBC	3.6	4.5–5.4 × 10^{12}/L
HB	75	130–160 g/L
Hct	0.23	0.33–0.43 L/L
MCV	91	83–101 fL
MCH	27	27–32 pg
MCHC	333	315–345 g/L
RDW	14	11.6–14.6%
PLT	15	130–430 × 10^9/L
MPV	10	7–11 fL
Poly #	4.5	1.7–6 × 10^9/L
Lymp#	1.9	1–3 × 10^9/L
Mono#	0.4	0.2–1.0 × 10^9/L
EO#	0.2	0.02–0.5 × 10^9/L
Baso#	0	0.02–0.1 × 10^9/L
RETIC%	12	0.5–1.5%
ESR	32	0–20 mm 1st h Westergren

A. Gupta, *Decision Making Through Problem Based Learning in Hematology*, https://doi.org/10.1007/978-981-99-8933-1_15

15.1 Questions

Q1. Interpret the CBC result given above and suggest investigations for further evaluation in such case.

Answer: The result of CBC shows normal total leucocytic count, low number of RBCs, decreased hemoglobin level and hematocrit with normal MCV, MCH, and MCHC values. Reticulocyte % is increased. There is severe thrombocytopenia. ESR value is also little high. So there is normocytic normochromic anemia (N/N Anemia). Causes of normocytic normochromic anemia include:

1. *Decreased production from marrow (will have low reticulocyte count)*: Chronic pathological conditions (such as chronic inflammations, neoplastic pathologies, and infections), chronic renal failure, chronic liver disease, endocrinopathies, marrow infiltration, and hypoplastic anemias.
2. *Increased destruction (will have increased reticulocytes with normal marrow):*
   (a) Red cell defects: Defects of red cell membrane, enzymes, or hemoglobin.
   (b) Without any defect of red cells (defects lie outside red cells): Autoimmune hemolytic anemia, micro-angiopathic hemolytic anemia (DIC/TTP/HUS).
3. *Sequestration: splenomegaly.*
4. *Hemorrhage.*

This patient has reticulocytosis. In the presence of high reticulocyte%, the possible cause of anemia is peripheral destruction, sequestration, or bleeding.

There is no splenomegaly. So the other causes of N/N anemia need to be considered first.

Next best investigation will be examination of blood film, assessment of hemolytic markers, and exclusion of bleeding from sites other than skin. Baseline serum chemistry for functions of liver, kidney, and thyroid is also indicated for evaluation. Routine urine for hematuria and stool examination for occult blood are also suggested. A CT scan of brain to assess any acute intracranial pathology is also required.

Q2. Given is image from blood film (Fig. 15.1). Also result of tests for hemolytic profile including liver, kidney, thyroid functions(Table 15.2), examination of urine and stools (Table 15.3), and result of CT scan are provided. Interpret these results and suggest a differential diagnosis? what further investigations should be done to exclude various possibilities?

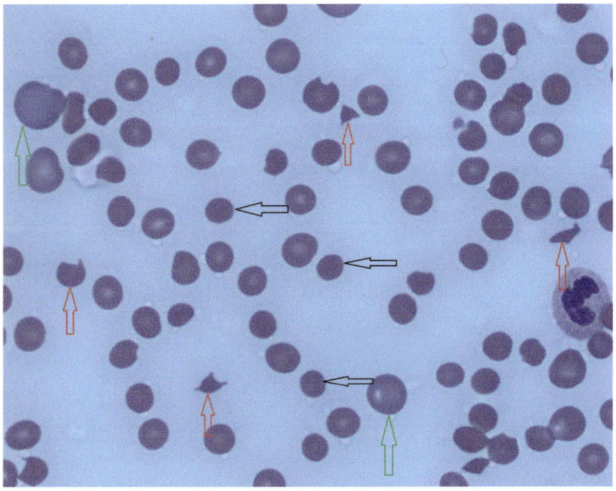

Fig. 15.1 PBF. Red cell fragments (red arrows), polychromatic cells (green arrows), spherocytes (black arrows). Leishman stain × 100

Table 15.2 Biochemical tests

Test	Patient's result	Ref range
Glu	5.4	3.9–6.1 mmol/L
Urea	5.9	2.5–6.6 mmol/L
Creat	99	60–120 μmol/L
Na+	142	136–146 mmol/L
K^+	4.9	3.7–5.0 mmol/L
Ca^+	2.3	2.2–2.6 mmol/L
Mg^+	1.0	0.08–1.1 mmol/L
T. Prot	78	63–80 mmol/L
Alb	44	35–47 mmol/L
Choles	3.5	1.5–5.2 mmol/L
TG	0.9	0.4–1.7 mmol/L
Urates	350	150–400 mmol/L
T Bil	63	3–20 μmol/L
D. Bil	5	0–5 μmol/L
I Bil	58	5–15 μmol/L
Alk Ph	60	26–88 IU/L
ALT	54	10–60 IU/L
AST	33	10–42 IU/L
GGT	55	7–64 IU/L
LDH	480	90–180 IU/L
Hapto	0.02	0.2–2.0 g/L
T4	10.6	7.8–16 pmol/L
TSH	3.99	0.27–4.2 μlU/mL
Amylase	20	28–100 IU/L

Table 15.3 Urine and stool examination

Urine examination	Patient's result	Reference range
SG	1.021	1.005–1.030
Ph	6.1	5–7
Leu	Neg	Neg
Nit	Neg	Neg
Pro	Neg	Neg
Glu	Neg	Neg
Ket	Neg	Neg
Uro	Present	Neg
Bil	Neg	Neg
Hemosiderin	Neg	Neg
Hemoglobin	Neg	Neg
Stool examination		
Occult blood	Neg	Neg
Ova/cysts	Neg	Neg

CT SCAN: No evidence of any acute intracranial insult

Answer: The blood film shows low density of red cells. Many red cell fragments and polychromatic cells are noted. Few spherocytes are also seen. There is marked thrombocytopenia. No immature cells are seen.

The biochemical tests show indirect hyperbilirubinemia, high levels of LDH, and reduced level of haptoglobin, which suggest a hemolytic process. The urine shows urobilinogen and stools examination is normal. The CT scan result does not show any acute intracranial disease process.

Presence of hemolytic biochemical parameters with red cell fragments and severe thrombocytopenia suggest many possibility, some of which include:

1. MAHA (DIC, TTP, HUS)
2. Autoimmune disease with vasculitis
3. Pre-eclampsia/eclampsia
4. March hemoglobinuria
5. Malignant hypertension

However, last three conditions are excluded as there is no hemoglobinuria, history of strenuous exercise, pregnancy, or hypertension [1].

Further tests required for evaluation are coagulation profile, direct antiglobulin test (DAT), and an immunology profile.

Q3. Given are results of coagulation profile (Table 15.4), direct antiglobulin test (DAT), and immunology profile (Table 15.5). Suggest a final diagnosis. How this diagnosis be confirmed and what other tests can be done to exclude close differential diagnosis?

Table 15.4 Coagulation profile

Test	Patient's result	Reference range
PT	11.5	9.6–13.6 s
INR	0.9	0.85–1.15
APTT	31	25–37 s
Fibrinogen/ Clauss	4.0	2.34–4.45 g/L
D-D dimer	280	Below 255 ng/mL

Table 15.5 DAT and immunology screen

Test	Patient's result	Ref range
Direct antiglobulin test	Negative	Negative
Anti ds-DNA antibody	Negative	0–20 Iu/mL
ANA screen	Negative	Negative
AnA pattern	Negative	Negative
ANA titer	Negative	Negative
Sm B	Negative	Negative
RNP A and C	Negative	Negative
SS-A	Negative	Negative
SS-B	Negative	Negative
Scl-70	Negative	Negative
Jo-1	Negative	Negative
Ribosomal P	Negative	Negative
Histone	Negative	Negative
MPO ab	Negative	Negative
Proteinase ab	Negative	Negative

Answer: Coagulation profile is within normal limits. The DAT is negative, and immunology profile is normal. These results exclude possibility of DIC and autoimmune diseases.

Based on other results of hemolytic anemia with red cell fragments and severe thrombocytopenia, the most likely possibilities are TTP and HUS. HUS is also excluded as there is no history of diarrhea, and renal functions are not impaired. So based on constellation of clinical and laboratory findings, a final diagnosis of TTP is suggested. For further evaluation and confirmation of diagnosis, serum levels of enzyme ADAMTS-13 are recommended.

Q4. Result of ADAMTS13 enzyme activity is given. Interpret the result?

ADAMTS 13 activity of patient: 3% (Normal 50% to 160%)

Answer: The activity of the enzyme is severely reduced (less than 5%). This confirms the diagnosis of TTP in this patient.

Q5. How is TTP classified?

Answer: A simplified classification is as follows: [2, 3].

(a) Congenital/inherited (Upshaw–Schulman syndrome).
(b) Acquired:

1. Primary (idiopathic or autoantibody-mediated)
2. Secondary (approximately 70%) to a variety of conditions like autoimmune disorders, solid organ or hematopoietic cell transplant, malignancy, drugs, and pregnancy. Secondary TTP has a worse prognosis than idiopathic TTP.

Q6. What is etiology of TTP/HUS?

Answer: In congenital/inherited TTP (Upshaw–Schulman syndrome), seen in approximately 2% patients, the deficiency is either due to homozygous or compound heterozygous (recessive) mutations of the *ADAMTS13* gene.

In more than 90% adults, ADAMTS13 deficiency is acquired—either idiopathic or caused by destruction of this enzyme in the other disease conditions or destruction secondary to development of auto antibodies.

Secondary causes include a variety of conditions like autoimmune disorders, solid organ or hematopoietic cell transplant, malignancy, drugs (such as mitomycin C, cyclosporine, quinine, clopidogrel, ticlopidine), pregnancy, and some infections like hepatitis and pneumococcal infections [2, 3].

Q7. What is pathogenesis of TTP?

Answer: In majority of cases, the cause is of TTP is unknown. There is severe deficiency of ADAMTS-13 enzyme either from auto antibody production or gene mutation.

Intravascular thrombi formation takes place in microvasculature with ischemia of multiple organs especially involving brain. Hematological abnormalities with red cell fragments and thrombocytopenia are present. Positive anti-ADAMTS13 IgG antibodies are seen in about 75% of TTP during an acute phase. Degradation by sepsis enzymes such as calpains, elastases, thrombin, or plasmin and inhibition of ADAMTS13 by free hemoglobin or interleukins are some of the pathogenetic mechanisms quoted in literature [4].

Under normal physiologic conditions, ultra-large VWF multimers are released from endothelial cells. These have high affinity to bind platelets in circulation and need to be cleaved down into smaller fragments which are less adhesive to platelets. This cleaving function is done by ADAMTS 13 enzyme. In TTP, functional ADAMTS13 is absent or very deficient. As such, ultra-large VWF multimers are released into blood and bind spontaneously to platelets. Microthrombi formation occurs in smaller blood vessels (arteries and capillaries). The VWF-platelet aggregates are large enough to obstruct lumen of blood vessels and induce tissue ischemia. This also results in consumption of platelet and microangiopathic hemolytic anemia (fragmented red cells) [5].

Q8. what are precipitating and predisposing factors for TTP?

Answer: Some conditions are considered as risk factors for TTP. These include: female sex, black ethnicity, HLA-DRB, and obesity. A few factors can precipitate TTP. These conditions increase level of VWF and include pregnancy, infection, and inflammation. Drugs such as quinine, Plavix, chemotherapy, and infections such as HIV, pneumococcal, and hepatitis as well as autoimmune diseases like SLE are also associated with TTP [6].

Q9. How is TTP different from DIC and HUS/atypical HUS?

Answer: Both conditions cause microvascular thrombosis, thrombocytopenia, and bleeding tendency associated with organ failure. In DIC, initial event is activation of coagulation with depletion of coagulation factors and hyperfibrinolysis. On the other hand, thrombosis is main initial event in TTP resulting from deficiency of ADAMTS-13 enzyme. (HUS is associated with Shiga toxin producing *E. coli,* and abnormalities of complement system are required for atypical HUS).

Q10. How the laboratory investigations help to differentiate TTP from DIC (and HUS)?

Answer: Similar to TTP, in a typical case of DIC also, the blood film will show red cell fragments and thrombocytopenia. However, the coagulation profile will be abnormal. Given is blood film image (Fig. 15.2) from a 30-year-old female patient who had septicemia following urinary tract infection. She developed anemia and thrombocytopenia with abnormal coagulation profile (prolonged PT, APTT, TT, low levels of fibrinogen, and high d-dimer). The blood film shows red cell fragments, a nucleated red cell, and thrombocytopenia, all of these along with abnormal coagulation are diagnostic of DIC. Please refer to table below for similarities and differences between DIC and TTP (Tables 15.6 and 15.7).

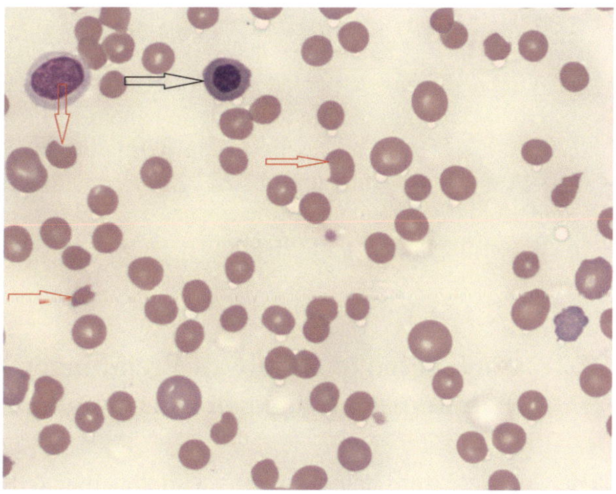

Fig. 15.2 PBF. Red cell fragments (red arrows), nucleated red cells (black arrows). Leishman stain × 100

Table 15.6 Similarities between DIC and TTP

Test	DIC	TTP
CBC and blood film		
Hemoglobin	Low (decreased)	Low(decreased)
Platelets	Low(decreased)	Low(decreased)
Reticulocyte %	High (increased)	High (increased)
Red cell fragments	Present (+++)	Present (+++)
Biochemical tests		
Indirect bilirubin	High	High
LDH	High	High
Haptoglobin	Low	Low

Table 15.7 Differences between DIC and TTP

Test	DIC	TTP
Prothrombin time (PT)	Prolonged (+++)	Normal (N)
Activated thromboplastin time (aPPT)	Prolonged (+++)	Normal (N)
Thrombin time (TT)	Prolonged (+++)	Normal (N)
FDPs	High (+++)	Normal to slightly high
Fibrinogen	Low(decreased)	Normal (N)
Antithrombin	Low (decreased)	Normal (N)

Q11. What is a typical presentation of TTP, DIC, and HUS?

Answer: TTP usually presents with fever, fatigue, pallor, and jaundice (signs of hemolytic anemia) and purpura, petechiae spots on skin, or mucosal bleeding (signs of thrombocytopenia). The central nervous and renal systems are most frequently affected. Neurological manifestations are seen in form of headache, confusion, focal neurological deficits, seizures, and coma. Mild renal impairment is also observed. Similar symptoms are seen in HUS but there is history of bloody diarrhea and severe renal dysfunction. In DIC, bleeding associated with multiorgan failure (renal, hepatic, respiratory, CNS) and shock are prominent features [7].

Q12. What is diagnostic pentad of TTP/HUS?

Answer: Microangiopathic hemolytic anemia (70–100%), thrombocytopenia (70–100%), renal dysfunction (approximately 50%), neurological dysfunction (50–90%), and fever (approx. 25%) are considered diagnostic pentad. Current guidelines recommend only presence of MAHA and thrombocytopenia sufficient for diagnosis of TTP/HUS [7].

15.2 Correlation of Results of Preliminary Investigations with Symptoms and Signs in Microangiopathic Hemolytic Anemia

Q13. Correlate signs and symptoms with the clinical diagnosis in this patient.

Answer: This patient has history of exertional dyspnea and lethargy for the past 1 week suggesting development of anemia. Symptoms of confusion, giddiness, and headache indicate CNS involvement. She had observed few petechial spots on chest, abdomen, and upper arms, due to thrombocytopenia. She also had fever prior to presentation. All these symptoms are indicative of TTP.

Q14 How do CBC, blood film, and biochemical tests guide in evaluation of this case?

Answer: The CBC result shows low number of RBCs, decreased hemoglobin level and hematocrit with normal MCV, MCH, and MCHC values. Reticulocyte % is increased. Severe thrombocytopenia is present. The blood film shows red cell fragments. The biochemical tests show indirect hyperbilirubinemia, high levels of LDH, and reduced level of haptoglobin, which suggest a hemolytic process.

Presence of hemolytic biochemical parameters with red cell fragments and severe thrombocytopenia indicate possibility of MAHA (DIC, TTP, HUS). Absence of history of diarrhea and normal renal functions excludes HUS. A normal coagulation profile makes DIC unlikely. So all these laboratory findings with markedly reduced levels of ADAMTS-13 confirm diagnosis of TTP in this case.

Q15. How does estimation of ADAMTS 13 help in confirmation of TTP and exclude other possibilities with MAHA?

For confirmation of TTP, the following tests are done, of which most commonly asked is ADAMTS 13 activity [8, 9].

1. ADAMTS 13 activity and antigen assays: Less than 10% activity is diagnostic of TTP. The levels of the ADAMTS 13 antigen can be measured by an enzyme-linked immunosorbent assay (ELISA).
2. ADAMTS 13 autoantibody and inhibitor assays: Patients with idiopathic TTP will have an autoantibody. The detection of an acquired inhibitor is essential to differentiate idiopathic TTP from congenital TTP. Most of the autoantibodies against ADAMTS 13 are of the immunoglobulin G (IgG) isotype.
3. ADAMTS 13-specific circulating immune complexes: Anti-ADAMTS 13 autoantibodies can circulate freely in plasma or bind to ADAMTS13, forming a complex that can be detected by an ELISA.

In appropriate clinical setting, ADAMTS 13 activity of <10% confirms the diagnosis of TTP. Additional studies to detect antigen levels and the presence of an inhibitor help to differentiate idiopathic TTP and congenital TTP. ADAMTS 13 is moderately decreased in other thrombotic microangiopathies such as DIC as well as in severe sepsis, solid organ transplantation, malignancy, autoimmune diseases, and malignant hypertension.

Q16. When is mutational analysis required for confirmation of TTP?

Answer: In newborn, if antigen level is very low and no inhibitor is detected, it is consistent with congenital TTP. In such cases, an ADAMTS 13 mutational analysis should be considered for confirmation.

Q17. How does ADMTS 13 help in follow-up of patients with TTP?

Answer: During follow-up of patients of TTP, possibility of relapse is indicated if:

1. Persistently severe decrease in ADAMTS 13 activity during course of disease is observed.
2. Positive inhibitors continue to persist.
3. During clinical remission, persistence of autoantibodies are observed.

15.3 Quick Information for Practicing Clinicians and Students

References [1–12]:

1. Thrombotic thrombocytopenic purpura is a life-threatening thrombotic microangiopathy. Rapid recognition is crucial to initiate appropriate management.
2. Approximately 50% of TTP cases are idiopathic. Bacterial infections and autoimmune diseases are most frequent clinical conditions associated with TTP in addition to other causes such as pregnancy, drugs, HIV infection, pancreatitis, and organ transplantation.
3. Diagnostic pentad for TTP are microangiopathic hemolytic anemia, thrombocytopenia, neurological dysfunction, renal dysfunction and fever.
4. Current guidelines recommend only presence of MAHA and thrombocytopenia (platelet count less than 30x 10^9/L) sufficient for diagnosis of TTP.
5. Presence of schistocytes on the blood smear is the morphologic hallmark of the disease.
6. Point-based TTP prediction scores are available in literature which help in prediction of an acquired ADAMTS13 deficiency. These scores are based on platelet count, serum creatinine level, antinuclear antibodies, d-dimer, reticulocytes, and indirect bilirubin.
7. ADAMTS 13 activity less than 10% usually confirms diagnosis of TTP.
8. ADAMTS 13 is the only specific marker to predict TTP relapses during the follow-up in clinical remission.
9. Thrombosis is main initial event in TTP resulting from deficiency of ADAMTS-13 enzyme. In DIC, the initial event is activation of coagulation with depletion of coagulation factors and hyperfibrinolysis. HUS is associated with Shiga toxin producing E. coli, and abnormalities of complement system are required for diagnosis of atypical HUS .
10. A presumptive diagnosis of TTP in the appropriate clinical setting can be made by using PLASMIC score. In appropriate clinical setting, a score of greater than 5 suggests a high probability of TTP and a score lower than 5 suggests a low probability of TTP. Details are in reference 12.

To acquire further knowledge on the subject, following sources are advised:

1. BCSH guidelines
2. Br Jr. Hematology
3. ASH education book
4. Blood
5. NEJM
6. Int Jr. Lab Hematology

References

1. Noris M, Remuzzi G. Atypical hemolytic-uremic syndrome. N Engl J Med. 2009;361(17):1676–87.
2. Amin Asnafi A, Jalali MT, Pezeshki SMS, Jaseb K, Saki N. The association between human leukocyte antigens and ITP, TTP, and HIT. J Pediatr Hematol Oncol. 2019 Mar;41(2):81–6.
3. Gavriilaki E, Anagnostopoulos A, Mastellos DC. Complement in thrombotic microangiopathies: Unraveling Ariadne's thread into the labyrinth of complement therapeutics. Front Immunol. 2019;10:337.
4. Verbij FC, Fijnheer R, Voorberg J, Sorvillo N. Acquired TTP: ADAMTS 13 meets the immune system. Blood Rev. 2014;28(6):227–34.
5. Lotta LA, Valsecchi C, Pontiggia S, et al. Measurement and prevalence of circulating ADAMTS13-specific immune complexes in autoimmune thrombotic thrombocytopenic purpura. J Thromb Haemost. 2014;12(3):329–36.
6. Mannucci PM, Canciani MT, Forza I, Lussana F, Lattuada A, Rossi E. Changes in health and disease of the metalloprotease that cleaves von Willebrand factor. Blood. 2001;98(9):2730–5.
7. Scully M, Yarranton H, Liesner R, et al. Regional UK TTP registry: correlation with laboratory ADAMTS 13 analysis and clinical features. Br J Haematol. 2008;142(5):819–26.
8. Ono T, Mimuro J, Madoiwa S, et al. Severe secondary deficiency of von Willebrand factor-cleaving protease (ADAMTS13) in patients with sepsis-induced disseminated intravascular coagulation: its correlation with development of renal failure. Blood. 2006;107(2):528–34.
9. Thouzeau S, Capdenat S, Stépanian A, Coppo P, Veyradier A. Evaluation of a commercial assay for ADAMTS13 activity measurement. Thromb Haemost. 2013;110(4):852–3.
10. Bentley MJ, Wilson AR, Rodgers GM. Performance of a clinical prediction score for thrombotic thrombocytopenic purpura in an independent cohort. Vox Sang. 2013;105(4):313–8.
11. Hie M, Gay J, Galicier L, et al. French thrombotic microangiopathies reference Centre. Preemptive rituximab infusions after remission efficiently prevent relapses in acquired thrombotic thrombocytopenic purpura. Blood. 2014;124(2):204–10.
12. Jamme M, Rondeau E. The PLASMIC score for thrombotic thrombocytopenic purpura. Lancet Haematol. 2017;4(4):e148–9.

Chapter 16
Aplastic Anemia

A 46-year-old lady presents with history of pruritic spots on thighs and legs of 5 days duration. There were few spots to begin with which are now increasing in number. Also, one day before, she had an episode of epistaxis. She had upper respiratory tract infection 1 week back, for which antibiotics were given by local physician. For the past 3 months, she had been experiencing progressive weakness with dyspnea on exertion in recent days. There is no other significant history in past, social life, or in family. She has no history of exposure to chemicals, radiations, or intake of medicines for long time.

Physical examination revealed pallor without jaundice. No organomegaly was detected. A palpable rash was observed involving both thighs and legs. Nothing abnormal was observed on chest or abdomen examination. Result of CBC done in this case is presented (Table 16.1).

A. Gupta, *Decision Making Through Problem Based Learning in Hematology*, https://doi.org/10.1007/978-981-99-8933-1_16

Table 16.1 CBC result

CBC parameter	Patient's result	Reference range
WBC	1.6	3.7–10 × 10^9/L
RBC	1.56	4.5–5.4 × 10^{12}/L
HB	58	130–160 g/L
Hct	0.16	0.33–0.43 L/L
MCV	98	83–101 fL
MCH	30	27–32 pg
MCHC	340	315–345 g/L
RDW	15	11.6–14.6%
PLT	9	130–430 × 10^9/L
MPV	12	7–11 fL
Poly#	0.9	1.7–6 × 10^9/L
Lymp#	0.5	1–3 × 10^9/L
Mono#	0.2	0.2–1.0 × 10^9/L
EO#	00	0.02–0.5 × 10^9/L
BASO#	00	0.02–0.1 × 10^9/L
RETIC%	0.01	0.5–1.5%
Absolute ret count	15	50–150 10^9/L
ESR	56	0–20 mm 1st h Westergren

16.1 Questions

Q1. Interpret the CBC result given above and suggest investigations for further evaluation in such case.

Answer: The CBC result shows decreased WBC count with markedly decreased neutrophils and lymphocytes. No eosinophils or basophils are counted. RBC count is low with decreased hemoglobin level and hematocrit and borderline high value for RDW. Platelet count is markedly reduced. ESR value is high. Reticulocyte percentage and absolute values are markedly decreased.

So, there is pancytopenia with reticulocytopenia.

Some of the possible causes of pancytopenia with low reticulocyte count include:

1. Pathologies involving bone marrow such as aplastic anemia, myelodysplastic syndrome, myelofibrosis, leukemia, lymphoma, storage disorders, and metastasis.
2. Infections (especially hepatitis A/B/C, HIV, EBV, parvovirus, and CMV infections).
3. Toxic substances, chemotherapy, and radiotherapy.
4. Nutritional deficiencies (vitamin B12, folate, copper, zinc, etc.).
5. Chronic renal failure, chronic liver disease, and endocrine disorders.
6. Immunological disorders.
7. Rarely inherited bone marrow failure syndromes also present in adult life.
8. PNH is a rare cause.
9. Idiopathic aplastic anemia is a diagnosis by exclusion [1–3].

Next best investigation will be examination of blood film. Baseline tests for renal, hepatic, pancreatic, and thyroid functions are recommended. In addition to viral screening, direct antiglobulin test (DAT) and immunology screen should also be done. Levels of serum B12, folic acid, ferritin, copper, and zinc should be estimated. A bone marrow examination for assessment of cellularity and flowcytometric analysis of peripheral blood for CD55 and CD59 is important to ascertain diagnostic possibilities. However, as BM examination is invasive procedure, it can be considered at later stages based on blood film findings.

Q2. Given are image of blood film (Fig. 16.1), renal, hepatic, pancreatic, and thyroid functions (Table 16.2); serum B12/, folic acid, copper, zinc, and ferritin levels (Table 16.3); virology screen(Table 16.4); DAT, immunology screening (Table 16.5); and urine routine examination (Table 16.6). Interpret these results and suggest provisional diagnosis. What further tests should be done for confirmation of final diagnosis?

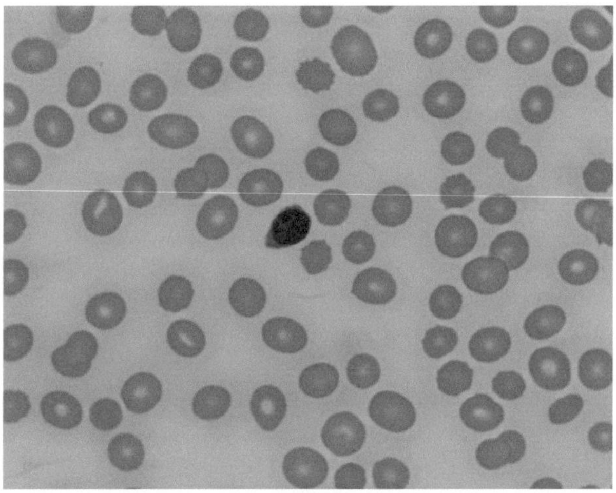

Fig. 16.1 PBF. Normocytic Normochromic red cells. Leishman stain ×100

Table 16.2 Biochemical tests

Test	Patient's result	Ref range
Glu	5.1	3.9–6.1 mmol/L
Urea	5.0	2.5–6.6 mmol/L
Creat	100	60–120 μmol/L
Na^+	141	136–146 mmol/L
K^+	4.4	3.7–5.0 mmol/L
Ca^+	2.4	2.2–2.6 mmol/L
Mg^+	1.0	0.08–1.1 mmol/L
T. Prot	70	63–80 mmol/L
Alb	42	35–47 mmol/L
Choles	3.5	1.5–5.2 mmol/L
TG	0.9	0.4–1.7 mmol/L
Urates	295	150–400 mmol/L
T Bil	15	3–20 μmol/L
D. Bil	2	0–5 μmol/L
Alk Ph	60	26–88 IU/L
ALT	66	10–60 IU/L
AST	40	10–42 IU/L
GGT	55	7–64 IU/L
LDH	140	90–180 IU/L
Hapto	1.6	0.2–2.0 g/L
T4	10.6	7.8–16 pmol/L
TSH	3.99	0.27–4.2 μlU/mL
Amylase	20	28–100 IU/L
Lipase	30	0–160 U/L

Table 16.3 Biochemical tests for iron, vitamins, and trace elements

Lab test	Patient's result	Reference range
Ferritin	80	24–336
Serum B12	250	50–700 pmol/L
Serum folic acid	30	10–42 nmol/L
Red cell folate	1500	1187–2854 nmol/L
Serum copper	80	60–140 mcg/dL
Serum zinc	110	70–180 μg/100 mL

Table 16.4 Serological tests for viruses

Test name	Result	Ref range
CMV-DNA	Not detected by real-time PCR	Non-reactive
CMV-IgG	Reactive	Non-reactive
CMV-IgM	Non-reactive	Non-reactive
EBV-DNA	Not detected by real-time PCR	Non-reactive
EBV-IgG	Reactive	Non-reactive
EBV-IgM	Non-reactive	Non-reactive
HBs Ag	Non-reactive	Non-reactive
HCV-Ab	Reactive	Non-reactive
HCV-Ag	Not detected	Non-reactive
HIV Ag/Ab	Non-reactive	Non-reactive
Parvovirus B19 IgG	Non-reactive	Non-reactive
Parvovirus B19 IgM	Non-reactive	Non-reactive

Table 16.5 Immunological tests

Test	Patient's result	Ref range
Direct antiglobulin test	Negative	Negative
Anti ds-DNA antibody	Negative	Negative
ANA	Negative	Negative
ANCA	Negative	Negative
Anti-LKM antibodies	Neg	Negative
Antimitochondrial antibodies	Neg	Negative
Anti-CCP antibodies	Neg	Negative
Rh-factor	Negative	Negative
Rh titer	10	0–20 IU/mL
CRP	10	0–10 mg/L
C3	0.899 g/L	0.83–1.77 g/L
C4	0.46 g/L	0.20–0.8 g/L
IgG	16	6–16 g/L
IgM	1.8	0.5–2.0 g/L
IgA	3	0.8–4.0 g/L

Table 16.6 Urine routine examination

Urine examination	Patient's result	Reference range
SG	1.021	1.005–1.030
Ph	6.1	5–7
Leu	Neg	Neg
Nit	Neg	Neg
Pro	Neg	Neg
Glu	Neg	Neg
Ket	Neg	Neg
Uro	Neg	Neg
Bil	Neg	Neg
Hemosiderin	Neg	Neg
Hemoglobin	Neg	Neg

Answer: The blood film shows low density of red cells, reduced leukocytes, and decreased platelets. Leukocytes are morphologically normal. No immature cells are seen. The red cells are normocytic normochromic. No tear drop cells, nucleated cells, or any other abnormality of red cells are noted. There is no polychromasia. The renal, hepatic, pancreatic, and thyroid functions are within normal limits. Serum B12, folic acid, copper and zinc levels are also normal. DAT and immunology profiles are negative. Virology screen does not show any evidence of active viral infection. The result of urine examination is normal.

These investigations exclude systemic diseases, immunological, viral, and nutritional causes of pancytopenia. Most likely cause of pancytopenia in this case is bone marrow pathology for which bone marrow biopsy is important.

Q3. Given are images from bone marrow aspirate and biopsy (Figs. 16.2, 16.3 and 16.4, 16.5), result of flowcytometry performed on peripheral blood (Table 16.7) and cytogenetics on bone marrow aspirate sample are provided. Interpret the findings and suggest final diagnosis.

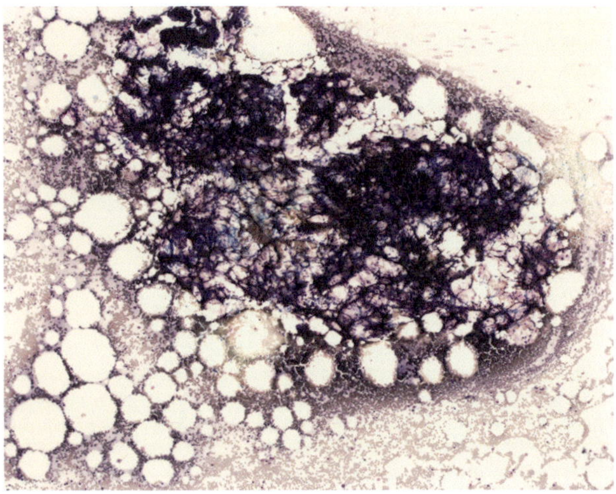

Fig. 16.2 BM aspirate. Hypocellular marrow. Leishman stain × 40

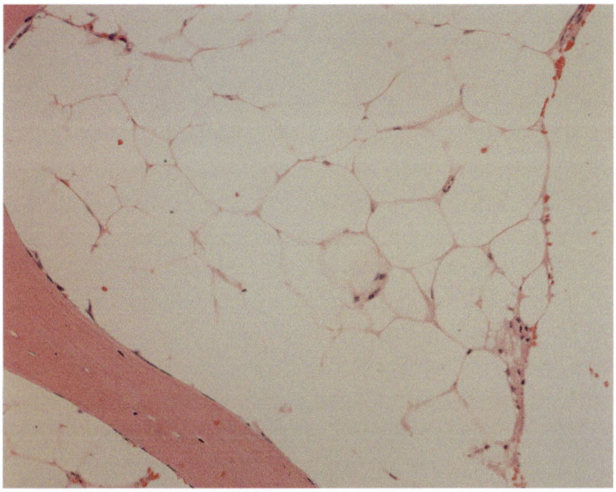

Fig. 16.3 BM trephine biopsy. Hypocellular marrow. H/E stain × 40

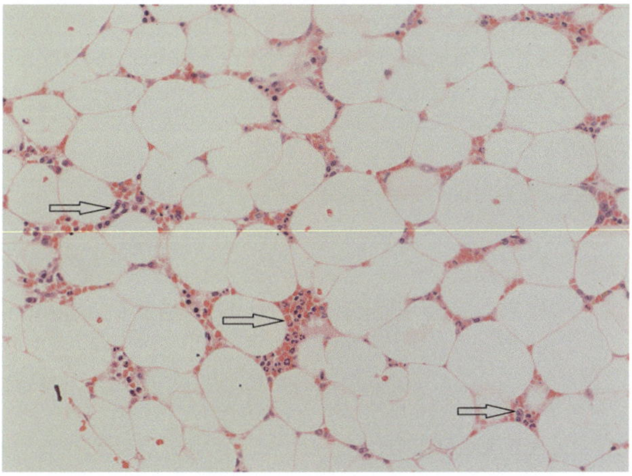

Fig. 16.4 BM trephine biopsy. Hypocellular marrow with few tiny collections of residual cells (arrows) H/E stain × 40

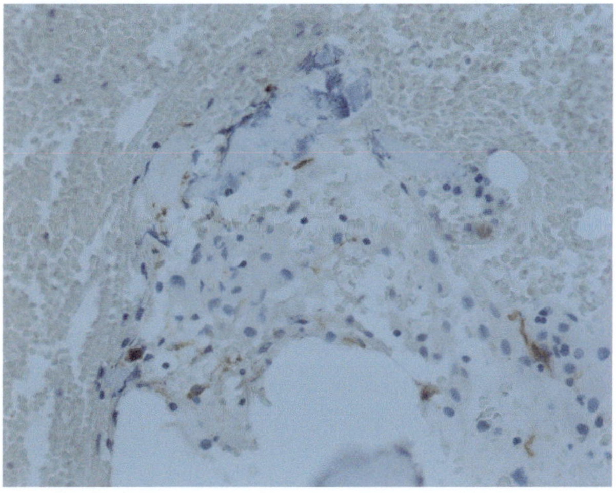

Fig. 16.5 BM trephine biopsy. No collections of immature cells. CD34 Immunohistochemical stain × 40

Table 16.7 Flowcytometric analysis of red cell and granulocyte anchoring proteins on peripheral blood

Cell type	Anchoring protein	Deficiency%
Red cells	CD55 and CD59	00% deficient
Neutrophils	CD24	00% deficient

Answer: The bone marrow aspirate and sections of the trephine biopsy show markedly hypocellular marrow for age with overall cellularity of less than 10%. All three cell lines are markedly reduced. All spaces are replaced by fat. Only few areas with tiny collections of residual cells are seen, which consist of few granulocytes, plasma cells, lymphocytes, and erythroid precursors. No immature cell collections, evidence of fibrosis, metastatic pathology, or dysplastic features are seen. Immunostain does not show any CD34+ cells. The flow cytometric analysis of the sample did not show any evidence of PNH as no deficiency of CD55, CD59, or CD24 is detected. Also, no cytogenetic abnormality was detected.

All these results exclude diagnosis of myelodysplastic syndrome (hypoplastic), myelofibrosis, leukemia, metastasis, or any other specific pathology in this case. So, a final diagnosis of idiopathic severe aplastic anemia is suggested.
Cytogenetic Analysis : Normal karyotype. No cytogenetic abnormality detected.

Q4. What additional investigations may be considered in patients of aplastic anemia during course of disease?

Answer:

1. HLA typing: Determine HLA profile in case the patient has to undergo bone marrow transplantation.
2. Myeloid malignancy gene sequencing /next-generation sequencing from peripheral blood or bone marrow: to confirm in case of suspected hypocellular MDS [4].
3. MicroRNAs: Three microRNAs have a disease monitoring role in acquired aplastic anemia and could be used in diagnosis. These are miR-150-5p, miR-146b-5p, and miR-1. Plasma levels of miR-150-5p and miR-146b-5p are elevated in aplastic anemia, whereas levels of miR-1 are decreased. Authors propose that miR-150-5p could be used for disease monitoring [5].Next-generation sequencing (NGS) may help differentiate aplastic anemia from MDS and also identify a subset of patients with a susceptibility for future progression to MDS/AML [6].

4. In young patients (under 40 years) suspected to have inherited bone marrow failure syndrome or those in whom BMT is to be done, the following tests are also considered: [7].

   (a) Chromosome breakage (if test is positive, it is consistent with a diagnosis of Fanconi anemia)).
   (b) Lymphocyte telomere length measurement from peripheral blood .
   (c) Inherited BMF gene panel sequencing.
   (d) Erythrocyte adenosine deaminase (Diamond -Blackfan Anemia).
   (e) Serum pancreatic isoamylase (Shwachman-Diamond syndrome-SDS).
   (f) Fecal elastase (SDS).
   (g) Immunoglobulins IgA, IgG, and IgM quantification.

   Some patients may require radiological investigations to assess organomegaly under appropriate clinical setup.

Q5. What are the important points in history?

Answer: A family history, nutritional habits, occupation, drug intake, exposure to toxins, chemicals, ionizing radiation, pregnancy, autoimmune disorders, and drug abuse should be taken as part of exploration for cause of aplastic anemia. Past history of receiving transfusion/ graft is also important.

In addition, duration of symptoms of anemia, recurrent infections, bleeding episodes, weight loss, etc. are important. Also, family history of cancers or long standing pancytopenia (especially if patient is under 40 years) should be taken.

Q6. What is the criteria for diagnosis of AA?

Answer: Criteria most followed for diagnosis of AA is tabulated [3, 7–9] (Table 16.8).

Table 16.8 Criteria for diagnosis of aplastic anemia

	Classification		
	Severe	Very severe	Non severe
Criteria	BM cellularity <25% and two or > of the following:	Same as severe except neutrophil count must be $<0.2 \times 10^9/L$	Hypocellular marrow not meeting the criteria for severe AA
	(a) Peripheral blood neutrophils $<0.5 \times 10^9/L$		
	(b) Peripheral blood platelets $<20 \times 10^9/L$		
	(c) Peripheral blood reticulocytes $<20 \times 10^9/L$		

Q7. What are the situations where pancytopenia is accompanied with hypercellular marrow?

Answer: Among various causes are nutritional deficiencies like B12/ folic acid, copper deficiency, MDS, PNH, hypersplenism, leukemia, lymphoma, metastasis, histiocytic disorders, storage disorders, and rarely viral diseases [2].

Q8. What is the pathogenesis of aplastic anemia?

Answer: [10–15].

The cause of aplastic anemia is usually multifactorial. There is intrinsic defect in hemopoietic cells and effect of external injury to these cells or defective stroma responsible for normal proliferation and function of hematopoietic cells.

1. In majority of the cases, defect in stem cell is the central mechanism for aplastic anemia. The stem cells and early progenitors cells are CD 34+. Their number is markedly reduced due to Fas-mediated apoptosis.
2. Hematopoiesis is suppressed due to increased number of CD8+ HLA-DR+ and cytotoxic T lymphocytes (CTLs). These cells produce inhibitory cytokines, such as gamma-interferon and tumor necrosis factor, which can suppress progenitor cell growth. In addition, these cytokines induce nitric oxide production by marrow cells, which results in immune-mediated cytotoxicity. Another mechanism by which these cytokines suppress hematopoiesis is by affecting the mitotic cycle.
3. The progenitor cells exhibit functional loss and become unresponsive to the effect of hemopoietic growth cells factors.
4. The transcription factors FOXP3 and NFAT1 have key roles in regulatory T-cell (also abbreviated as Treg) development and function. Tregs play an important role in autoimmunity. They are decreased at presentation in almost all patients with aplastic anemia.
5. Variations in telomere length in peripheral blood cells (neutrophils) have been reported in severe aplastic anemia, and it has been associated with the risk of relapse, clonal evolution, and overall survival in patients with severe aplastic anemia.

16.2 Correlation of Results of Preliminary Investigations with Symptoms and Signs in Aplastic Anemia

Q9. How do symptoms and signs in this patients correlate with the diagnosis of aplastic anemia?

Answer: This lady presented with history of pruritic spots on thighs and legs and epistaxis indicating thrombocytopenia. She had experienced progressive weakness with dyspnea on exertion and physical examination revealed pallor which suggested anemia. She also had history of upper respiratory tract infections, which indicated possibility of leukopenia. All these findings suggest pancytopenia in this patient which correlates with diagnosis of aplastic anemia.

Q10. How do CBC, blood film, and biochemical tests correlate and guide in evaluation of this case? what was the confirmatory test?

Answer: The CBC showed pancytopenia with reticulocytopenia. The blood film did not show any specific cause of pancytopenia. The biochemical tests were also normal. No specific cause of pancytopenia could be reached by all relevant investigations done in this case. The bone marrow was markedly hypocellular. Its cellularity is less than 10%. The platelet count is less than 20×10^9/L and reticulocyte count less than 20×10^9/L. All these features correlate with the diagnosis of idiopathic severe aplastic anemia.. This is a diagnosis by exclusion.

Q11. This patient may require long-term transfusion support in future. What lab investigations may be required in follow-up and what complications can occur in such patients?

Answer: Complete RBC phenotypic assessment, a hepatitis screen, and human leukocyte antigen (HLA) typing are recommended before initiation of blood transfusion therapy. Patients on regular blood products may develop alloantibodies and also refractoriness to platelet transfusion. Other complications inherent to long-term transfusion such as hepatitis, etc. may be kept in consideration.

16.3 Quick Information for Practicing Clinicians and Students

References [1–15]:

1. Most important initial tests in a patient with pancytopenia are reticulocyte count and examination of blood film. So do it quickly. Reticulocyte counting will differentiate if the cause of pancytopenia is peripheral (high reticulocyte count with reactive hypercellular bone marrow) or bone marrow (low reticulocytes count with suppression with or without replacement of normal hemopoietic cells).
2. Review finer details in history especially family history, skeletal abnormalities, repeated infections, symptoms, and signs suggestive of autoimmune disorders, nutritional history, exposure to chemicals, radiations and toxins, etc.
3. Confirm absence of splenomegaly by either manual examination or radiological tests.
4. In patients above 40 years age, preliminary tests for B12/folic acid, systemic diseases, autoimmune disorders are ordered if active infection is excluded.
5. In patients less than 40 years, inherited bone marrow failure syndromes must be excluded.
6. In febrile patient, viral screen should be requested. Blood and urine cultures should be considered provided the patient has not been started on antibiotics.
7. HLA typing is done to determine HLA profile in case the patient is considered for bone marrow transplantation in future.
8. In cases suspected to have hypocellular MDS, myeloid malignancy gene sequencing from peripheral blood or bone marrow should be done.
9. In young patients (under 40 years) suspected to have inherited bone marrow failure syndrome or those in whom BMT is to be done, the following tests should be considered:

    (a) Chromosome breakage.
    (b) Lymphocyte telomere length measurement.

(c) Inherited BMF gene panel sequencing.
(d) Erythrocyte adenosine deaminase.
(e) Serum pancreatic isoamylase.
(f) Fecal elastase.
(g) Immunoglobulins IgA, IgG, and IgM quantification.

10. Remember, diagnosis of idiopathic aplastic anemia is by exclusion of other causes.

To acquire further knowledge on the subject, following sources are advised:

1. BCSH guidelines
2. Br Jr. Hematology
3. ASH education book
4. Blood
5. NEJM
6. Int Jr. Lab Hematology

References

1. Bennett JM, Orazi A. Diagnostic criteria to distinguish hypocellular acute myeloid leukemia from hypocellular myelodysplastic syndromes and aplastic anemia: recommendations for a standardized approach. Haematologica. 2009;94:264–8.
2. Elizabeth PW, Daniel AA. The differential diagnosis and bone marrow evaluation of new-onset pancytopenia. Am J Clin Pathol. 2013;139:9–29.
3. Killick SB, Bown N, Jamie CJ. Guidelines for the diagnosis and management of adult aplastic anaemia. Br J Haematol. 2016;172:187–207.
4. Yoshizato T, Dumitriu B, Hosokawa K, et al. Somatic mutations and clonal hematopoiesis in aplastic anemia. N Engl J Med. 2015;373(1):35–47.
5. Hosokawa K, Kajigaya S, Feng X. A plasma microRNA signature as a biomarker for acquired aplastic anemia. Haematologica. 2017;102(1):69–78.
6. Boddu PC, Kadia TM. Molecular pathogenesis of acquired aplastic anemia. Eur J Haematol. 2019;102(2):103–10. https://doi.org/10.1111/ejh.13182.
7. DeZern AE, Churpek JE. Approach to the diagnosis of aplastic anemia. Blood Adv. 2021;5(12):2660–71.
8. Camitta BM, Rappeport JM, ParkmanR NDG. Selection of patients for bone marrow transplantation in severe aplastic anemia. Blood. 1975;45:355–63.
9. Bacigalupo A, Hows J, Gluckman E, Nissen C, et al. Bone marrow transplantation (BMT) versus immunosuppression for the treatment of severe aplastic anaemia (SAA): a report of the EBMT SAA working party. Br J Haematol. 1988;70:177–82.
10. Ogawa S. Clonal hematopoiesis in acquired aplastic anemia. Blood. 2016;128(3):337–47.
11. Wu L, Mo W, Zhang Y, et al. Impairment of hematopoietic stem cell niches in patients with aplastic anemia. Int J Hematol. 2015;102:645–53. https://doi.org/10.1007/s12185-015-1881-2.
12. Young NS, Calado RT, Scheinberg P. Current concepts in the pathophysiology and treatment of aplastic anemia. Blood. 2006;108:2509–19.
13. Dufour C, Ferretti E, Bagnasco F, et al. Changes in cytokine profile pre- and post-immunosuppression in acquired aplastic anemia. Haematologica. 2009;94:1743–7.
14. Zaimoku Y, Takamatsu H, Hosomichi K, et al. Identification of an HLA class I allele closely involved in the autoantigen presentation in acquired aplastic anemia. Blood. 2017;129:2908–16.
15. Brummendorf TH, Maciejewski JP, Mak J, et al. Telomere length in leukocyte subpopulations of patients with aplastic anemia. Blood. 2001;97:895–900.

Chapter 17
Pure Red Cell Aplasia

A 10-year-old boy presented with history of progressive weakness of 1 week duration. Two weeks ago, he had high grade fever, runny nose, headache, and diarrhea. It was associated with rash on face, arms, and thighs. A local medical practitioner had given him antibiotics for 5 days. Fever had subsided but it was followed by appearance of slapped cheek type rash on face. There was no other significant history in the past, social life, or in family. Examination revealed pallor without jaundice. Rash was observed on both cheeks and thighs. Few tiny upper cervical lymph nodes were palpated. There was no hepato- or splenomegaly. Chest examination was unremarkable. Result of CBC done in this case (Table 17.1) is presented.

A. Gupta, *Decision Making Through Problem Based Learning in Hematology*, https://doi.org/10.1007/978-981-99-8933-1_17

Table 17.1 CBC

CBC parameter	Patient's result	Reference range
WBC	8	3.7–10 × 10^9/L
RBC	1.48	4.5–5.4 × 10^{12}/L
HB	60	130–160 g/L
Hct	0.18	0.33–0.43 L/L
MCV	93	83–101 fL
MCH	30	27–32 pg
MCHC	320	315–345 g/L
RDW	13.2	11.6–14.6%
PLT	190	130–430 × 10^9/L
MPV	10	7–11 fL
Poly#	5	1.7–6 × 10^9/L
Lymp#	2.4	1–3 × 10^9/L
Mono#	0.4	0.2–1.0 × 10^9/L
EO#	02	0.02–0.5 × 10^9/L
BASO#	00	0.02–0.1 × 10^9/L
RETIC%	0.02	0.5–1.5%
Absolute ret count	22	50–150 10^9/L
ESR	60	0–20 mm 1st h Westergren

17.1 Questions

Q1. Interpret the CBC result given above and suggest investigations for further evaluation in such case

Answer: The CBC result shows normal values for total WBC with normal differential count. RBC count is low with decreased hemoglobin level and hematocrit. MCV, MCH, and MCHC are within normal range. RDW and platelet count are also normal. ESR value is high. Reticulocyte percentage and absolute values are markedly decreased.

So, there is normocytic normochromic anemia with reticulocytopenia. Causes of anemia with decreased reticulocyte count include:

1. Nutritional deficiencies like combined deficiency iron and B12/folic acid.
2. ACD- (inflammation and systemic disorders).
3. Most cases of aplastic anemia.

4. Infiltrative and fibrotic disorders of bone marrow, including leukemia, lymphoma, and solid tumors.
5. MDS.
6. Autoimmune disorders.
7. Viral and bacterial infections, drugs.
8. Acute bleeding episode.
9. Pure red cell aplasia (PRCA).

Next best investigation will be examination of blood film. Tests for renal, hepatic, pancreatic, and thyroid functions are recommended. In addition, serum iron profile, B12/folic acid levels, CRP, viral screening, direct antiglobulin test (DAT) and immunology screen should also be done. Bone marrow examination and radiological tests for organomegaly can be considered at later stage. Stool examination for occult blood and urine examination for hematuria are optional tests at this stage which form a part of panel of tests for any case of anemia.

Q2. Given are image of blood film (Fig. 17.1); renal, hepatic, pancreatic, and thyroid functions (Table 17.2); CRP, serum iron profile, and B12/folic acid levels(Table 17.3); virology screen (Table 17.4); DAT and immunology screening (Table 17.5). Interpret these results and suggest possible provisional diagnosis. What further tests should be done to confirm final diagnosis?

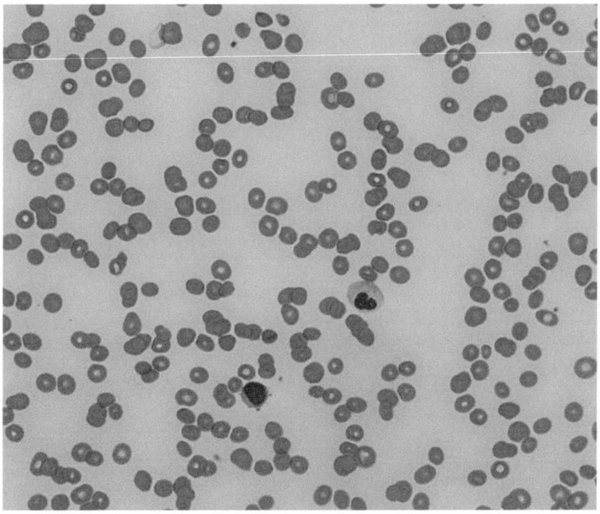

Fig. 17.1 PBF. Low density of normocytic normochromic red cells. Leishman stain × 100

Table 17.2 Biochemical tests

Test	Patient's result	Ref range
Glu	5.6	3.9–6.1 mmol/L
Urea	5.1	2.5–6.6 mmol/L
Creat	99	60–120 μmol/L
Na^+	140	136–146 mmol/L
K^+	4.6	3.7–5.0 mmol/L
Ca^+	2.3	2.2–2.6 mmol/L
Mg^+	1.0	0.08–1.1 mmol/L
T. Prot	72	63–80 mmol/L
Alb	40	35–47 mmol/L
Choles	3.4	1.5–5.2 mmol/L
TG	0.9	0.4–1.7 mmol/L
Urates	350	150–400 mmol/L
T Bil	15	3–20 μmol/L
D. Bil	3	0–5 μmol/L
Alk Ph	63	26–88 IU/L
ALT	64	10–60 IU/L
AST	40	10–42 IU/L
GGT	50	7–64 IU/L
LDH	142	90–180 IU/L
Hapto	1.6	0.2–2.0 g/L
T4	10.6	7.8–16 pmol/L
TSH	3.99	0.27–4.2 μlU/mL
Amylase	20	28–100 IU/L
Lipase	30	0–160 U/L

Table 17.3 Serum iron profile, B12/folic acid, and CRP

Test	Patient's result	Ref range
S. Iron	16	11–31 μmol/L
Transferrin	0.7	2.1–3.6 g/L
Trans. Sat%	55.8	20–40%
Ferritin	521	11–307 ng/mL
S. B12	565	150–700 pmol/L
S. Folate	31.7	10–42 nmol/L
RBC folate	2554	1187–2854 nmol/L
CRP	79.5	0–10 mg/L

Table 17.4 Viral serology

Test	Result	Ref range
CMV-DNA	Not detected by real-time PCR	Non-reactive
CMV-IgG	Reactive	Non-reactive
CMV-IgM	Non-reactive	Non-reactive
EBV-DNA	Not detected by real time PCR	Non-reactive
EBV-IgG	Reactive	Non-reactive
EBV-IgM	Non-reactive	Non-reactive
HBs Ag	Non-reactive	Non-reactive
HCV-Ab	Reactive	Non-reactive
HCV-Ag	Not detected	Non-reactive
HIV Ag/Ab	Non-reactive	Non-reactive
Parvovirus B19 IgG	Reactive	Non-reactive
Parvovirus B19 IgM	Reactive	Non-reactive

Table 17.5 DAT and immunology profile

Test	Patient's result	Ref range
Direct antiglobulin test	Negative	Negative
Anti ds-DNA antibody	Negative	Negative
ANA	Negative	Negative
ANCA	Negative	Negative
Anti-LKM antibodies	Neg	Negative
Anti-mitochondrial antibodies	Neg	Negative
Anti-CCP antibodies	Neg	Negative
Rh- factor	Negative	Negative
Rh titer	10	0–20 IU/mL
CRP	10	0–10 mg/L
C3	0.899 g/L	0.83–1.77 g/L
C4	0.46 g/L	0.20–0.8 g/L
IgG	16	6–16 g/L
IgM	1.8	0.5–2.0 g/L
IgA	3	0.8–4.0 g/L

Answer: The blood film shows low density of red cells which are normocytic normochromic. No polychromatic cells are seen. The leukocytes and platelets are normal. No tear drop cells, nucleated cells, or any other abnormality of red cells is noted. No immature white cells are seen. The renal, hepatic, pancreatic, and thyroid functions are within normal limits. The iron profile, levels of serum B12, folic acid, and CRP are also normal. DAT and immunology profiles are negative. These investigations exclude systemic and immunological diseases, MDS, autoimmune disorders, and nutritional causes of anemia. Virology screen shows positive test result for parvovirus B19 IgG and IgM antibodies.

For confirmation, the test of choice is polymerase chain reaction on peripheral blood for parvovirus B19 antigen and a bone marrow examination which can support diagnosis and also used to exclude any other pathology associated with anemia under such situations.

Q3. Given are result of PCR for parvovirus B19 antigen and images from bone marrow biopsy (Figs. 17.2, 17.3, 17.4, and 17.5) Interpret the findings and suggest final diagnosis in this case.

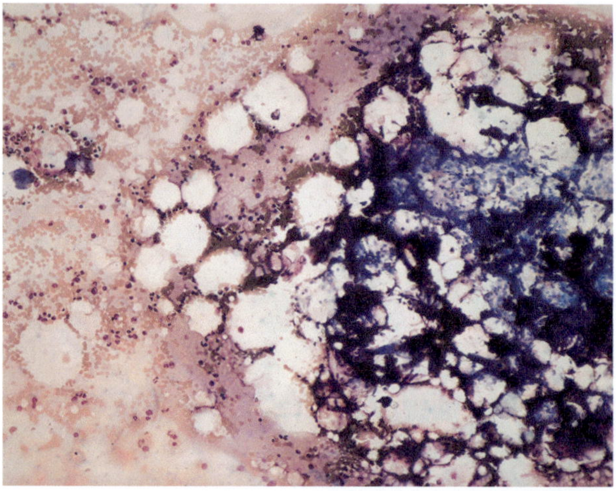

Fig. 17.2 BM aspirate. Hypocellular marrow. Leishman stain x 40

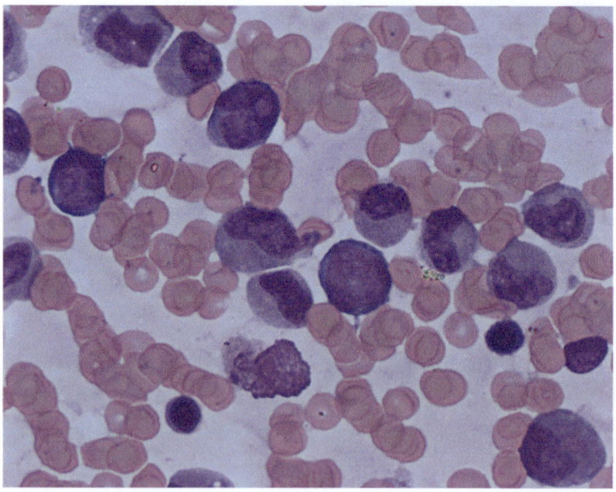

Fig. 17.3 BM aspirate. Markedly reduced erythroid precursors. Only granulocytic cells and few mature lymphocytes are seen. Leishman stain × 40

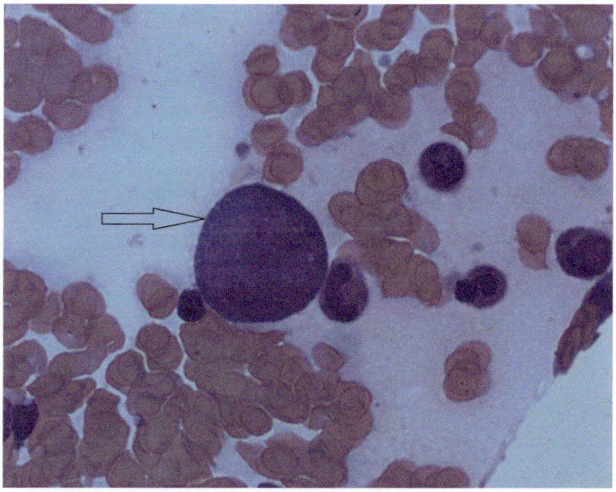

Fig. 17.4 BM aspirate. Giant pro-erythroblast with deeply blue cytoplasm. Leishman stain × 100

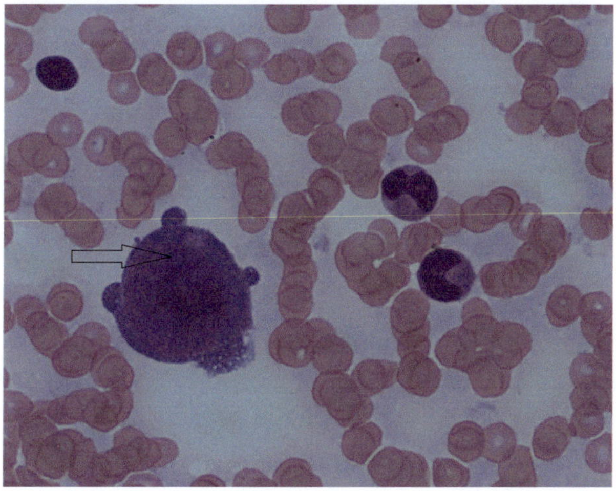

Fig. 17.5 BM aspirate. Giant pro-erythoblast with cytoplasmic blebs and vacoulations, frequently seen in parvovirus B19 infection. An intranuclear inclusion is also seen (arrow). Leishman stain × 100

Parvovirus DNA by PCR	Positive

Cytogenetic analysis on bone marrow aspirate: No cytogenetic abnormality was detected.

Answer: The bone marrow aspiration smears show a hypocellular marrow. The cellular part of trails show normal granulocytic precursors with sufficient maturation. Normal megakaryocytes were seen. However, there was marked decrease in number of erythroid precursors (erythroblastopenia). Few proerythroblasts were seen, some of which were giant in size. A conspicuous observation was blebbing, fine vacuolation, and intranuclear inclusions in erythroblasts, these changes are consistent with parvovirus B19 infection. There was no evidence of dysplastic features in granulocytic cell lines, immature cell collection, evidence of fibrosis, or metastatic pathology.

The PCR showed parvovirus B19 DNA in serum. This finding along with bone marrow changes is confirmatory for diagnosis of pure red cell aplasia due to parvovirus B19 infection in this patient.

So a final diagnosis of pure red cell aplasia secondary to parvovirus infection is established.

Q4. What is the criteria for diagnosis of PRCA?

Answer: By definition, the criteria for pure red cell aplasia (PRCA) is presence of a normocytic normochromic anemia associated with severe reticulocytopenia and absence or marked reduction of erythroid precursors (erythroblastopenia) in bone marrow [1, 2].

Q5. How is PRCA classified?

Answer: PRCA is usually classified as below: [3].

1. Congenital PRCA: DBA (congenital form of PRCA).
2. Acquired PRCA: It is further categorized into:

   (a) Primary;

   - Primary autoimmune and Transient erythroblastopenia of childhood.
   - Primary MDS.

   (b) Secondary associated with:

   - Autoimmune and collagen vascular disorders.
   - Lymphoproliferative disorders including multiple myeloma.
   - Myeloproliferative disorders.
   - Solid tumors like thymoma, thyroid, breast, and renal cell carcinoma.
   - Viral and bacterial infections.
   - Drugs including erythropoietin.
   - Pregnancy.
   - Riboflavin deficiency.

Q6. What additional investigations may be considered in patients of PRCA during course of disease?

Answer: Those cases where definite cause is not clear, additional investigations may be requested based on appropriate clinical setting. In all cases with cytopenia, a search for abnormal cytogenetics and clonal T cell receptor should be considered. Characteristic bone marrow changes of PRCA with abnormal cytogenetics may indicate myelodysplastic variant of PRCA. Similarly, BM changes consistent with PRCA with increased lymphocytes and plasma cells should be further analyzed for polyclonal nature of these cells to diagnose acquired immune PRCA. If monoclonal lymphocytes are noted, TCR gene rearrangement is mandatory to exclude lymphoproliferative disorders [4].

In adult patients, if there is no evidence of infection or cause of secondary PRCA, thymoma needs to be excluded by appropriate radiological tests [5].

It is difficult to differentiate inherited PRCA from acquired PRCA if the patient is young. Under such situation, a thorough history, including family history, physical examination, and bone marrow evaluation, helps in establishing a diagnosis.

Q7. What are the important things in history and physical examination?

Answer: History of recent infection, symptoms suggestive of autoimmune disorders, known malignancy, and history of drug intake are important points in history. Skin exam is necessary to look for erythema infectiosum, which correlates with parvovirus B19 [6].

In Diamond-Blackfan syndrome, physical anomalies should be looked for. Craniofacial dysmorphism and thumb abnormalities are classic in DBA. In addition to this, short stature, web neck, skeletal, and cardiac defects can also be seen in such patients [7].

Q8. What is the pathogenesis of PRCA?

Answer: Patients with inherited hematological disorders such as thalassemia, sickle cell anemia, and hereditary spherocytosis are more prone to parvovirus B19 induced transient aplastic crisis. IgM antibodies and antibody-virus immune complex are responsible for arthritis, arthralgia, and slapped cheek appearance seen mostly in children [8].

1. *Congenital PRCA (DBA)-* seen as autosomal dominant/ sporadic: Mechanism—defective ribosomal gene cannot mount an antibody response against the parvovirus [3, 9, 10].
2. *Acquired primary.*
   - (a) Autoimmune diseases as RA, SLE, myasthenia gravis, autoimmune hemolytic anemia, acquired hypogammaglobulinemia, autoimmune polyglandular syndrome, and thymoma: Mechanism—immune process disturbs erythroid differentiation at erythroid precursor level.
   - (b) MDS associated: Mechanism—activating point mutations in N-RAS and loss of the *RPS-14* gene (in patients with 5q deletion) lead to PRCA in patients with MDS.
   - (c) Transient erythroblastopenia of childhood: Mechanism—both IgG and T-cell mediated mechanisms appear to play a role self-limited occurring between the ages of 3 months and 4 years.
3. *Acquired Secondary PRCA.*
   - (a) Parvovirus B19 infection: Mechanism—directly infects human erythroid progenitors through the red cell surface P antigen.
   - (b) EPO associated: Mechanism—anti-Epo antibodies (seen in patients with renal failure who have received recombinant human Epo).
   - (c) LPD: Chronic lymphocytic leukemia and large granular lymphocyte leukemia: Mechanism—T-cell-mediated mechanism – suppression of erythropoiesis.
   - (d) Drug induced: Mechanism—most cases linked to IgG-mediated inhibition of erythropoiesis.
   - (e) Immunodeficiency secondary to viruses, e.g., (HIV): Mechanism—cannot mount an antibody response against the parvovirus.

Q9. Which other diseases have immune based failure of bone marrow erythropoiesis similar to PRCA?

Answer: Cause of anemia similar to PRCA is seen in patients with autoimmune diseases (Immune-mediated) like SLE, RA, myasthenia gravis, autoimmune hemolytic anemia, acquired hypogammaglobulinemia, autoimmune polyglandular syndrome, and thymoma.

17.2 Correlation of Results of Preliminary Investigations with Symptoms and Signs in Pure Red Cell Aplasia

Q10. How do symptoms and signs in this patients corelate with diagnosis?

Answer: This child had fever, runny nose, headache, diarrhea, and rash which corelate well with a viral infection. A slapped cheek type rash is highly suggestive of parvovirus infection. For the preceding 1 week, he was progressively feeling weak and tired, all of which suggest possibly decreased hemoglobin with symptoms of anemia. There are no specific signs for parvovirus infection.

Q11. How do CBC, blood film, and biochemical tests guide in evaluation of this case?

Answer: The CBC result shows low RBC count with decreased hemoglobin level and hematocrit. Reticulocyte percentage and absolute values are markedly decreased. WBC and platelet counts are normal with normal differential count. So, there is anemia with reticulocytopenia. Blood film shows evidence of anemia only. The bone marrow revealed marked erythroid hypoplasia (erythroblastopenia) and virology screen and DNA testing confirmed diagnosis of parvovirus B19 infection.

17.3 Quick Information for Practicing Clinicians and Students

References [1–11]:

1. Fever with rash, especially slapped cheek rash, in a child with anemia and reticulocytopenia should raise suspicion of parvovirus B19 infection. Blood film examination is must to exclude other causes (mentioned above) of anemia with reticulocytopenia.
2. A thorough history and general physical examination are important.
3. A viral screen and immunology profile are very helpful in reaching early diagnosis.
4. Erythroid hypoplasia in bone marrow is hallmark features of red cell aplasia. Arrest at pronormoblast stage in bone marrow is characteristic. Large proeryth-

roblasts with vacuolated cytoplasm and pseudopodia ("giant pronormoblasts") are suggestive of parvovirus B19 infection [11].
5. Patients with inherited hematological disorder (e.g., thalassemia, sickle cell anemia, hereditary spherocytes) are more prone to parvovirus-induced transient aplastic crisis.
6. Those patients who have immunodeficiency secondary to viruses like HIV, drugs especially chemotherapy, immunosuppressive drugs or have congenital immunodeficiency, cannot mount an antibody response against the parvovirus. This results in persistent infection and leads to chronic red cell aplasia.
7. Diamond-Blackfan syndrome is associated with increased activity of erythrocyte adenosine deaminase. Very few centers perform this test.
8. Transient erythroblastopenia of infancy resolves within a few weeks, but anemia may persist for months.
9. Radiological tests are required to diagnose thymoma as a cause, if other conditions are excluded.

To acquire further knowledge on the subject, following sources are advised:

1. BCSH guidelines
2. Br Jr. Hematology
3. ASH education book
4. Blood
5. NEJM
6. Int Jr. Lab Hematology

References

1. Sawada K, Fujishima N, Hirokawa M. Acquired pure red cell aplasia: updated review of treatment. Br J Haematol. 2008;142(4):505–14. https://doi.org/10.1111/j.1365-2141.2008.07216.x.
2. Fisch P, Handgretinger R, Schaefer HE. Pure red cell aplasia. Br J Haematol. 2000;111(4):1010–22.
3. Lipton J, Glader B, Means RT. Red cell aplasia: acquired and congenital disorders. In: Greer JP, Arber DA, Glader BE, List A, Means RT, Paraskevas F, Rodgers GM, editors. Wintrobe's clinical hematology. 13th ed. Philadelphia, PA: Lippincott Williams & Wilkins; 2013. p. 975–89.
4. Masuda M, Teramura M, Matsuda A, et al. Clonal T cells of pure red-cell aplasia. Am J Hematol. 2005;79(4):332–3.
5. Bernard C, Frih H, Pasquet F, et al. Thymoma associated with autoimmune diseases: 85 cases and literature review. Autoimmun Rev. 2016;15(1):82–92.
6. Lipton JM, Atsidaftos E, Zyskind I, Vlachos A. Improving clinical care and elucidating the pathophysiology of diamond Blackfan anemia: an update from the diamond Blackfan Anemia registry. Pediatr Blood Cancer. 2006;46(5):558–64.
7. Da Costa L, Willig TN, Fixler J, Mohandas N, Tchernia G. Diamond-Blackfan anemia. Curr Opin Pediatr. 2001;13(1):10–5.
8. Frickhofen N, Chen ZJ, Young NS, Cohen BJ, Heimpel H, Abkowitz JL. Parvovirus B19 as a cause of acquired chronic pure red cell aplasia. Br J Haematol. 1994;87(4):818–24.

9. Hirokawa M. RPS19 mutations in patients with diamond-Blackfan anemia. Br J Haematol. 2008;142:911–20.
10. Robert TM. Pure red cell aplasia. Blood. 2016;128(21):2504–9.
11. Au WY, Cheng VC, Wan TS, Ma SK. Myelodysplasia masquerading as parvovirus-related red cell aplasia with giant pronormoblasts. Ann Hematol. 2004;83(10):670–1.

Chapter 18
Myelofibrosis

A 40-year-old female patient presents with complaints of 2 months history of feeling tired and weak. Recently, she was feeling short of breath even after minor physical exertion. In addition, she had observed easy bruising and menorrhagia for the past 3 months. She also gave history of fever off and on, sometimes excessive sweating at night, vague bony pains, and a sense of fullness on upper left side of abdomen under the ribs. Her socio-economic status was good, and there was no significant past history of any specific illness. There was no exposure to drugs, chemicals, or radiation. Examination revealed moderate pallor. There was no jaundice. The liver was palpable 2 cm and spleen 5 cm below costal margin. No lymphadenopathy was observed.

Given is CBC result done at presentation (Table 18.1).

A. Gupta, *Decision Making Through Problem Based Learning in Hematology*,
https://doi.org/10.1007/978-981-99-8933-1_18

Table 18.1 CBC

CBC parameter	Patient's result	Reference range
WBC	16	3.7–10 × 10^9/L
RBC	3.1	4.5–5.4 × 10^{12}/L
HB	8.5	130–160 g/L
Hct	0.25	0.33–0.43 L/L
MCV	83	83–101 fL
MCH	27	27–32 pg
MCHC	320	315–345 g/L
RDW	26	11.6–14.6%
PLT	400	130–430 × 10^9/L
MPV	15	7–11 fL
Poly#	10	1.7–6 × 10^9/L
Lymp#	4.5	1–3 × 10^9/L
Mono#	1.0	0.2–1.0 × 10^9/L
EO#	05	0.02–0.5 × 10^9/L
BASO#	00	0.02–0.1 × 10^9/L
RETIC%	0.5	0.5–1.5%
Absolute ret count	50	50–150 × 10^9/L
ESR	50	0–20 mm 1st h Westergren

18.1 Questions

Q1. Interpret the CBC result and suggest further investigations in such case.

Answer: The CBC shows leukocytosis with neutrophilia. Moderate normocytic normochromic anemia with high RDW and inappropriately low reticulocyte response is present. ESR is also high. Platelet count is within normal range.

So, there is normocytic normochromic anemia with high RDW.

Normocytic normochromic anemia can be seen in the following conditions: [1, 2].

(a) *Decreased production from marrow (will have low reticulocyte count)*: Chronic pathological conditions (such as chronic inflammations, neoplastic pathologies, and infections), chronic renal failure, chronic liver disease, endocrinopathies, marrow infiltration, myelofibrosis, and hypoplastic anemias.

(b) *Increased destruction (will have increased reticulocytes with normal marrow)*:

1. Red cell defects: Defects of red cell membrane (HS HE), hemoglobin (structural hemoglobinopathies), or enzymes deficiency (G6PD, pyruvate kinase, NADPH, glutathione).
2. Without any defect of red cells (defects lies outside red cells): Autoimmune hemolytic anemia, micro-angiopathic hemolytic anemia (DIC/TTP/HUS).
3. PNH.

(c) *Sequestration: splenomegaly.*
(d) *Hemorrhage.*

The patient does not have a history of chronic inflammatory disorder or infection. She has a history of menorrhagia, and spleen is also palpable.

Next best investigations will be examination of blood film and perform tests for renal, hepatic, and pancreatic functions.

Q2. Given are images from blood film (Figs. 18.1 and 18.2) and results of tests for kidney, liver, pancreas, and thyroid functions (Table 18.2). Interpret these results and suggest a differential diagnosis. What further tests should be done to arrive at final diagnosis?

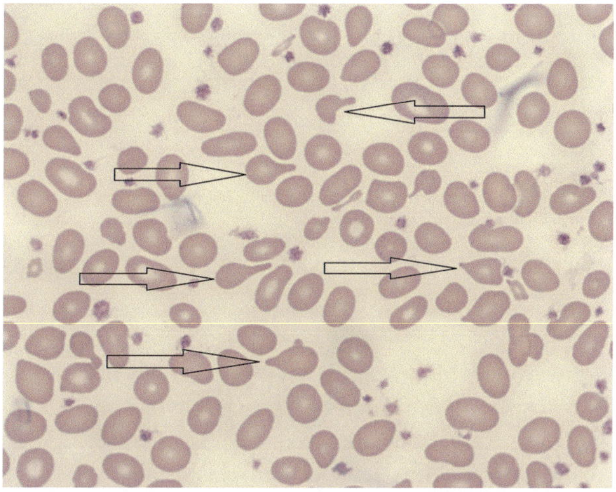

Fig. 18.1 Peripheral blood film. Anisopoikilocytosis with tear drop cells (arrows). Leishman stain × 100

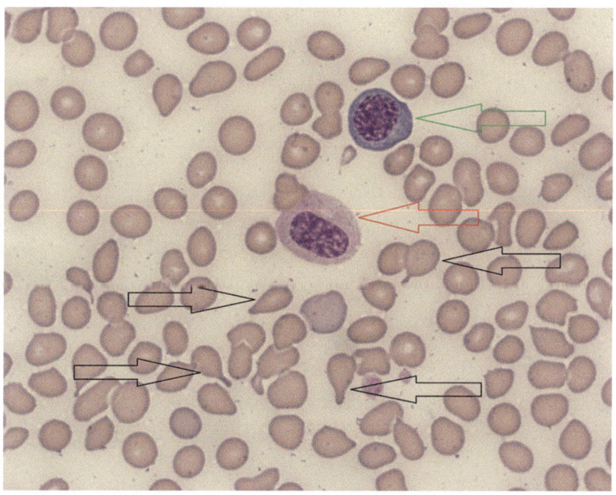

Fig. 18.2 Peripheral blood film. Anisopoikilocytosis with tear drop cells (black arrows), myelocyte (red arrow), and nucleated red cell (green arrow). Leishman stain × 100

Table 18.2 Biochemical tests

Test	Patient's result	Ref range
Glu	4.2	3.9–6.1 mmol/L
Urea	3.9	2.5–6.6 mmol/L
Creat	102	60–120 μmol/L
Na^+	139	136–146 mmol/L
K	4.5	3.7–5.0 mmol/L
Ca^+	2.3	2.2–2.6 mmol/L
Mg^+	1.0	0.08–1.1 mmol/L
T. Prot	68	63–80 mmol/L
AIb	39	35–47 mmol/L
Choles	2.5	1.5–5.2 mmol/L
TG	0.9	0.4–1.7 mmol/L
Urates	370	150–400 mmol/L
I Bil	18	3–20 μmol/L
D. Bil	5	0–5 μmol/L
I Bil	13	5–15 μmol/L
AIkPh	80	26–88 IU/L
ALT	54	10–60 IU/L
AST	32	10–42 IU/L
GGT	20	7–64 IU/L
LDH	450	90–180 IU/L
TSH	3.99	0.27–4.2 μIU/mL

Answer: The blood film shows reduced density of red cells. There is anisopoikilocytosis with few microcytes, macrocytes, ovalocyte, and many tear drop poikilocytes. Rare nucleated red cell is seen in addition to few myelocytes and metamyelocytes- leucoerythroblastic picture. The biochemical tests show high LDH. Other test results are within normal limits.

So, there is normocytic normochromic anemia with high RDW, leuko-erythroblastic picture in blood film and high LDH.

Important causes of leuko-erythroblastic picture in peripheral blood are as follows:

1. Severe infection
2. Bleeding
3. Severe cobalamin deficiency
4. Hemolytic crises
5. Bone marrow involvement with infections like tuberculosis, metastatic cancers, lymphoma, and storage disorders
6. Myeloproliferative disorders as primary MF, CML, ET, and PV.

Based on constitutional symptoms, hepatosplenomegaly, blood film findings, and high LDH, a possibility of myeloproliferative disorder is suggested.

Next best investigation will be a bone marrow biopsy.

Q3. Given are results of mutational analysis (Table 18.3) and images from bone marrow biopsy (Figs. 18.3, 18.4, 18.5, 18.6, and 18.7). Interpret the findings and suggest final diagnosis.

Table 18.3 Mutational analysis

1. JAK2 mutational analysis	POSITIVE
2. CALR and MPL mutations	Negative
3. BCR-ABL	Negative

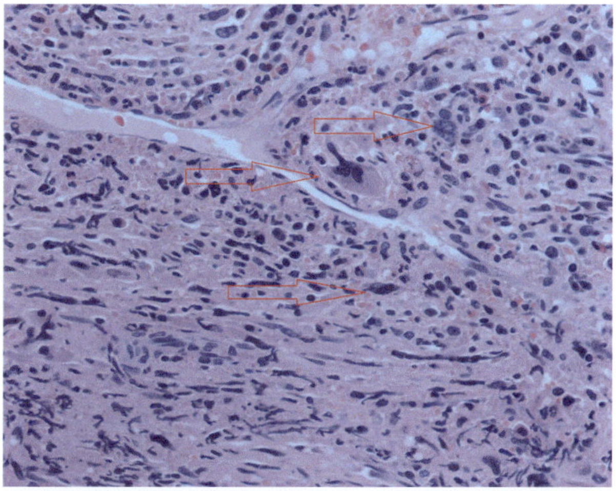

Fig. 18.3 Trephine biopsy. Myelofibrosis with variable sized megakaryocytes (arrows). H/E × 40

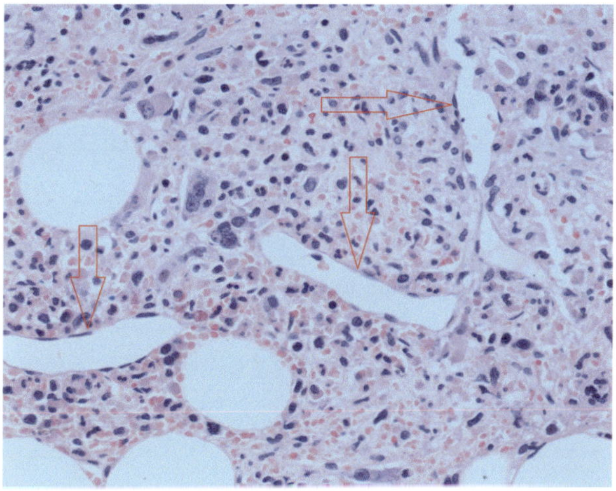

Fig. 18.4 Trephine biopsy. Myelofibrosis with few diated capillaries (arrows). H/E × 40

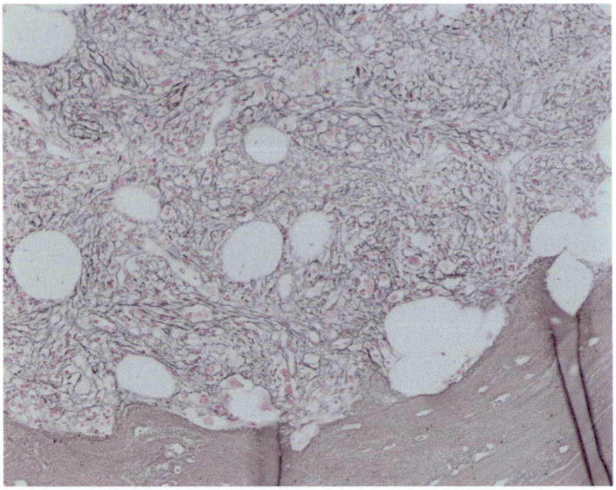

Fig. 18.5 Trephine biopsy. Grade 3 Myelofibrosis. Reticulin stain × 40

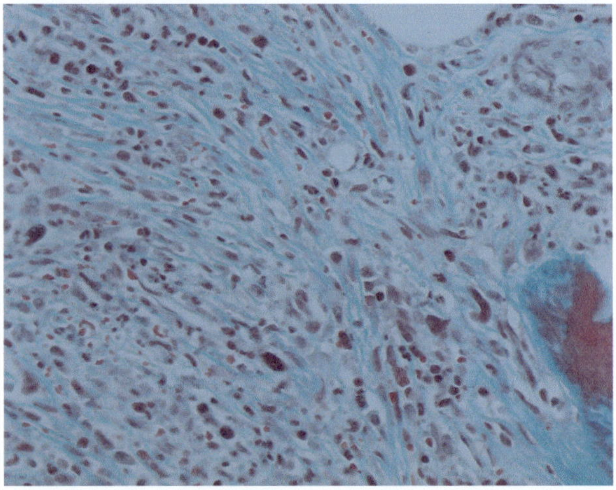

Fig. 18.6 Trephine biopsy. Mild background (bluish) collagenization. Masson's trichome stain × 40

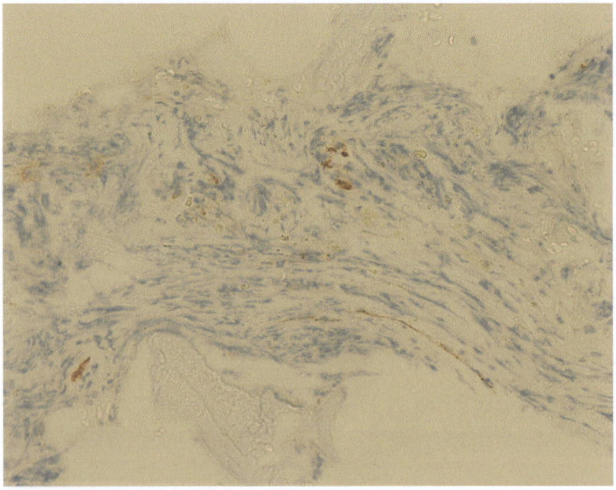

Fig. 18.7 Trephine biopsy. CD34 immunostain × 40

Answer: The trephine biopsy shows marked fibrosis of bone marrow with fibrous bands seen running in all spaces with thin strands throughout the biopsy. The normal hematopoietic cells are reduced in number. However, megakaryocytes are seen embedded in fibroblastic background. There is no evidence of tuberculosis, hematological, or non-hematological malignancy or storage disorder. The reticulin stain showed grade 3 fibrosis on a scale of 0–4 (no thick bands were seen in any space). The Masson trichome stain shows bluish background indicating formation of collagen. Negative CD34 immunostain excludes possibility of any immature cell collections. The mutational analysis shows JAK2 mutation. All these findings suggest a final diagnosis of primary myelofibrosis in this patient.

Q4. What is etiopathogenesis of primary myelofibrosis?

Answer: Primary MF results from hematopoietic stem cell defect due to abnormalities of JAK/STAT signaling pathway which causes abnormal proliferation of megakaryocytes and granulocytes. Release of inflammatory cytokines, such as transforming growth factor beta (TGF-β), platelet derived growth factor (PDGF), and fibroblast growth factor (FGF) from their alpha granules of granulocytes produces fibrosis and extramedullary hematopoiesis. Approximately 60–65% patients have JAK2 mutation while CALR and MPL mutations are seen in approximately 25% and 10% cases, respectively. Around 10% have no mutation. Based on degree of myelofibrosis, it is categorized into pre-MF and overt MF stages. Fibrosis of grade 2 or < is categorized as pre-MF while more than 2 as overt MF. For more details on diagnostic criteria and prognostic factors, refer to guidelines on primary MF [3–5].

Q5. What is the cause of anemia and hepatosplenomegaly?

Answer: Ineffective erythropoiesis and extramedullary hematopoiesis are the main causes of anemia and organomegaly. There is reduction in erythroid precursors, ineffective medullary as well as extramedullary erythropoiesis, splenic sequestration of red cells, and their destruction in spleen [6, 7].

Extramedullary hematopoiesis is seen not only in the liver and spleen but also in the lymph nodes, serosal surfaces, urogenital system, and epidural and paraspinal spaces.

Q6. What is the cause of constitutional symptoms.

Answer: Abnormal cytokine production by clonal cells causes ineffective erythropoiesis, extramedullary hematopoiesis, and constitutional symptoms [6].

Q7. Which diseases come in close differential diagnosis of primary myelofibrosis and what are the causes of secondary myelofibrosis?

Answer: Following disease should be considered in differential diagnosis of primary MF:

1. Other myeloproliferative disease: Essential thrombocythemia, polycythemia rubra vera, chronic myeloid leukemia.
2. Hairy cell leukemia.
3. Metastasis by non-hematological cancers.
4. Infections like tuberculosis and fungal infections.
5. Sarcoidosis.

18.2 Correlation of Results of Preliminary Investigations with Symptoms and Signs in Myelofibrosis

Q8. Correlate the symptoms and signs in this patient with final diagnosis.

Answer: This patient had symptoms of anemia related to low hemoglobin, an easy bruising and menorrhagia related to thrombocytopenia and constitutional symptoms (fever off and on, sometimes excessive sweating at night) which are part of disease. Vague bony pains are related to bone marrow pathology, and a sense of fullness in upper left side of abdomen under the ribs was due to splenomegaly. All these symptoms correlate well with diagnosis of myelofibrosis. High LDH is due to extramedullary hematopoiesis in these patients. Since all other causes of fibrosis in bone narrow are excluded, a diagnosis of primary myelofibrosis is confirmed.

Q9. What additional tests should be done in such patients?

Answer: Myelofibrosis can occur secondary to other myeloproliferative disorders such as ET, PV, and CML. Cytogenetic analysis and molecular studies for exclusion of these conditions must be done from bone marrow aspirate samples or peripheral blood. Detailed radiological investigations like CXR, bone scan for bony metastasis, and MRI for marrow infiltration are optional.

Rarely, non-clonal bone marrow fibrosis is seen in association with autoimmune disorders and has been designated as "autoimmune myelofibrosis. An autoimmune profile is also optional based on other clinical symptoms and signs.

Q10. What is the cause of high LDH?

Answer: Increased cell turnover due to clonal myeloproliferation, i.e., leukocytosis and extramedullary hematopoiesis in the liver result in high LDH.

Q11. What is the cause of leukoerythroblastic picture in myelofibrosis?

Answer: Myeloproliferation with increased leukocytes and megakaryocytes produces packed marrow in initial stages. When fibrosis develops, the hematopoietic cells are squeezed out of marrow. In this process, some immature cells—both granulocytic and erythroid—appear in peripheral blood. Shape abnormalities appear in red cells- tear drop poikilocytes.

Q12. What are the causes of anemia in MF?

Answer: There is reduction in erythroid precursors, ineffective medullary as well as extramedullary erythropoiesis and splenic sequestration and destruction of red blood cells.

Q13. What are prognostic factors in primary myelofibrosis?

Answer: Degree of constitutional symptoms, anemia, leukocytosis, number of immature cells especially blasts and some cytogenetic abnormalities have prognostic role in MF. PMF carries the worst prognosis among the MPNs [8, 9].

18.3 Quick Information for Practicing Clinicians and Students

References [1–10]:

1. Anemia, constitutional symptoms and huge splenomegaly should raise a suspicion of myelofibrosis.
2. Leuko-erythroblastic blood film with high serum LDH are further pointers toward this entity.
3. Bone marrow aspirate is frequently aparticulate – dry tap.
4. JAK2, CALR, and MPL mutational analysis is supportive of diagnosis of MF (seen in 90% cases) but not diagnostic as these can also be seen in evolution of myelofibrosis following PV and ET. These tests can be done on peripheral blood also.
5. Pre-MF needs to be distinguished from ET.
6. Some mutations have prognostic significance. These include *SRSF2*, *ASXL1*, and *U2AF1*-Q157. Detection of these mutations predicts inferior survival.
7. It is important to distinguish between myelofibrotic and overt fibrotic stages as treatment modalities may differ.
8. The World Health Organization (WHO) classification system(2016) distinguishes “prefibrotic” from “overtly fibrotic” PMF. The prefibrotic MF might mimic ET in its presentation.

To acquire further knowledge on the subject, following sources are advised:

1. BCSH guidelines
2. Br Jr. Hematology
3. ASH education book
4. Blood
5. NEJM
6. Int Jr. Lab Hematology

References

1. Ward PC. Investigation of nonpoikilocytic normochromic normocytic anemia. Postgrad Med. 1979;65(3):233–5, 238, 241–3
2. Ford J. Red blood cell morphology. Int J Lab Hematol. 2013;35:351–7. https://doi.org/10.1111/ijlh.12082.
3. Schmitt A, Jouault H, Guichard J, et al. Pathologic interaction between megakaryocytes and polymorphonuclear leukocytes in myelofibrosis. Blood. 2000;96:1342–7.
4. Mudireddy M, Shah S, Lasho T, et al. Prefibrotic versus overtly fibrotic primary myelofibrosis: clinical, cytogenetic, molecular and prognostic comparisons. Br J Haematol. 2017;182:594–7. https://doi.org/10.1111/bjh.14838.
5. Arber DA, Orazi A, Hasserjian R, et al. The 2016 revision to the World Health Organization classification of myeloid neoplasms and acute leukemia. Blood. 2016;127:2391–405.

6. Tefferi A. Pathogenesis of myelofibrosis with myeloid metaplasia. J Clin Oncol. 2005;23:8520–30.
7. Tefferi A. Myelofibrosis with myeloid metaplasia. N Engl J Med. 2000;342:1255–65.
8. Komrokji RS, Verstovsek S, Padron E, et al. Advances in the management of myelofibrosis. Cancer Control. 2012;19:4–15.
9. Guglielmelli P, Vannucchi AM, Investigators A. The prognostic impact of bone marrow fibrosis in primary myelofibrosis. Am J Hematol. 2016;91:E454–5.
10. Tefferi A. Annual clinical updates in Hematological malignancies. Am J Hematol. 2021;96:145–62. https://doi.org/10.1002/ajh.26050.

Chapter 19
Myelodysplastic Syndrome

A 60-year-old lady presented with complaints of progressive weakness, fatigue difficulty in performing routine activities, and breathlessness on mild exertion. For the last 1 year, these symptoms were getting worse. During the previous 6 months, she also had observed repeated upper respiratory tract infections for which she had been prescribed antibiotics twice. In addition, most recently she was experiencing easy bruisability and had observed petechial spots on arms, both thighs and buttocks. She is on anti-diabetic medications for last 10 years.

In past, she was diagnosed as a case of carcinoma breast 5 years back for which she had received chemotherapy. One year back, she was given radiotherapy. Currently she was taking only multivitamins which included vitamin B12. On physical examination, she had pallor without evidence of jaundice or cyanosis. The general physical examination did not reveal any lymphadenopathy or organomegaly. The examination of chest and abdomen was unremarkable. Result of CBC done at presentation is given in Table 19.1.

A. Gupta, *Decision Making Through Problem Based Learning in Hematology*,
https://doi.org/10.1007/978-981-99-8933-1_19

Table 19.1 CBC

CBC parameter	Patient's result	Reference range
WBC	3.2	3.7–10 × 10^9/L
RBC	2.10	4.5–5.4 × 10^{12}/L
HB	78	130–160 g/L
Hct	0.22	0.33–0.43 L/L
MCV	105	83–101 fL
MCH	32	27–32 pg
MCHC	340	315–345 g/L
RDW	18	11.6–14.6%
PLT	40	130–430 × 10^9/L
MPV	14	7–11 fL
Poly#	1.6	1.7–6 × 10^9/L
Lymp#	0.5	1–3 × 10^9/L
Mono#	1.2	0.2–1.0 × 10^9/L
EO#	0.8	0.02–0.5 × 10^9/L
BASO#	00	0.02–0.1 × 10^9/L
RETIC%	1.0	0.5–1.5%
Absolute ret count	105	50–150 10^9/L
ESR	53	0–20 mm 1st h Westergren

19.1 Questions

Q1. Interpret the CBC result given above and suggest investigations for further evaluation in such case

Answer: The CBC result shows decreased WBC count with markedly decreased neutrophils and lymphocytes. RBC count is low with decreased hemoglobin level and hematocrit and borderline high value for RDW. MCV is slightly high. Platelet count is markedly reduced. ESR value is high. Reticulocyte percentage and absolute values are within normal range.

So, there is pancytopenia. Anemia is mildly macrocytic. Possible causes of pancytopenia in this age group are as follows: [1].

1. Ineffective erythropoiesis as it happens in nutritional causes such as megaloblastic anemia, dual deficiency anemia, copper deficiency or zinc toxicity, and myelodysplastic syndrome.
2. Bone marrow infiltration/ replacement as in leukemia, lymphomas, myeloma, or metastasis.
3. Bone marrow suppression by autoimmune disorders, CRF, hemophagocytic syndromes, PNH, aplastic anemia, myelofibrosis, and following chemotherapy for malignancies.

4. Infections such as fungal, tubercular, and viral infections such as HIV, hepatitis, and Epstein–Barr virus.
5. Consumption as it happens in DIC or sequestration into spleen due to splenomegaly (portal HT with cirrhosis, myelofibrosis, storage diseases, etc.).

So all these diseases need to be excluded through history, physical examination, and appropriate investigations.

Next best investigation will be examination of blood film. Tests for renal, hepatic, pancreatic, and thyroid functions are recommended. Coagulation profile is mandatory. Levels of serum B12, folic acid, ferritin, copper, and zinc should be estimated. In addition to viral screening, direct antiglobulin test (DAT) and immunology screen should also be done.

A bone marrow examination as well as assessment with flowcytometric analysis of CD55 and CD59 on peripheral blood are important to ascertain diagnostic possibilities. However, these can be considered at later stage based on blood film findings.

Q2. Given are images from blood films (Figs. 19.1 and 19.2) and results of kidney, liver, pancreas, and thyroid function tests (Table 19.2). Also results of serum B12, folic acid, ferritin, copper, zinc (Table 19.3), coagulation profile (Table 19.4); DAT, immunology (Table 19.5) and viral screen (Table 19.6) Interpret the results. What are the possible differential diagnoses? What further investigations will be required to exclude various possibilities and suggest a final diagnosis?

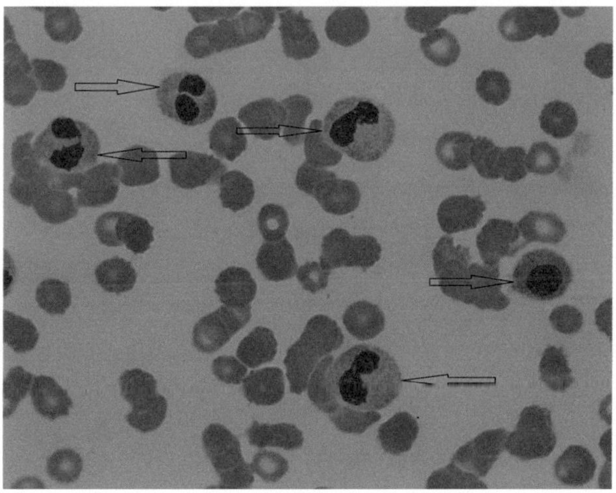

Fig. 19.1 PBF. Low density of red cells and many pseudo–Pelger-Huet neutrophils (arrows). Leishman stain × 100

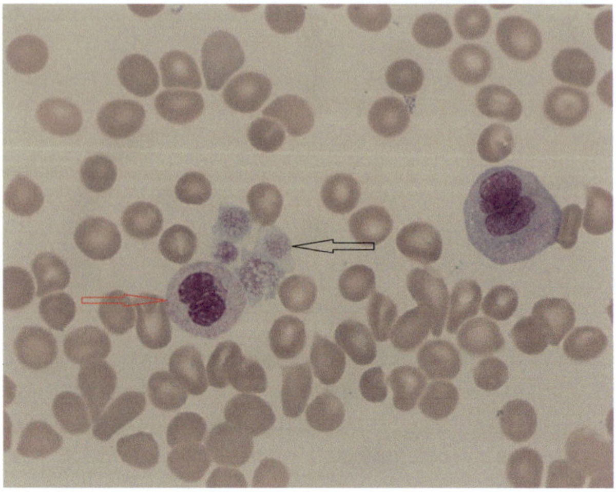

Fig. 19.2 PBF. Pseudo–Pelger-Huet neutrophils (red arrow) and large platelets(black arrow). Leishman stain × 100

Table 19.2 Biochemical tests

Test	Patient's result	Ref range
Glu (F)	8.1	3.9–6.1 mmol/L
Urea	2.9	2.5–6.6 mmol/L
Creat	101	60–120 μmol/L
Na^+	141	136–146 mmol/L
K^+	4.6	3.7–5.0 mmol/L
Ca^+	2.3	2.2–2.6 mmol/L
Mg+	1.0	0.08–1.1 mmol/L
T. Prot	67	63–80 mmol/L
Alb	41	35–47 mmol/L
Choles	2.9	1.5–5.2 mmol/L
TG	0.9	0.4–1.7 mmol/L
Urates	300	150–400 mmol/L
T Bil	41	3–20 μmol/L
Indirect Bil	32	5–20 μmol/L
D. Bil	9	0–5 μmol/L
Alk Ph	80	26–88 IU/L
ALT	56	10–60 IU/L
AST	34	10–42 IU/L
GGT	30	7–64 IU/L
LDH	400	90–180 IU/L
Hapto	0.4	0.2–2.0 g/L
T4	10.2	7.8–16 pmol/L
TSH	3.90	0.27–4.2 μLU/mL
Amylase	20	28–100 IU/L
Lipase	33	0–160 U/L

Table 19.3 Serum B12, folic acid, iron profile, zinc, and copper

Test	Patient's result	Ref range
S. B12	780	150–700 pmol/L
S. Folate	31.7	10–42 nmol/L
RBC folate	2554	1187–2854 nmol/L
Ferritin	380	20–340 mcg/L
s. Iron	29	11–31 μmol/L
Transferrin	3.2	2.1–3.6 g/L
Tran sat%	45%	20–40%
Zinc	0.84	0.66–1.10 mcg/mL
Copper	100	65–140 mcg/dL

Table 19.4 Coagulation profile

	Patient's result	Reference range
PT	11.5	9.6–13.6 s
INR	0.9	0.85–1.15
APTT	31	25–37 s
Fibrinogen/Clauss	4.0	2.34–4.45 g/L
D–D dimer	155	Below 255 ng/mL

Table 19.5 DAT and immunological tests

Test	Patient's result	Ref range
Direct antiglobulin test	Negative	Negative
Anti-ds-DNA antibody	Negative	0–20 Iu/mL
ANA screen	Negative	Negative

Table 19.6 Viral screen

Test name	Result	Ref range
HBs Ag	Not detected	Not detected
HCV-Ab	Non-reactive	Non-reactive
HCV-Ag	Not detected	Not detected
HIV Ag/Ab	Non-reactive	Non-reactive

Answer: The blood film shows low density of red cells and few clumps with mild rouleaux formation. Few macrocytes and many pseudo–Pelger–Huet cells (bilobed and hypogranular) are noted, which is a sign of dysplasia. There is true thrombocytopenia. No immature cell is noted. Few large platelets are also seen.

The biochemical tests show high values for total bilirubin, indirect bilirubin, and LDH. Rest of the tests for Liver, kidney, thyroid, and pancreatic functions are within normal range except for fasting blood glucose.

Serum B12 is high (she is on oral vitamin B12). Serum folate and red cell folate levels are normal. Serum ferritin and transferrin saturation are also raised. Levels of zinc and copper are within normal range.

The coagulation profile is normal, and immunological and virology screens are negative.

Pseudo—Pelger–Huet neutrophils are observed in myelodysplastic syndrome, acute leukemia, severe infections, myeloma, secondary to metastasis, and myxedema. The observations so far indicate possibility of myelodysplastic syndrome. However, a bone marrow examination with cytogenetic analysis is required for definite confirmation of the diagnosis and exclusion of other differential diagnoses [2].

Q3. Given are images from bone marrow aspirate (Figs. 19.3, 19.4, 19.5, 19.6, 19.7) and biopsy (Fig. 19.8). Result of genetic analysis is also provided. Interpret the findings and suggest final diagnosis.

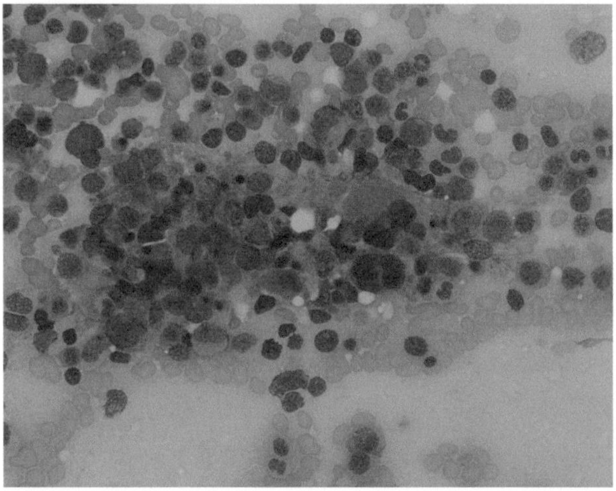

Fig. 19.3 BM aspirate. Hypercellular marrow. Leishman stain × 40

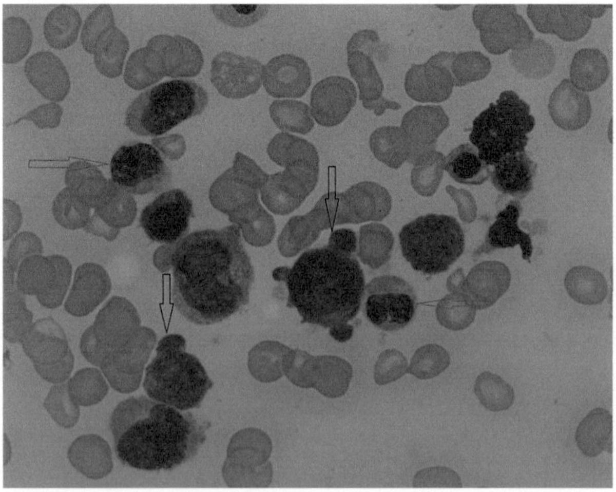

Fig. 19.4 BM aspirate. Dysplastic erythroblasts (black arrows) . Hyposegmented neutrophils (red arrows) Leishman stain × 100

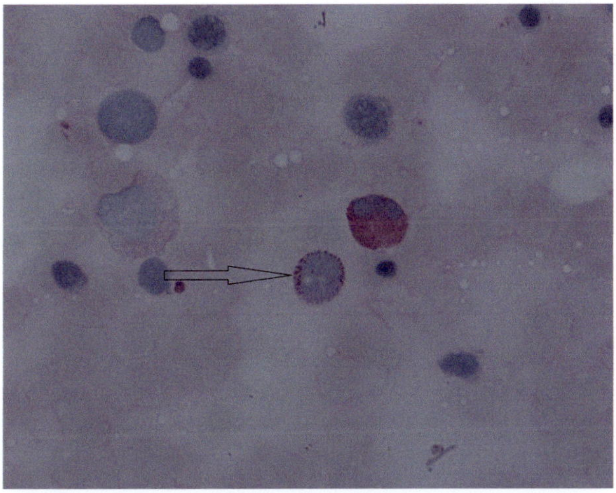

Fig. 19.5 BM aspirate. PAS positive dysplastic erythroblast. (arrow) PAS stain × 100

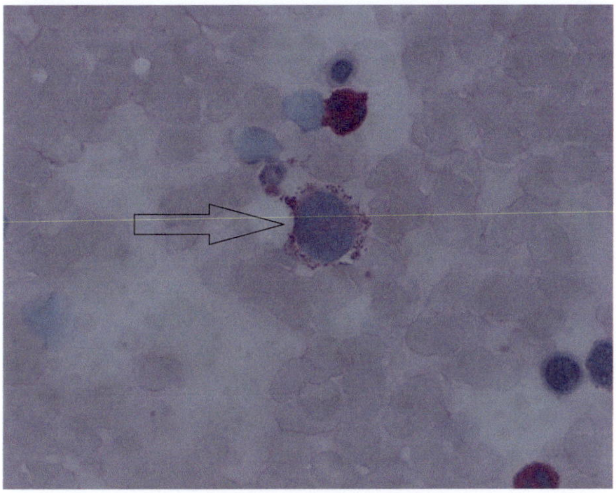

Fig. 19.6 BM aspirate. Dysplastic megakaryocyte (arrow). PAS stain × 100

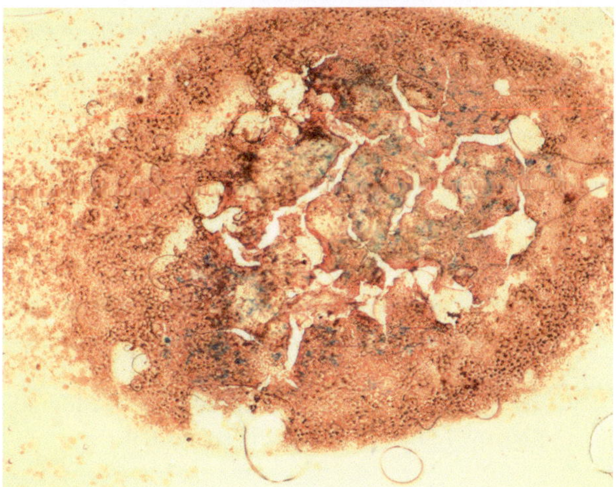

Fig. 19.7 BM aspirate. Adequate iron stores in BM particle. Prussian blue stain × 40

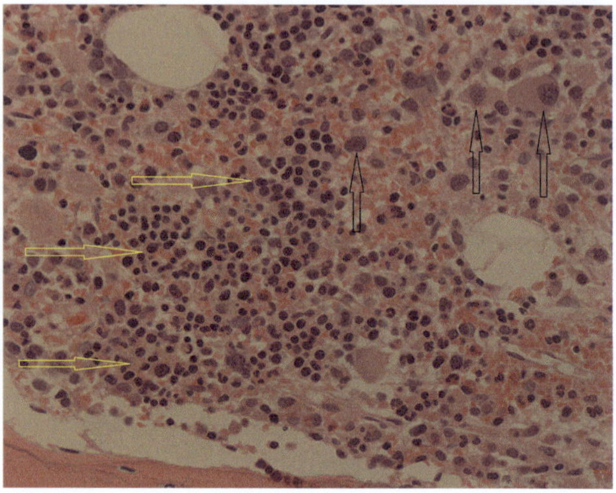

Fig. 19.8 BM biopsy. Erythroid hyperplasia (yellow arrows) and mononuclear dysplastic megakaryocytes (black arrows). H/E × 40

FISH analysis for MDS: Monosomy 7 in 80% (Probe D7S486/CEP7).

Answer: The smears from aspirated sample of bone marrow show a hypercellular marrow. Dysplastic changes are seen in erythroid precursors (cytoplasmic blebs) and granulocytes (pseudo–Pelger-Huet neutrophils). In addition, dysplastic changes are also seen in megakaryocytes which show hypolobation of nuclear lobes. When counted, the blast count was less than 5% and pseudo–Pelger-Huet neutrophils were more than 20%. PAS stain on bone marrow aspirate shows PAS positive dysplastic erythroid precursors. The Prussian blue stains does not show any ring sideroblasts. The sections from biopsy confirm hyperplastic bone marrow with many areas of erythroid collections and many hyposegmented megakaryocytes. There is no evidence of leukemia/lymphoma or metastatic pathology. FISH analysis shows monosomy 7.

All these findings of hypercellular marrow, panhyperplasia, and trilineage (Multilineage) dysplasia confirm a diagnosis of myelodysplastic syndrome with multilineage dysplasia (MDS-MLD)-post chemo/radiotherapy. All other differential diagnoses are excluded.

Pseudo– Pelger-Huet neutrophils are dysplastic neutrophils which are bilobed connected through a thin band of chromatin or have mononuclear appearance. Also, hypo- and hyper-granulation is a feature of dysplastic feature in neutrophils [2].

Q4. What more investigations are required in such patients which may help later in management?

Answer:

1. Serum erythropoietin level.
2. Fluorescence in situ hybridization (FISH) to detect chromosomal abnormalities which are not detected by standard cytogenetic analysis.
3. HLA typing.
4. Telomere length analysis should be considered if late onset Inherited bone marrow failure syndrome is suspected.

Q5. Once MDS is diagnosed, next step is to stage it to assess prognosis according to International Prognostic Scoring System (IPSS)? What are the general principles of this staging system?

Answer: International prognostic scoring system-revised is used to assess prognosis in patients with MDS. It takes into account peripheral blood cytopenias, BM blast percentage, and cytogenetic abnormalities . Based on these parameters, points are given. This system gives fairly accurate estimates of the risk of evolving AML in patients with primary MDS. It is divided into very low risk<1.5 score; low risk>1.5 to 3.0 score; intermediate>3 to 4.5 score; high risk >4.5–6 score; very High risk >6 score. For details see reference [3].

Q6. What are the different classification systems for MDS in general?

Answer: Three classifications systems are used- FAB (1982), WHO (2016, 2022), and ICC of myeloid neoplasm and acute leukemia. Only important points are highlighted below. Readers are suggested to go through references [4–7].

The Who classification (June 2022).

1. MDS with defining genetic abnormalities: Subcategorized into two categories based on bone marrow blasts percentage, 5q-, monosomy7, complex karyotyping, **and** mutations involving SF3B1 and TP53.
2. MDS, morphologically defined: Subcategorized into 5 categories based on percentage of blasts in peripheral blood and bone marrow (MDS with low blasts, MDS with increased blasts-IB1 and IB2, MDS hypocellular and MDS with fibrosis).

Note: Detection of $\geq$15% ring sideroblasts may substitute for *SF3B1* mutation. For hypocellular MDS- $\leq$25% bone marrow cellularity expected for age.

International Consensus Classification of Myeloid Neoplasms and Acute Leukemias: integrating morphologic, clinical, and genomic data-2022: Premalignant clonal cytopenias and myelodysplastic syndromes:

1. Clonal cytopenia of undetermined significance.
2. Myelodysplastic syndrome with mutated *SF3B1*.
3. Myelodysplastic syndrome with del(5q).
4. Myelodysplastic syndrome with mutated *TP53*.
5. Myelodysplastic syndrome, not otherwise specified (MDS, NOS).
   (a) MDS, NOS without dysplasia.
   (b) MDS, NOS with single lineage dysplasia.
   (c) MDS, NOS with multilineage dysplasia.
6. Myelodysplastic syndrome with excess blasts.
7. Myelodysplastic syndrome/acute myeloid leukemia (MDS/AML).
   (a) MDS/AML with mutated *TP53*.
   (b) MDS/AML with myelodysplasia-related gene mutations.
   (c) MDS/AML with myelodysplasia-related cytogenetic abnormalities.
   (d) MDS/AML, not otherwise specified.

Nowadays including a panel of molecular abnormalities is mandatory [8].

Q7. Which cytogenetic anomalies have prognostic role in patients with MDS?
Answer:

1. Good prognosis: -Y,del(11q),-5q,-12p,-20q.
2. Intermediate prognosis: -7q,+8,+19, t(17q).
3. Poor: -7, inv3, complex abnormalities.

Cytogenetic abnormalities are detected in about half of de novo MDS cases and in approximately 90% of secondary MDS cases, the most frequent are −5/del(5q), −7/del(7q), trisomy 8, and monosomy 18. del(5q) is more frequent in radiation induced t-MDS, while monosomy 7 is more frequent with alkylating agents [4, 5].

Q8. Which mutations have prognostic role in MDS? [9–11].
Answer: Mutations of TET2, SF3B1, ASXL1, SRSF2, DNMT3A, and RUNX1 are very frequent in MDS.
Mutations in SF3B1 are seen mostly in refractory anemia with ringed sideroblasts and have a favorable clinical prognosis. The risk of transformation to AML is low.
Mutations in PRPF8 are associated with a more aggressive clinical course.
Mutations in SRSF2 are associated with a high risk of AML transformation.
TET2 mutation is detected in approximately 25% of MDS patients.
NPM1 mutation is associated with poor survival in MDS.
TP53 mutation and del(5q) are seen in approximately 15% of MDS cases. Such cases show resistance to treatment.

Q9. Which mutations are considered predisposition factor for MDS?
Answer: Many mutations are thought to predispose to MDS. These include RUNX1, ANKRD26, DDX41, ETV6, GATA2, and SRP72 [9–11].

Q10. What is pathogenesis of cytopenia in MDS? [12, 13].
Answer: Myelodysplastic syndromes are clonal acquired diseases of the hematopoietic stem cell accompanied with increased (and rarely normal or hypocellular) bone marrow cellularity and peripheral blood cytopenias.
It developed as a result of genetic abnormalities with recurrent mutations which damage DNA and subsequent dysregulation of growth factor pathways. Over 90% cases result from somatic mutations. These mutations have an effect at stem cell level and are responsible for clonal evolution of myeloid cells.
Progenitors especially erythroid progenitors are affected resulting in partial resistance to hematopoietic cytokines. There is, however, normal expression and function of erythropoietin receptors.
In addition, there is an increased susceptibility to apoptosis which is also due to associated deregulated Fas/Fas ligand system and affects all three hematopoietic lineages, which may result in bicytopenia or pancytopenia. Increased apoptosis is also thought to be due to increased quantity of stromal inhibitory cytokines such as TNF-α and IFN-γ secreted by activated T cells, formation of which is

triggered by expression of new antigens on progenitor cells which have mutations. Since MDS is clonal, it is categorized as a premalignant condition.

1. Approximately 80% of patients are classified as primary or idiopathic MDS, as there is no obvious cause. Complex karyotypes are seen in 30% cases.
2. About 20% are classified as secondary MDS, in which there is history of exposure to cytotoxic chemotherapy, radiations, viral infections, or chemicals like benzene. Complex karyotype is seen in 50% cases.

19.2 Correlation of Results of Preliminary Investigations with Symptoms and Signs in Myelodysplastic Syndrome

Q11. What are the common symptoms and signs of MDS and how do they corelate with our patient?

Answer: Myelodysplastic syndrome can have variable presentations. Most commonly the patients present with symptoms of anemia like progressive generalized weakness fatigue, malaise, lethargy giddiness, dyspnea on exertion, pale appearance, etc. If there is thrombocytopenia, patients are prone to develop bruises, purpuric spots, or episodes of bleeding from mucosal surfaces. In presence of leukopenia and neutropenia, there is preceding history of recurrent infections. Examination usually does not show any organomegaly except in cases of CMML [14].

This patient also had progressive weakness, fatigue difficulty in performing routine activities and breathlessness on mild exertion, which are symptoms of anemia. She also had observed repeated upper respiratory tract infections due to neutropenia and easy bruising indicating thrombocytopenia. All these correlate well the symptoms of MDS.

Q12. CBC shows pancytopenia, mild macrocytosis and inappropriately low reticulocyte count. What is cause of these changes in MDS?

Answer: Myelodysplasia is a clonal acquired diseases of the hematopoietic stem cell due to mutations leading to DNA damage. These mutations result in production of clonal myeloid cells. Morphologically there is hyperplasia of all three cell lines. There is abnormal maturation with dysplastic changes. Most of the cell die in bone marrow due to this defective maturation—resulting in ineffective hematopoiesis, which, in addition, is also due to apoptosis from increased stromal cytokines like TNF-alfa and Interferon-gamma. This results in peripheral blood pancytopenia [12, 13].

Due to defective DNA, maturation of erythroid cells is affected, which results in mild megaloblastic change in erythroblasts and macrocytes in peripheral blood in spite of normal B12 and folic acid level. Similarly, ineffective erythropoiesis in bone marrow due to death of maturing erythroblasts results in low reticulocyte count in peripheral blood.

Q13. What are the dysplastic changes seen in MDS and how do these correlate in our patient?

Answer: Dysplastic changes can be seen in one hemopoietic lineage or multiple lineages. In erythroid series, presence of binucleation or multi-nucleation, cytoplasmic blebs, internuclear and intercytoplasmic bridges, abnormal karyorrhexis, and megaloblastic changes (in absence of B12/FA deficiency) are considered dysplastic changes. In granulocytic series hypo- as well as hyper segmentation of nuclear lobes and hypo- or hypergranulation of granulocytic cells is a feature of dysplasia. The dysplastic megakaryocytes show that hypo-lobation of the nuclei, micro megakaryocytes, and abnormal budding of platelets (which is reflected as large sized platelets in peripheral blood), are also features of dysmegakaryopoiesis [15].

In our patient, presence of hyposegmented neutrophils (pseudo–Pelger-Huet) and mild macrocytosis in peripheral blood with dysplastic changes in all three cell lines in bone marrow (dysplastic erythroblasts, granulocytic precursors, and megakaryocytes) correlated well with diagnosis of MDS.

Q14. This patient has high indirect bilirubin and LDH. How do these correlate with the diagnosis of MDS?

Answer: High LDH and high indirect bilirubin are main indicators of ineffective erythropoiesis seen in MDS. High LDH results from accelerated turnover of bone marrow cells during which this enzyme is released from dividing and dying cells. High indirect bilirubin comes from metabolism of hemoglobin released from dead cells. Other indicators which can be associated with ineffective erythropoiesis and hemolysis are reduced haptoglobins, raised urine urobilinogen, positive urine hemosiderin, and raised serum iron and ferritin.

Q15. In which conditions other than classical MDS, dysplastic changes may be seen in Bone marrow?

Answer: Mild dysplastic changes especially in erythroid precursors, are noted in megaloblastic anemia, copper deficiency or zinc excess, infections like HIV and parvovirus, toxins such as ethanol and heavy metals, following treatment with growth factors like GMCSF and erythropoietin, certain chemotherapeutic agents such as antifolate agents, immunological disorders, and congenital causes like CDA [16, 17].

Q16. What are the salient features of MDS-RS?

Answer: MDS-RA is seen in approximately 3–11% of all MDS cases and affects older age-group. There can be single- or multi-lineage dysplasia.

In FAB classification, MDS-RARS is one of the categories which is diagnosed when blast count is less than 5%in bone marrow but there is trilineage dysplasia and presence of ring sideroblasts (>15%) in bone marrow.

In WHO classification, for diagnosis of MDS with ring sideroblasts (MDS-RS), there should be ≥15% erythroid precursors should be ring sideroblasts in bone marrow or presence of *SF3B1* mutation if ≥5% ring sideroblasts are observed. Dysplasia can be single lineage (RARS) or multilineage (MDS-MLD-RS). There should be no isolated del (5q). Clinical course of RARS is prolonged with low incidence of progression to acute leukemia. Mutations in *SF3B1* are seen in ≥80% of patients with MDS-RS-SLD [18].

Given are images of peripheral blood (Fig. 19.9) and bone marrow aspirate (Figs. 19.10 and 19.11) from a 60-year-old lady, who had chronic anemia and was subjected to bone marrow examination when other investigations were non-conclusive. The peripheral blood showed anemia and dysplastic neutrophils. The bone marrow aspirate shows dysplastic erythroblasts, and Prussian blue stain on bone marrow aspirate shows many ring sideroblasts, confirming a diagnosis of MDS-RARS in this patient.

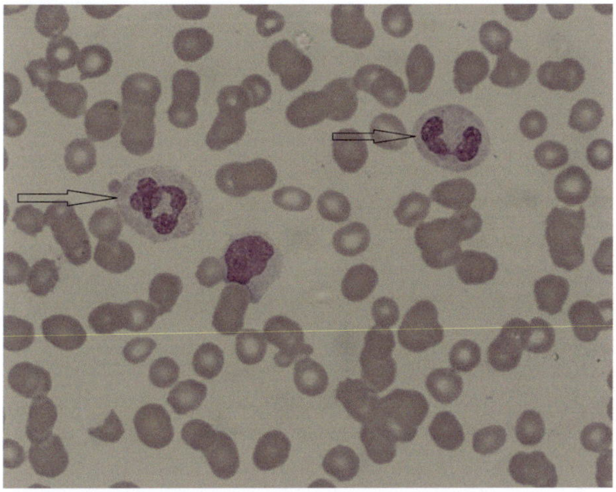

Fig. 19.9 PBF. Low density of red cells and dysplastic neutrophils. Leishman stain × 40

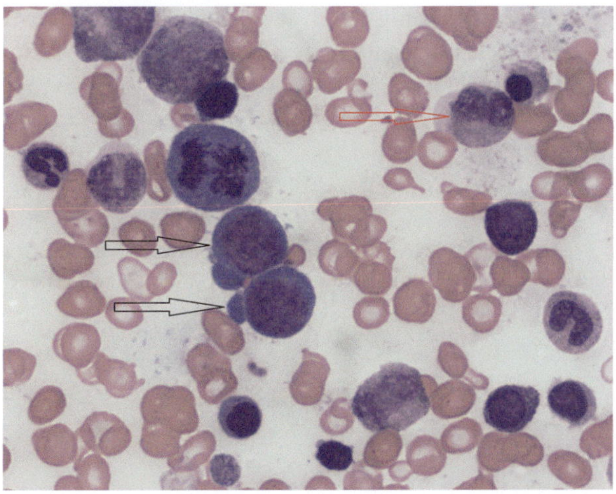

Fig. 19.10 BM aspirate. Dysplastic erythroid cells (black arrows) Hyposegmented neutrophil (red arrow). H/E stain × 100

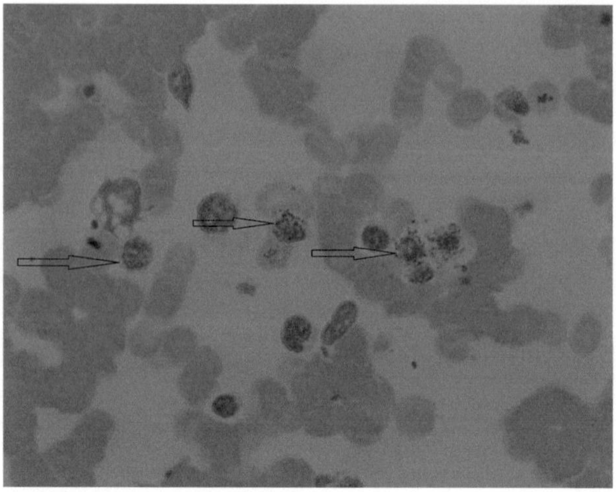

Fig. 19.11 BM aspirate. Ring sideroblasts. Prussian Blue stain × 100

Ring sideroblasts are abnormal sideroblasts where iron accumulates around the nucleus in mitochondria giving appearance of ring. The ring generally covers more than 1/3 of the circumference.

Q17. What are the salient points in diagnosis of hypocellular MDS? what clinical course can such cases take place?

Answer: Classical MDS is hypercellular. In approximately 10% cases, bone marrow is hypocellular. This is designated as hypocellular MDS. The dysplastic changes are not that florid and this makes the diagnosis a bit challenging (Figs. 19.12 and 19.13). In ICC classification, it is categorized as MDS-h under MDS-morphologically defined category. There should be equal or less than 25% of cellularity. The differential diagnoses of aplastic anemia and aleukemic leukemia need to be excluded. In classical aplastic anemia, cytogenetics are normal. Although presence of dysplasia and macrocytosis favor MDS, in 50% cases cytogenetics is normal. If there is PNH clone, it favors AA (seen in 30% to 60%) whereas it is extremely rare to see this in MDS. Few points of differentiation are provided in Table 19.7.

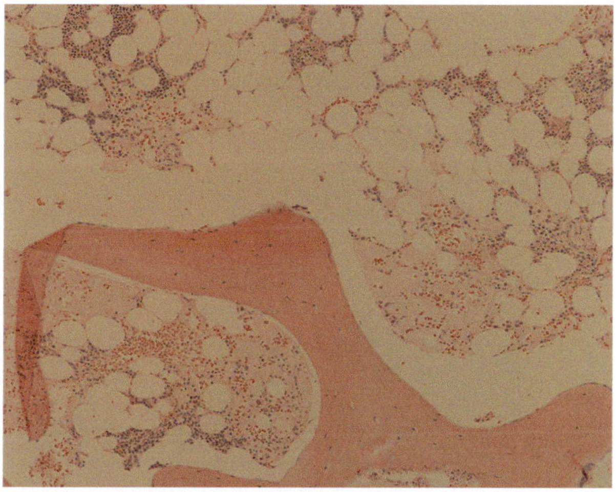

Fig. 19.12 Bone marrow biopsy. Hypocellular marrow. HE stain × 20

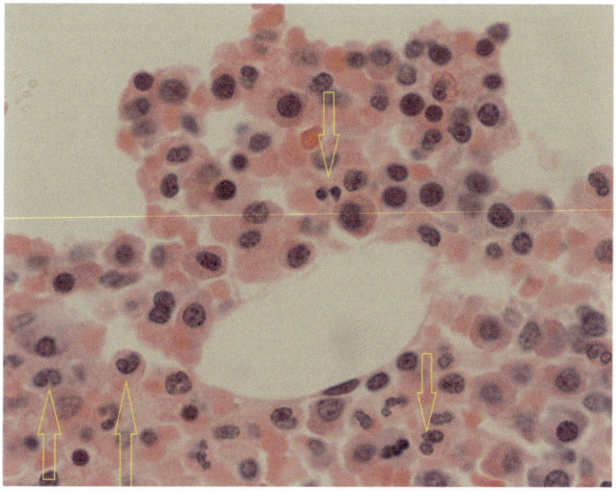

Fig. 19.13 Bone marrow biopsy. Dysplastic neutrophils. HE stain × 100

Table 19.7 Differentiation between aplastic anemia and hypocellular MDS

BM finding	Aplastic anemia	Hypoplastic MDS
Cellularity	Decreased	Decreased
Dysgranulopoiesis (abnormal PMN)	No	Yes
Dysmegakaryopoiesis (abnormal megs)	No	Yes
Blasts	No	+/–
Megakaryocyte number	Decreased	Present
LGLs	Absent	Present
Cytogenetics	Normal	Abnormal in 50%
PNH clone	20–30%	Absent

Flowcytometry or Immunocytometry should be done to assess number of CD43+ cells and exclude PNH clone. Mutational analysis for mutated telomere genes is also recommended to exclude inherited BM failure syndrome presenting in late life.

As the bone marrow is hypocellular, based on morphology and genetics, clinical course may differ. Cases in which there is evidence of monoclonality are likely to transform to leukemia and the others may follow benign course and have better prognosis [19].

Given below are images from a 45-year-old female patient who was being investigated for pancytopenia. Few dysplastic neutrophils were seen in peripheral blood. The bone marrow aspirate was pauci-cellular. However, the trephine biopsy showed hypocellularity and on close examination, hyposegmented, and occasional Pelger-Huet neutrophils were observed. Cytogenetic analysis revealed monosomy 7. No PNH clone was detected.

Q18. What are the salient points in diagnosis of 5q- syndrome?

Answer: 5q – syndrome is seen in approximately 10% of case of MDS. It affects primarily females and is considered as low-risk MDS with less than 10% chances of transformation to leukemia. It is characterized by anemia, usually macrocytic, and normal or elevated platelets [20].

Given are images from a case of 5q- syndrome. The peripheral blood (Fig. 19.14) shows anemia, pseudo–Pelger-Huet neutrophils and many large and few giant platelets. The bone marrow is hypercellular and shows erythroid hyperplasia with dysplastic megakaryocytes (Fig. 19.15). Many dysplastic megakaryocytes with abnormal platelet budding are seen (Fig. 19.16). Blasts are less than 5%. The FISH analysis on aspirated BM sample showed deletion of 5q31 in 50% cells using D7S486 probe (5q-). These observations confirmed the diagnosis of MDS 5q- syndrome.

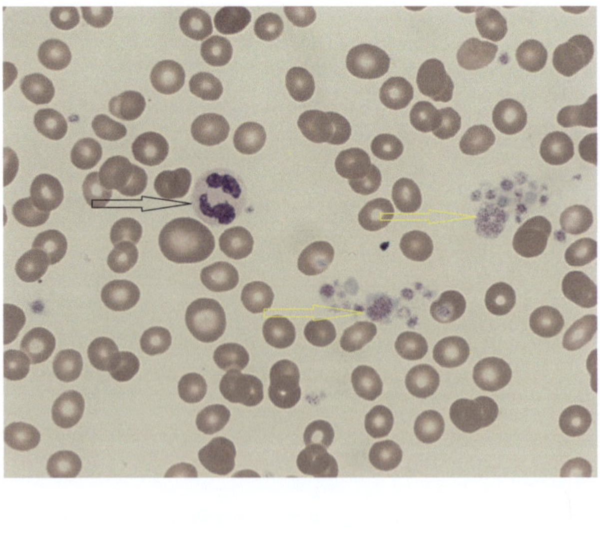

Fig. 19.14 PBF. Anemia, Pelger-Huet neutrophils (black arrow) and large-sized platelets (yellow arrows). Leishman stain × 100

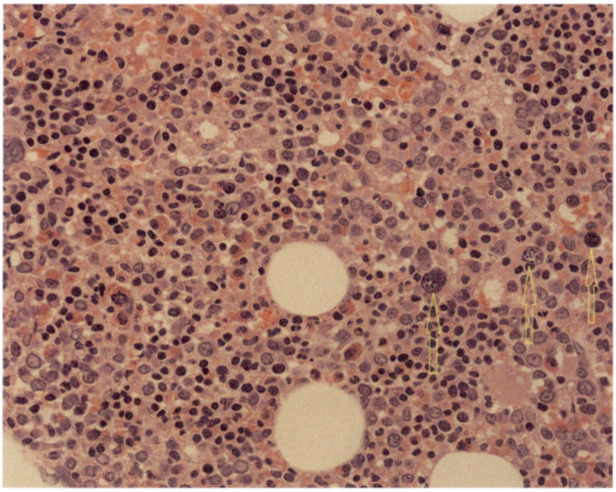

Fig. 19.15 BM biopsy. Hypercellular marrow with dysplastic megakaryocytes (yellow arrows). H/E × 40

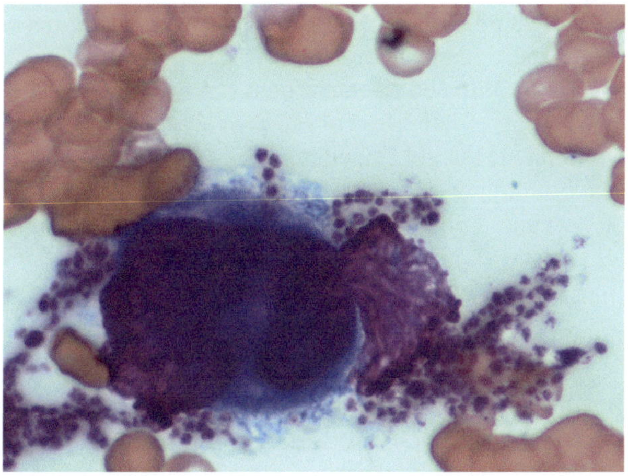

Fig. 19.16 BM aspirate. Dysplastic megakaryocytes with platelet budding. PAS stain × 100

19.3 Quick information for Practicing Clinicians and Students

References [1–21]:

1. Most commonly, patients present with anemia followed by bicytopenia and/or pancytopenia.
2. Macrocytic anemia (or bicytopenia/pancytopenia) with high RDW, peripheral blood findings of dysplasia, and evidence of ineffective erythropoiesis (high LDH, indirect bilirubin, and low reticulocyte count) must alert for possible diagnosis and further workup to exclude MDS.

3. Bone marrow examination is done to confirm and subcategorize MDS.
4. Approximately 30% cases can transform to acute myeloblastic leukemia (AML).
5. In indeterminate cases, emerging and increasing population of CD34, CD117, and myeloperoxidase positive cells in bone marrow, identified by flow cytometry, immunohistochemistry, or immunophenotyping are suggestive of transformation.
6. Chromosomal abnormalities are seen in approximately 50% of patients with de novo MDS and about 80–90% cases of therapy induced-MDS.
7. Molecular genetic analysis is important as it has both therapeutic and prognostic significance.
8. The presence of paroxysmal nocturnal hemoglobinuria (PNH) in patients with MDS has important implications for prognosis and treatment. Patients with MDS and increased PNH-type cells may present with severe thrombocytopenia but less pronounced blood cell-morphologic abnormality, less karyotypic abnormalities, and lower rates of progression to acute leukemia.. Patients with PNH and MDS may benefit from anticomplement C5 monoclonal antibody treatment.
9. In patients with close differential diagnosis between hypocellular MDS and aplastic anemia, bone marrow samples should be subjected to mutational analysis for mutated telomere genes to exclude inherited BM failure syndrome presenting in late life. For Fanconi anemia, a positive chromosomal breakage test remains the gold standard.
10. Both hypocellular MDS and AA can show dys-erythropoiesis. More than 10% pseudo–Pelger-Huet cells in the peripheral blood and marrow granulocytic dysplasia, abnormal localization of immature precursors (ALIP), dysmegakaryopoiesis, fibrosis, and increased blasts are in favor of hypocellular MDS.
11. Family history of hematologic disorders and dysmorphic physical features may help to diagnose inherited bone marrow failure syndrome.

According to BCSH guidelines for diagnosis and evaluation of prognosis of adult myelodysplastic syndrome, myelodysplastic syndromes should be considered in all patients with otherwise unexplained cytopenia(s). World Health Organization (WHO) thresholds for cytopenias are hemoglobin <100 g/L, absolute neutrophil count $<1.8 \times 10^9$/L, and platelets $<100 \times 10^9$/L. [21].

WHO-defined diagnosis of MDS requires either (i) morphological dysplasia (involving ≥10% of bone marrow cells in ≥1 lineage); (ii) increased myeloblasts (≥5%, but <20%); or (iii) evidence of clonality with a typical MDS-associated cytogenetic abnormality.

In MDS-RA-MLD category, either >15% ring sideroblasts or >5% ring sideroblasts If *SF3B1* mutation should be present. *SF3B1* mutations are found in >95% of MDS cases with ring sideroblasts and are associated with a relatively favorable prognosis.

At diagnosis, the prognosis for all patients should be calculated using IPSS-R & IPSS.

To acquire further knowledge on the subject, following sources are advised:

1. BCSH guidelines
2. Br Jr. Hematology
3. ASH education book
4. Blood
5. NEJM
6. Int Jr. Lab Hematology

References

1. Elizabeth PW, Daniel AA. The differential diagnosis and bone marrow evaluation of new-onset pancytopenia. Am J Clin Pathol. 2013;139:9–29.
2. Shetty VT, Mundle SD, Raza A. Pseudo Pelger-Huet anomaly in myelodysplastic syndrome: hyposegmented apoptotic neutrophil? Blood. 2001;98:1273–5.
3. Greenberg P, et al. International scoring system for evaluating prognosis in myelodysplastic syndromes. Blood. 1997;89:2079–88.
4. Montalban-Bravo G, Garcia-Manero G. Myelodysplastic syndromes: 2018 update on diagnosis, risk-stratification and management. Am J Hematol. 2018;93(1):129–47.
5. Ming H, Guangsheng H. The 2016 revision to the World Health Organization classification of myelodysplastic syndromes. J Transl Int Med. 2017;5(3):139–43. https://doi.org/10.1515/jtim-2017-0002.
6. Daniel AA, Attili O, Robert P, Hasserjian JB, et al. International consensus classification of myeloid neoplasms and acute Leukemias: integrating morphologic, clinical, and genomic data. Blood. 2022;140(11):1200–28. https://doi.org/10.1182/blood.2022015850.
7. Vardiman J. The classification of MDS: From FAB to WHO and beyond. Leuk Res. 2012;36(12):1453–8. https://doi.org/10.1016/j.leukres.2012.08.008.
8. Haferlach T, Nagata Y, Grossmann V, et al. Landscape of genetic lesions in 944 patients with myelodysplastic syndromes. Leukemia. 2014;28(2):241–7.
9. Bejar R, Stevenson K, Abdel-Wahab O, et al. Clinical effect of point mutations in myelodysplastic syndromes. N Engl J Med. 2011;364:2496–506.
10. Bersanelli M, Travaglino E, Meggendorfer M, et al. Classification and personalized prognostic assessment on the basis of clinical and genomic features in myelodysplastic syndromes. J Clin Oncol. 2021;39:1223–33.
11. Nazha A, Komrokji R, Meggendorfer M, et al. Personalized prediction model to risk stratify patients with myelodysplastic syndromes. J Clin Oncol. 2021;39:3737–46.
12. Alex A, Peter LG. Molecular pathophysiology of the myelodysplastic syndromes: insights for targeted therapy. Blood Adv. 2018;2(20):2787–97.
13. Valeria V, Ramon VT, Heesun JR. Pathogenesis of myelodysplastic syndromes: an overview of molecular and non-molecular aspects of the disease. Blood Res. 2014;49(4):216–27. https://doi.org/10.5045/br.2014.49.4.216.
14. James MF, Jamile MS. Clinical presentation, diagnosis, and prognosis of myelodysplastic syndromes. Am J Med. 2012;125(7 Suppl):S6–13. https://doi.org/10.1016/j.amjmed.2012.04.015.
15. Francisco PT, Daphne CA, Guang F. Myelodysplastic syndrome: diagnosis and screening. Diagnostics. 2022 Jul;12(7):1581. https://doi.org/10.3390/diagnostics12071581.
16. Wickramasinghe SN, Wood WG. Advances in the understanding of the congenital dyserythropoietic anaemias. Br J Haematol. 2005;131(4):431–46.
17. Amos RJ, Deane M, Ferguson C, Jeffries G, Hinds CJ, Amess JA. Observations on the haemopoietic response to critical illness. J Clin Pathol. 1990;43(10):850–6.

18. Arber DA, Orazi A, Hasserjian R, et al. The 2016 revision to the World Health Organization classification of myeloid neoplasms and acute leukemia. Blood. 2016;127:2391–405.
19. Valeria S, Daniela MG, Elisa M, et al. Myelodysplastic syndromes with hypocellular marrow: clinical characteristics and evaluation of outcome. Blood. 2018;132(Supplement 1):1829.
20. Jacqueline B, Andrea P, Andrew NJK, James SW. Advances in the 5q− syndrome. Blood. 2010;116(26):5803–11.
21. Sally BK, Daniel HW, Lynn Q. British Society for Haematology guidelines for the diagnosis and evaluation of prognosis of adult myelodysplastic syndromes. Br J Haematol. 2021;194:282–93. https://doi.org/10.1111/bjh.

Chapter 20
Secondary Hemochromatosis

A 30-year-old male patient known case of sickle cell/ beta-thalassemia presents with progressive weakness, lethargy, and dyspnea on exertion. He has received multiple blood transfusions over the past 20 years, the last one was 3 weeks back. Recently, he has observed increased frequency of micturition, easy fatiguability even after blood transfusion and appearance of brownish hyperpigmentation of skin all over body, more marked over face and arms. He also complained of bony pains in small joints of hands. There was no history of fever or any other relevant symptoms. His mother had been diagnosed with beta-thalassemia trait and father has sickle cell anemia.

Examination showed pallor with mild jaundice. Mild enlargement of liver and spleen was observed on palpation. There was no lymphadenopathy. Result of CBC is presented (Table 20.1).

Table 20.1 CBC

CBC parameter	Patient's result	Reference range
WBC	7.4	3.7–10 × 10^9/L
RBC	2.9	4.5–5.4 × 10^{12}/L
HB	6.5	130–160 g/L
Hct	0.190	0.33–0.43 L/L
MCV	68	83–101 fL
MCH	19	27–32 pg
MCHC	305	315–345 g/L
RDW	19	11.6–14.6%
PLT	170	130–430 × 10^9/L
MPV	10	7–11 fL
Poly#	3.9	1.7–6 × 10^9/L
Lymp#	2.7	1–3 × 10^9/L
Mono#	0.5	0.2–1.0 × 10^9/L
EO#	0.3	0.02–0.5 × 10^9/L
BASO#	00	0.02–0.1 × 10^9/L
RETIC%	5	0.5–1.5%
Absolute ret count	225	50–150 × 10^9/L
ESR	59	0–20 mm 1st h Westergren

A. Gupta, *Decision Making Through Problem Based Learning in Hematology*, https://doi.org/10.1007/978-981-99-8933-1_20

20.1 Questions

Q1. Interpret the result of CBC and suggest further investigations?

Answer: The CBC shows anemia with low MCV, MCH, and MCHC. RDW is high. Reticulocyte count and ESR are also high. So there is microcytic hypochromic anemia with reticulocytosis. As the patient is known SCA/beta-thalassemia and has persistent anemia in spite of recent blood transfusion, further tests will be required to see for hemolysis and bleeding. Bone marrow suppression is unlikely as the reticulocyte count is high, which indicates adequate response of bone marrow. Next best investigation will be examination of blood film, tests for liver and kidney functions with hemolytic profile, and examination of urine and stools for blood. A rare possibility of delayed hyperhemolysis syndrome is unlikely as reticulocyte count is high but still presence of alloantibodies should also be checked.

Q2. Given is image from blood film (Fig. 20.1). Results of biochemical tests (Table 20.2), urine and stool examination (Table 20.3) are also provided. Interpret the results and suggest further investigations in such case.

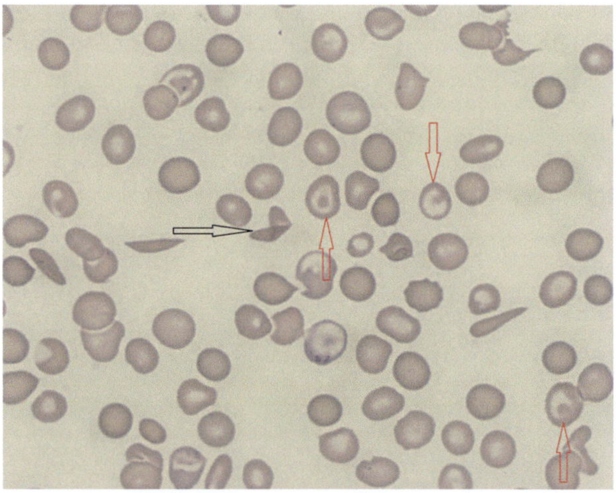

Fig 20.1 PBF. Microcytic hypochromic cells, sickle cells (black arrow), and target cells (red arrows). Leishman × 100

Table 20.2 Biochemical tests

Test	Patient's result	Ref range
Glu	8.5	3.9–6.1 mmol/L
Urea	2.9	2.5–6.6 mmol/L
Creat	101	60–120 μmol/L
Na^+	139	136–146 mmol/L
K^+	4.8	3.7–5.0 mmol/L
Ca^+	2.5	2.2–2.6 mmol/L
Mg^+	1.0	0.08–1.1 mmol/L
T. Prot	69	63–80 mmol/L
Alb	37	35–47 mmol/L
Choles	2.5	1.5–5.2 mmol/L
TG	0.9	0.4–1.7 mmol/L
Urates	370	150–400 mmol/L
T Bil	80	3–20 μmol/L
D. Bil	20	0–5 μmol/L
I Bil	60	5–15 μmol/L
Alk Ph	112	26–88 IU/L
ALT	210	10–60 IU/L
AST	190	10–42 IU/L
GGT	60	7–64 IU/L
LDH	280	90–180 IU/L
Hapto	0.1	0.2–2.0 g/L
T4	10.6	7.8–16 pmol/L
TSH	3.99	0.27–4.2 μlU/mL
Amylase	20	28–100 IU/L
Lipase	30	0–160 U/L

Table 20.3 Urine and stool examination

Urine examination	Patient's result	Reference range
SG	1.020	1.005–1.030
Ph	6	5–7
Leu	Neg	Neg
Nit	Neg	Neg
Pro	Neg	Neg
Glu	Neg	Neg
Ket	Neg	Neg
Uro	Neg	Neg
Bil	Neg	Neg
Stool examination		
Occult blood	Neg	Neg
Ova/cysts	Neg	Neg

Answer: The blood film shows low density of red cells, anisopoikilocytosis with microcytic hypochromic red cells, sickle cells, and target cells. So the blood film findings confirm microcytic hypochromic anemia with evidence of sickle cell/thalassemia in this patient. The biochemical tests show increased levels of blood glucose, bilirubin (both direct and indirect), and LDH in addition to ALT and AST. Haptoglobin is decreased. The urine and stool examinations are unremarkable. No allo-antibodies were detected.

All these findings suggest a hemolytic process in already diagnosed case of SCA/beta-thalassemia.

As the patient has symptoms of joint pains (arthralgia) and brownish discoloration of skin, further evaluation will require a serum iron profile, hepatitis profile, CRP, and immunology profile.

Q3. Given are results of serum iron profile (Table 20.4), hepatitis profile (Table 20.5), immunology profile, and CRP (Table 20.6). Interpret the results and suggest differential diagnosis.

Table 20.4 Serum iron profile

Test	Patient's result	Ref range
S. Iron	40	11–31 µmol/L
Transferrin	2.2	2.1–3.6 g/L
Trans. Sat %	50	20–40%
TIBC	200	250–300 µg/dL
Ferritin	650	11–307 ng/mL

Table 20.5 Hepatitis and other viral serology

Test name	Result	Ref range
HBs Ag	Non-reactive	Non-reactive
HCV-Ab	Reactive	Non-reactive
HCV-Ag	Not detected	Non-reactive
HIV Ag/Ab	Non-reactive	Non-reactive
Parvovirus B19 IgG	Non-reactive	Non-reactive
Parvovirus B19 IgM	Non-reactive	Non-reactive
CMV-DNA	Not detected by real-time PCR	Non-reactive
CMV-IgG	Reactive	Non-reactive
CMV-IgM	Non-reactive	Non-reactive
EBV-DNA	Not detected by real-time PCR	Non-reactive
EBV-IgG	Reactive	Non-reactive
EBV-IgM	Non-reactive	Non-reactive

Table 20.6 CRP and Immunology profile

Test	Patient's result	Ref Range
CRP	10	0–10 mg/L
Anti-ds-DNA antibody	2	0–20 Iu/mL
ANA screen	Negative	Negative
Sm B	Negative	Negative
RNP A and C	Negative	Negative
SS-A	Negative	Negative
SS-B	Negative	Negative
Scl-70	Negative	Negative
Jo-1	Negative	Negative
Ribosomal P	Negative	Negative
Histone	Negative	Negative
MPO Ab	Negative	Negative
Proteinase Ab	Negative	Negative

Answer: The results show high serum level of iron, transferrin saturation, ferritin, and reduced iron binding capacity These suggest iron overload in this patient. There is no evidence of active infection or inflammation. Hepatitis and immunological profiles are normal.

Possible causes of iron overload include: [1].

1. Chronic blood transfusion therapy especially in patients of hemoglobinopathies such as sickle cell anemia, thalassemia, sideroblastic anemia, myelodysplasia, etc.
2. Hereditary hemochromatosis
3. Chronic liver disease (alcoholic liver disease)
4. Chronic inflammatory disorders including autoimmune diseases
5. Any cause of ineffective erythropoiesis with hyperplastic bone marrow such as sideroblastic anemia

This patient is a known case of sickle cell/beta-thalassemia with regular multiple transfusions for many years. So the most likely cause of iron overload is secondary to chronic transfusions. However, for confirmation of this diagnosis, hereditary hemochromatosis, sideroblastic anemia, and myelodysplasia should be ruled out. For this, genetic testing for HFE gene and a bone marrow biopsy should be done.

Q4. Given are images from bone marrow biopsy (Figs. 20.2, and 20.3), Prussian blue stain on bone marrow aspirate (Figs. 20.4 and 20.5), and result of genetic tests for HFE gene. Interpret the results and suggest a final diagnosis.

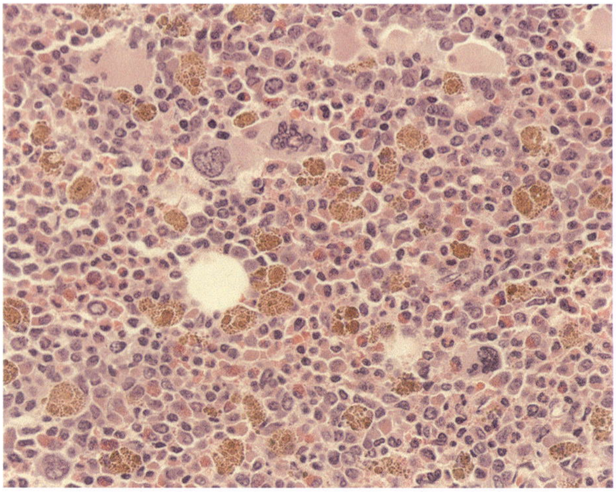

Fig. 20.2 BM trephine biopsy. Many hemosiderin laden macrophages are seen scattered in all spaces. H/E × 40

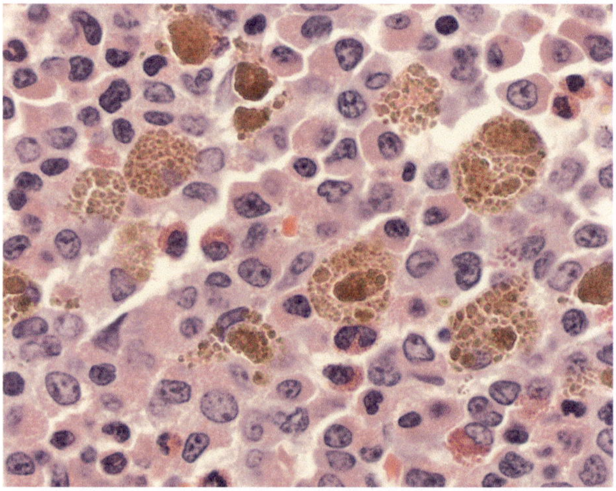

Fig. 20.3 .BM trephine biopsy. Hemosiderin laden macrophages- Golden brown colored pigment. H/E × 100

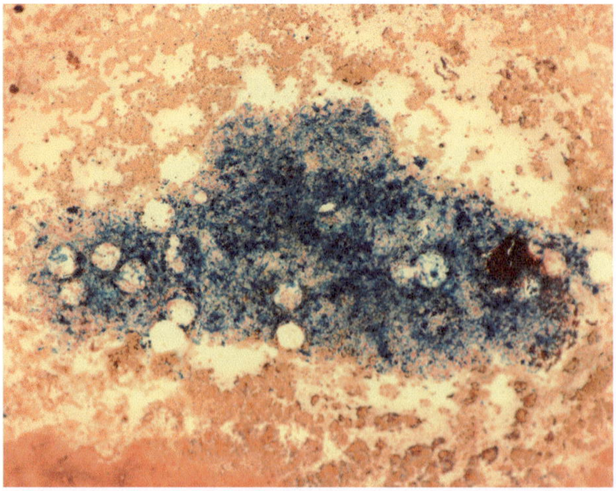

Fig. 20.4 BM aspirate. BM particle is loaded with iron. Prussian blue stain × 40

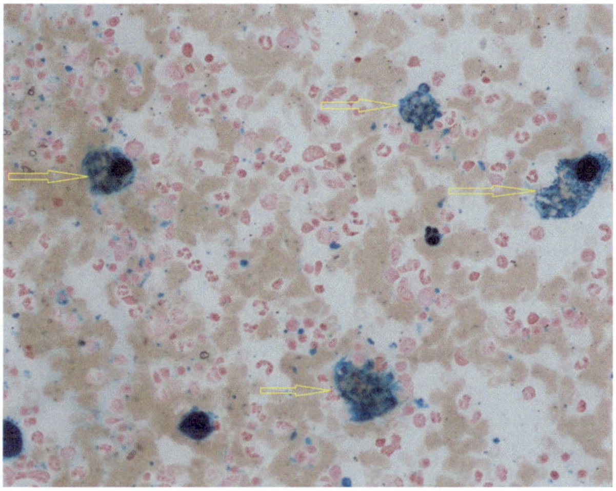

Fig. 20.5 BM aspirate. Many macrophages loaded with iron are seen (Yellow arrows). Prussian blue stain × 40

Genetic test for HFE gene mutation	No genetic mutation (C282Y and H63D) detected

Answer: The trephine biopsy shows hemosiderin laden macrophages in all spaces. The bone marrow aspirate shows many hemosiderin laden macrophages. The Prussian blue stain confirms the presence of hemosiderin in these macrophages. There are no dysplastic changes or any evidence of increased sideroblasts or ring sideroblasts. No genetic mutations are seen. These findings substantiate diagnosis of hemochromatosis secondary to chronic blood transfusion in this patient.

Q5. What additional investigations may be required in evaluation in such case which affects treatment and prognosis?
Answer: [2–4].

1. Tests for hepatitis B and C.
2. Liver biopsy for iron concentration (hepatic iron content). Liver biopsy with estimation of hepatic iron concentration is helpful in evaluation of liver status and prognosis. In secondary hemochromatosis, the iron deposition starts in Kupffer cell.
3. Skin biopsy from representative areas for evaluation of iron deposition.
4. CXR for cardiomegaly and ECHO cardiography.
5. CT scan and MRI for hepatomegaly and estimation of hepatic iron content (non-invasive method of measuring hepatic iron content).
6. In patients who have evidence of cirrhosis, endoscopy is advised.

20.2 Correlation of Results of Preliminary Investigations with Symptoms and Signs in Secondary hemochromatosis

Q6. Correlate the symptoms and signs in this patient with final diagnosis of hemochromatosis.

Answer: This patient had complaints of increased frequency of micturition possibly from development of diabetes mellitus due to pancreatic beta cell damage as a result of iron deposition. Brownish hyperpigmentation of skin is from iron deposition. Also joint pains results from iron deposition in bones and joint spaces. The increased requirements of transfusion were most likely from ineffective erythropoiesis resulting from non-utilization of iron in bone marrow. Deposition of iron in liver and spleen produces hepatosplenomegaly.

Patient had anemia, jaundice, and evidence of hemolysis due to pre-existing disease (SCA/beta-thalassemia). The liver functions are abnormal due to hepatic damage resulting from iron deposition.

Abnormal iron profile (with high transferrin saturation, ferritin, and low TIBC) suggested iron overload. The final diagnosis of secondary hemochromatosis was confirmed from presence of iron deposition in bone marrow and absence of genetic mutations of HFE gene.

Q7. What is etio-pathogenesis of hemochromatosis and what possible complications can arise in such patients.

Answer: Haemochromatosis refers to accumulation of iron in different organs of body resulting in organ damage.

Out of all causes referred above, the two most important causes are hereditary hemochromatosis and chronic transfusion related iron overload. Liver, heart, endocrine organs, joints, and skin are the most common organs affected leading to chronic liver disease, cirrhosis, heart failure, hypogonadism, pituitary dysfunction, diabetes, arthritis, and bronze discoloration of skin, respectively. Diabetes secondary to deposition of iron in beta cells of pancreas with brown discoloration of skin is also referred to as "Bronze diabetes" [5–8].

Hemochromatosis has been classified into primary (hereditary) and secondary. Primary hemochromatosis is autosomal recessive disorder seen in approximately 95% cases. It results from mutations of the HFE gene on chromosome 6. This gene regulates hepcidin which is involved in regulation of iron metabolism. Hepcidin controls iron absorption. Normally, it is up-regulated when iron stores are elevated and prevents excessive iron absorption and storage. Due to mutation in gene which regulates hepcidin, there is increased iron absorption from the gastrointestinal tract, leading to chronic deposition of iron in the tissues. The rest of cases result from mutations in genes coding for the iron regulatory proteins hemojuvelin, transferrin receptor-2, and ferroportin. Based on the types of mutation, hemochromatosis has been classified into 4 types—type 1 to type 4 [9–11].

Secondary hemochromatosis results from chronic hemolytic anemias and ineffective erythropoiesis such as thalassemia, myelodysplasia, etc. where patients receive repeated blood transfusions. Some conditions like alcoholic hepatitis and cirrhosis, long-term hemodialysis, and disease-like porphyria cutanea tarda can predispose to hemochromatosis [6].

Q8. What is the difference between hemochromatosis and hemosiderosis?

The hemochromatosis is the systemic deposition of iron and results in tissue damage, whereas hemosiderosis is only focal deposition of iron that does not cause any tissue damage.

Q9. What are the symptoms and signs of iron overload?

Answer: These include chronic fatigue, arthralgia, abdominal pain, hepatomegaly, hypogonadism, decreased libido, elevated blood glucose levels, hyperpigmentation (bronze skin), and depression [12].

20.3 Quick Information for Practicing Clinicians and Students

References [1–13]:

1. Hemochromatosis should be suspected in patients who are being investigated for anemia and are found to have transferrin saturation greater than 45%. This is the initial test of choice.
2. Hemochromatosis is suggested if persistently elevated transferrin saturation is observed in the absence of other causes of iron overload and should always be considered in the differential diagnosis of patients with elevated liver enzymes and abnormal iron study results.
3. The presence of the C282Y or H63D mutation is tested to confirm the diagnosis of hereditary hemochromatosis and in first degree relatives of diagnosed patients.
4. Hereditary hemochromatosis is usually diagnosed in the fourth or fifth decade of life.
5. Secondary hemochromatosis results from excessive iron deposition due to chronic blood transfusion as in hemoglobinopathies such as sickle cell anemia, thalassemia, sideroblastic anemia, myelodysplasia, and conditions like chronic liver disease and chronic inflammatory disorders including autoimmune diseases.
6. The most commonly involved organs are liver, pancreas, joints, heart, skin, and pituitary glands.
7. Hepatic iron content (liver biopsy or MRI) and cardiac status (ECHO cardiography) are used to assess functions of these organs and for assessment of prognosis in follow-up.
8. Cirrhosis following alcoholic hepatitis, porphyria cutanea tarda, and prolonged hemodialysis are considered predisposing risk factors for hemochromatosis.
9. Continuous alcohol intake, diabetes, high aspartate transaminase levels, and liver iron concentration over 2000 μmol/g increase risk of liver damage.

10. Risk of liver damage and cirrhosis increases If the serum ferritin is greater than 1000 μg/L at diagnosis. There is increased incidence of hepatocellular carcinoma in these patients.
11. Serum ferritin greater than 300 ng/mL in males and greater than 150–200 ng/mL in menstruating females can be indicative of iron overload.
12. Rarely, the patients who develop hyperhemolysis are those receiving chronic frequent blood transfusions and present clinically with fever, jaundice, and pain. The reticulocyte count is low with elevated lactate dehydrogenase and elevated bilirubin. Nucleated red blood cells can be seen on blood films.

To acquire further knowledge on the subject, following sources are advised:

1. BCSH guidelines
2. Br Jr. Hematology
3. ASH education book
4. Blood
5. NEJM
6. Int Jr. Lab Hematology

References

1. Gattermann N. The treatment of secondary hemochromatosis. Dtsch Arztebl Int. 2009;106(30):499–504.
2. Bacon BR, Adams PC, Kowdley KV, Powell LW, Tavill AS. Diagnosis and management of hemochromatosis: 2011 practice guideline by the American Association for the Study of Liver Diseases. Hepatology. 2011;54:328–43.
3. Ramm GA. Hemochromatosis. N Engl J Med. 2022;387(23):2159–70.
4. Pietrangelo A. Haemochromatosis. Gut. 2003;52(90002):1123–30.
5. Waalen J, Felitti VJ, Gelbart T, Beutler E. Screening for hemochromatosis by measuring ferritin levels: a more effective approach. Blood. 2008;111(7):3373–6.
6. McLaren GD, Muir WA, Kellermeyer RW. Iron overload disorders: natural history, pathogenesis, diagnosis, and therapy. Crit Rev Clin Lab Sci. 1983;19(3):205–66.
7. Lu JP. Selective iron deposition in pancreatic islet B cells of transfusional iron-overloaded autopsy cases. Pathol Int. 1994;44(3):194–9.
8. Pietrangelo A. Hereditary hemochromatosis: pathogenesis, diagnosis, and treatment. Gastroenterology. 2010;139(2):393–408. https://doi.org/10.1053/j.gastro.2010.06.013.
9. Queiroz-Andrade M, Blasbalg R, Ortega CD, et al. MR imaging findings of iron overload. Radiographics. 2009;29:1575–89.
10. Brandhagen DJ, Fairbanks VF, Batts KP, Thibodeau SN. Update on hereditary hemochromatosis and the HFE gene. Mayo Clin Proc. 1999;74(9):917–21.
11. Arthur CA, Howard LH, Robert JG. Secondary hemochromatosis: I. Transfusion (exogenous) hemochromatosis. Blood. 1953;8(9):824–36.
12. McLaren GD, McLaren CE, Adams PC, et al. Hemochromatosis and iron overload screen (HEIRS) study research investigators. Clinical manifestations of hemochromatosis in HFE C282Y homozygotes identified by screening. Can J Gastroenterol. 2008;22(11):923–30.
13. Banks M, Shikle J. Hyperhemolysis Syndrome in Patients With Sickle Cell Disease. Arch Pathol Lab Med. 2018;142:1425–7.

Chapter 21
Sickle Cell Anemia and Related Hemoglobinopathies

A 4-year-old male child was brought to pediatric casualty with complains of severe pain in legs and arms. He had mild fever for the last 2 days due to upper respiratory tract infection for which a local practitioner had prescribed antibiotics. The mother informed that the child had been suffering from repeated infections for the last 2 years with poor weight gain and was feeling excessively tired after playing with progressively decreasing stamina for physical activities. Also he was looking pale and was complaining of abdominal and bony pains in hands and feet off and on. Child was being given oral supplements with proteins and vitamins. Their socio-economic status was good. The father had been diagnosed as a case of sickle cell trait during his young age. The mother was never investigated for anemia.

Examination revealed pallor and mild icterus. Mild tachycardia and tachypnoea were observed. There was no organomegaly or evidence of delayed growth.

A CBC done at presentation is given below (Table 21.1).

A. Gupta, *Decision Making Through Problem Based Learning in Hematology*, https://doi.org/10.1007/978-981-99-8933-1_21

Table 21.1 CBC

CBC parameter	Patient's result	Reference range
WBC	6.2	3.7–10 × 10^9/L
RBC	3.10	4.5–5.4 × 10^{12}/L
HB	88	130–160 g/L
Hct	0.26	0.33–0.43 L/L
MCV	92	83–101 fL
MCH	29	27–32 pg
MCHC	320	315–345 g/L
RDW	18	11.6–14.6%
PLT	300	130–430 × 10^9/L
MPV	10	7–11 fL
Poly#	3.8	1.7–6 × 10^9/L
Lymp#	1.2	1–3 × 10^9/L
Mono#	0.6	0.2–1.0 × 10^9/L
EO#	0.6	0.02–0.5 × 10^9/L
BASO#	00	0.02–0.1 × 10^9/L
RETIC%	9.0	0.5–1.5%
Absolute ret count	390	50–150 × 10^9/L
ESR	25	0–20 mm 1st h Westergren

21.1 Questions

Q1. Interpret the CBC result given above and suggest investigations for further evaluation in such case

Answer: The CBC result shows anemia (low values for red cells, hemoglobin, and hematocrit), reticulocytosis, and elevated ESR. The values for MCV, MCH, and MCHC are normal. RDW is slightly high. ESR is slightly higher than normal.

So, there is normocytic normochromic anemia with reticulocytosis. Causes of normocytic normochromic anemia with reticulocytosis in this age-group include: [1, 2].

1. Hemolytic anemias
2. Bleeding
3. Splenomegaly.

Examination has excluded splenomegaly as a cause. The hemolytic anemias presenting in this age-group include:

1. RBC membrane defects (i.e., HS HE),
2. Inherited defects of hemoglobin (i.e., thalassemia and structural hemoglobinopathies)
3. Enzyme deficiencies (i.e., G6PD and PK).
4. Also autoimmune hemolytic anemia and microangiopathic hemolytic anemia including disseminated intravascular coagulation (DIC) can present with normocytic normochromic anemia with reticulocytosis.

All causes of hypoplastic/aplastic anemia are excluded as reticulocyte count is high. Rarely bone marrow infiltration can have similar red cell parameters.

The next best tests will be to examine a blood film and do biochemical tests to establish hemolytic pathology (total and indirect bilirubin, LDH, haptoglobin). Routine examination of urine and stools are also recommended.

Q2. Given are images from blood film (Figs. 21.1 and 21.2), results biochemical tests with hemolytic profile (Table 21.2) and urine and stool examination (Table 21.3. What is interpretation and which further investigations will be required to arrive at final diagnosis?

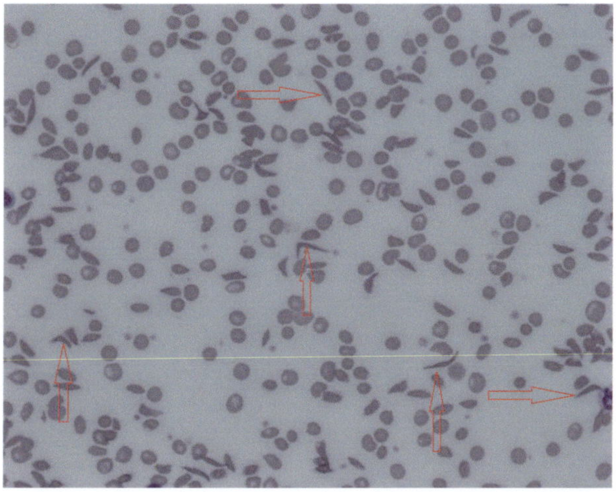

Fig. 21.1 Peripheral blood film. Low red cell density and sickle cells. Leishman stain × 40

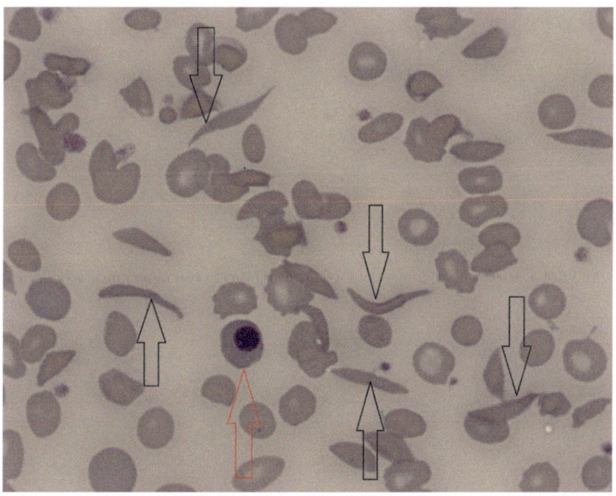

Fig. 21.2 Peripheral blood film. Sickle cells (black arrows) and nucleated red cell (red arrow). Leishman stain × 100

Table 21.2 Biochemical tests

Test	Patient's result	Ref range
Glu	4.5	3.9–6.1 mmol/L
Urea	2.9	2.5–6.6 mmol/L
Creat	90	60–120 μmol/L
Na^+	139	136–146 mmol/L
K^+	4.5	3.7–5.0 mmol/L
Ca^+	2.3	2.2–2.6 mmol/L
Mg^+	1	0.08–1.1 mmol/L
T. Prot	68	63–80 mmol/L
Alb	37	35–47 mmol/L
Choles	2.5	1.5–5.2 mmol/L
TG	0.9	0.4–1.7 mmol/L
Urates	370	150–400 mmol/L
T Bil	48	3–20 μmol/L
D. Bil	5	0–5 μmol/L
I Bil	43	5–15 μmol/L
Alk Ph	41	26–88 IU/L
ALT	54	10–60 IU/L
AST	32	10–42 IU/L
GGT	20	7–64 IU/L
LDH	290	90–180 IU/L
Hapto	0.01	0.2–2.0 g/L
T4	10.6	7.8–16 pmol/L
TSH	3.99	0.27–4.2 μIU/mL
Amylase	20	28–100 IU/L
Lipase	30	0–160 U/L

Table 21.3 Urine and stool examination

Urine examination	Patient's result	Reference range
SG	1.020	1.005–1.030
Ph	6	5–7
Leu	Neg	Neg
Nit	Neg	Neg
Pro	Neg	Neg
Glu	Neg	Neg
Ket	Neg	Neg
Uro	Positive	Neg
Bil	Neg	Neg
Hemosiderin	Positive	Neg
Stool examination		
Occult blood	Neg	Neg
Ova/cysts	Neg	Neg

Answer: The peripheral blood smears show low density of red cells, anisopoikilocytosis with few ovalocytes, few fragmented cells, and many sickle-shaped cells. One nucleated red cell is also seen. The biochemical tests show indirect hyperbilirubinemia, high LDH, and reduced haptoglobin. The urine examination shows urobilinogen and hemosiderin. There is no hematuria. Stool examination is normal.

All these findings suggest a diagnosis of sickle cell anemia with hemolytic crisis. For confirmation of SCD, hemoglobin analysis is required.

Q3. Given is image from hemoglobin analysis by capillary electrophoresis Sebia (Fig. 21.3)). Interpret the result and suggest final diagnosis.

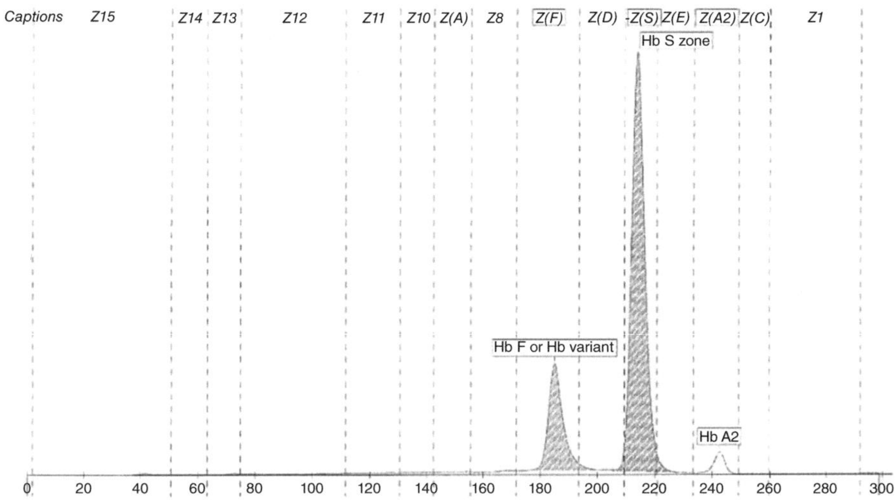

Fig. 21.3 Hb electrophoresis. SCA. Capillary electrophoresis. HbS 80%, HbF 17.9%, HbA2 2.1%

Answer: The result shows a prominent band in region of sickle hemoglobin calculated as 80%. In addition, there is also slightly raised HbF (17.9%). The HbA2 is within normal range. A diagnosis of sickle cell anemia (SCA) is confirmed.

Q4. What investigations are usually performed in SCA patients and how do these help in subsequent management?

Answer: The following tests are sensitive in identifying affected individuals. For definite diagnosis and differentiation of HbSS from HbS/β^0-thalassemia, genetic studies are required [3–9].

1. Sickling test: A positive sickling test is useful to differentiate Hb-S from Hb-D and Hb-G. It is not reliable if Hb-S is below 20%. False negative can be seen in patients with low Hb or following transfusion.
2. Hb A2 measurement by microcolumn chromatography: Done if microcytosis is present and there is possibility of coexistent beta-thalassemia. However, it is not always reliable to distinguish sickle cell/B^0 thalassemia because many times there is interaction with alfa-thalassemia. Genetic studies and family screening are more helpful.
3. Hb electrophoresis using alkaline and acid gels. These are getting obsolete now. Alkaline gel does not distinguish between hemoglobin variants such as HbD and HbG, which co-migrate with HbS. Similarly, HbE and Hb 0-Arab have identical migration pattern to Hb C molecules. However, many of these variants can be separated effectively using citrate agar electrophoresis. In presence of different Hb variants, capillary zone electrophoresis is even better than HPLC for quantifying HbA2.
4. HPLC: High pressure liquid chromatography is used to detect and quantify HbF, Hb A2, HbS, HbC, Hb Barts, and other Hb variants. It detects different types of hemoglobin based on the retention time.
5. Isoelectrophoresis: It is available in select laboratories This method can analyze whole blood samples and dried blood spots for analysis. This technique can detect HbS and HbA easily in a high concentration of HbF. It separates Hb D-Punjab from HbS.
6. Globin chain electrophoresis: This method can be used to assess which chain is effected (alfa-, beta, or gamma).
7. Genetic studies: These can assess homozygous or heterozygous state in combination with another hemoglobin mutation. Genetic studies of patient and family screening are quite helpful for management.
8. Grouping, antibody screening, red cell phenotyping, and HLA typing: These are required as the patient has to receive repeated blood transfusions and is also necessary if bone marrow transplant is considered.

In laboratories where advanced tests are not available, sickling test, HB electrophoresis on alkaline and acid gel, HPLC and HbA2 estimation by microcolumn chromatography are performed.

Q5. What is etiology of SCA?

Answer: Adult hemoglobin is made of two alfa- and two beta chains. The beta chains are controlled by genes on chromosome 11. Sickle cell disease is caused by a single base-pair point mutation (GAG to GTG) which results in substitution of the amino acid glutamic acid to Valine at sixth position of the beta chain. Both homozygous and compound heterozygote inheritance of a mutation in the beta chain can be seen. If the inheritance is homozygous (both alleles affected, i.e., HbS/HbS)), it is termed as sickle cell anemia (SCA-SS). This is the most common form of SCD. The next most common form is the co-inheritance of HbS and HbC (HbS/HbC). In other situations, there can be co-inheritance with beta-thalassemia (HbS/beta^{o} or HbS/beta^{+}). HbS/beta^{0} is usually as severe as homozygous SCA (HbS/HbS). However, those with HbS/beta^{+} thalassemia have mild to moderate phenotypes [10].

Q6. What is the pathogenesis of symptoms of SCA and how these mechanisms are related to complications?

Answer: Under normal de-oxygenated state in peripheral circulation, hemoglobin undergoes conformal change that enables binding of hemoglobin with carbon dioxide molecules. But under same conditions, hemoglobin S undergoes polymerization and becomes rigid. These rigid red cells obstruct the smaller blood vessels thus compromising blood flow to tissues resulting in ischemia, hypoxia, subsequent infarction, and ultimately organ damage. These rigid cells have reduced life span of 10–20 days as they undergo hemolysis. Hypoxia reduced nitric acid production and presence of free hemoglobin mop up the nitric oxide in circulation. Normally, nitric oxide acts as a vasodilator. Its reduction results in less relaxation of blood vessels which adds to vaso-occlusion. All these factors are responsible for symptoms, signs, and complications such as leg ulceration, stroke, pulmonary hypertension, and priapism [12].

Q7. What are the symptoms and signs of SCA?

Answer:

1. Vaso-occlusive crisis: Painful crises is the most common clinical manifestation of SCD and results from ischemia, necrosis, edema, and stimulation of nerve endings at these sites. Pain is triggered by dehydration, fever, infections, or sudden change in weather. Sites of pain are abdomen, bones, joints, and soft tissue. Repeated episodes result in organ damage like splenic infarction (auto splenectomy), liver infarcts, and papillary necrosis of kidneys.[13].
2. Anemia: All patients develop symptoms of anemia [14].
3. Infection: Patients are more susceptible to bacterial infections due to hyposplenism resulting from autosplenectomy which is due to repeated episodes of sickling and splenic infarction. The organisms are streptococcus pneumoniae, haemophilus influenzae, Neisseria meningitides, and salmonella. In addition, complement defects, neutrophil dysfunction, and defective opsonization also play a role in predisposition to infection. Respiratory infections can trigger the sickle cell acute chest syndrome [15, 16].
4. Aplastic crises: Parvovirus B-19 infects RBC progenitors in bone marrow, resulting in reduced cell division and is associated with fever, malaise, and a rash (Fifth disease). The condition is self-limiting [17].
5. Splenic sequestration: It occurs most frequently during the first 5 years of life and is characterized by the onset of life-threatening anemia with rapid enlargement of the spleen. It is a medical emergency [14].

6. Hand-foot syndrome: It is characterized by pain and soft tissue swelling of the dorsum of the hands and feet. It develops suddenly and lasts for 1–2 weeks. [18].
7. Acute chest syndrome: It is characterized by chest pain, fever, cough, tachypnea, leukocytosis, and pulmonary infiltrates in the lungs. Infections, pulmonary infraction, and fat embolism are some of the predisposing factors. Acute chest syndrome is a medical emergency [15].

21.2 Correlation of Results of Preliminary Investigations with Symptoms and Signs in SCA and Related Hemoglobinopathies

Q8. Correlate the symptoms and signs of SCA with symptoms in this patient.

Answer: This patient had presented with complains of severe pain in legs and arms suggesting vaso-occlusive crises. He had fever due to upper respiratory tract infection, which was possibly the precipitating factor. In past, he had complains of abdominal and bony pains in hands and feet, which were also possibly due to mild to moderate vaso-occlusion. The child was suffering from repeated infections for the last 2 years most likely due to functional hyposplenia. He had poor weight gain and had history of progressively decreasing stamina for physical activities, suggesting effect of anemia. Examination had revealed pallor, mild icterus, tachycardia, and tachypnoea, all these features are suggestive of anemia. The father had been diagnosed with sickle cell trait during his young age. This is a clue to hereditary causes of anemia, most likely SCD.

All these observations in our patient correlate well with classical symptoms of SCA with vaso-occlusive crises and hemolytic anemia.

Q9. How do the results of investigations done in this case correlate with diagnosis of SCA?

Answer: CBC showed anemia and reticulocytosis. The peripheral blood smears confirmed normocytic normochromic anemia with few fragmented and many sickle shaped cells. One nucleated red cell was also seen. The biochemical tests showed indirect hyper-bilirubinemia, high LDH, and reduced haptoglobin. The urine examination showed urobilinogen and hemosiderin. All these findings correlate well with intravascular hemolytic process in sickle cell anemia.

The result of capillary electrophoresis showed a prominent band in region of sickle hemoglobin calculated at 80% which confirmed the diagnosis of sickle cell anemia (SCA).

**Subsequently, the Hb analysis of parents showed that both father and mother had sickle cell traits.*

Q10. Both parents of this patient had sickle cell trait. How does this disease transmit to offsprings?

Answer: SCA is hemoglobinopathy which results from altered structure of hemoglobin molecule. Its inheritance is autosomal recessive. If both parents have sickle cell trait (HbAS):

Chances of child being SCA-25% (1/4).
Chances of child being normal-25% (1/4).
Chance of child being sickle cell trait-50% (2/4).

Q11. What are long-term complications in patients with SCA?
Answer:

1. Cholelithiasis: It is due to chronic hemolysis with hyper-bilirubinemia.
2. Central nervous system involvement: The manifestation includes stroke, resulting in varying degrees of neurological deficit effecting 10–30% cases. Hemiparesis, convulsions, and silent infarcts are some of other complications.
3. Many other complications with lesser incidence are cardiac involvement (dilated chambers), renal involvement (papillary necrosis and isosthenuria), eye involvement (proliferative retinitis), leg ulcers, priapism, avascular necrosis of the femoral or humeral head, and pulmonary hypertension [19].

Q12. What is genotypic-phenotypic correlation in cases of SCD?
Answer: [20–22].

1. The SCA is homozygous SS state (Hb SS) with over 50% HbS. There is no HbA. However, HbF may or may not be elevated. HbA2 is in normal range.
2. Sickle cell trait is the heterozygous carrier state (HbAS) with HbS less than 50% and HbA more than 50% (usually in ratio of 40:60).
3. HbS can exist in combination with other hemoglobinopathies in a double heterozygous state such as beta^0 or beta$^+$ thalassemia, Hb D, Hb G, Hb C, Hb E, Hb, O-Arab, etc.

Table 21.4 shows genotype-phenotype correlation when SCA is associated with other hemoglobinopathies.

Table 21.4 Association of SCD with other hemoglobinopathies

Genotype	Phenotype
HbS/beta^0 thalassemia	Similar to SCD but is slightly less severe
HbS/beta$^+$ thalassemia	Similar to SCD but is milder
Hb S/D disease	Mild to severe hemolytic anemia but overall less severe as compared to Hb SS
Hb S/G disease	Mostly asymptomatic (Philadelphia)
Hb S/C disease	Milder sickling disorder
Hb S/E disease	Milder than SCA—it may present with vaso-occlusive crisis (VOC) in the setting of precipitating factors

Q13. What is the approximate concentration of different types of hemoglobins required for diagnosis of hemoglobinopathies?

Answer: Percentage of hemoglobin required for diagnosis of different types of hemoglobinopathies are summarized below (Table 21.5) [20, 23–27].

Table 21.5 Distribution of types of hemoglobin in various sickle cell hemoglobinopathies

Hb variant	Hb A %	HbA2%	HbF%	HBS%	HBE%	HBC%	HBD%
Normal	95–98	2–3	<2				
HBSS	0	2–4	2–15	80–90			
HbAS	50–60	<3.5	<2	35–45			
HbS/B^0thal	0	>3.5	2–15	80–90			
HbS/B^+thal	5–30	>3.5	2–10	65–90			
HbS/HbC	0	<3.5	1–8	45–50		45–50	
HbS/HbD	0	<3.5	1–8	45–50			45–50
HbS/HbE	0	2–4	<2	60	30		

Q14. What are the molecular defects in major structural hemoglobinopathies?

Answer: Molecular defects in common structural hemoglobinopathies are summarized below (Table 21.6) [4, 10, 20, 21, 26, 27].

Table 21.6 Molecular defects in hemoglobinopathies

Molecular defect	Hemoglobinopathy
Beta^{6} Glu > Val	HbS
Beta^{6} Glu > lys	HbC
Beta^{26} Glu > lys	HbE
Beta^{121}Glu > Gln	HbD
Alfa^{68}Asn > Lys	Hb G-Philadelphia
Beta^{121}Glu > Lys	Hb O-Arab

Q15. Which heterozygous states associated with sickle cell disease have severe phenotypes?

Answer: Hb S/D disease, Hb S/beta^0 thalassemia, Hb S/C disease, hemoglobin S/O--Arab and HbS/Lepore diseases are more severe than other combinations.

Q16. What are the fundamental changes and diagnostic features in sickle cell trait (SCT)?

Answer: [2, 4, 8, 20, 26].

The sickle cell trait is milder form of sickle cell disease with same defect as in SCA, i.e., there is substitution of glutamic acid to valine due to mutation at position of sixth amino acid in beta chain. The patients are asymptomatic and are detected mostly when they have concomitant pathological conditions which require investigations for anemia or in situations like severe infections, extremes of exercise at high altitude or flying for long times in unpressurized airplanes. The CBC and blood films are usually normal. Sickling test is positive and confirmation requires Hb electrophoresis. Given below is hemoglobin electrophoresis result of a 15 years old patient with sickle cell trait (Fig. 21.4), diagnosed at time of hospital admission for high grade fever. The sickle hemoglobin is 35% (less than 50%) and adult hemoglobin 62.5%.

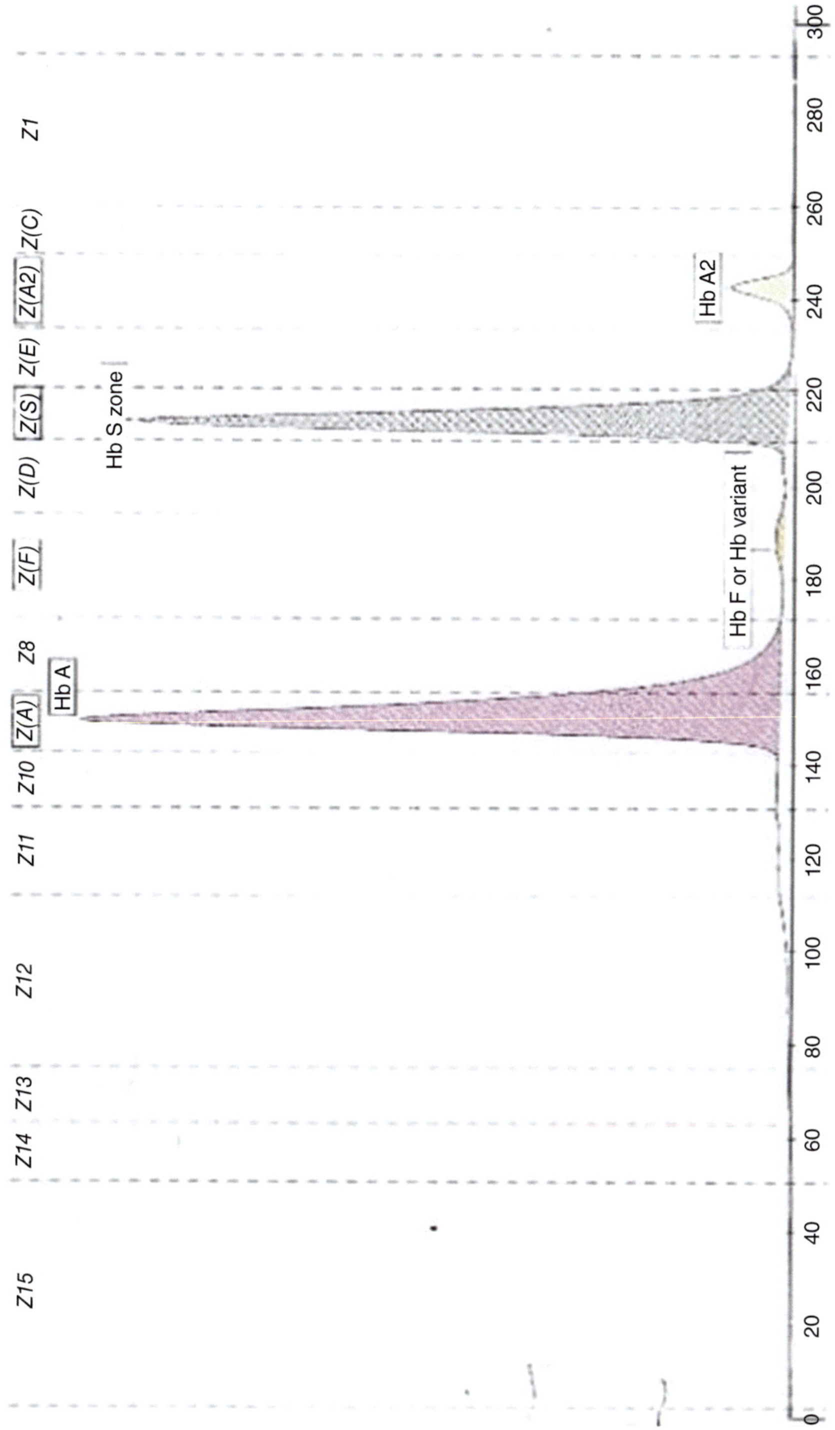

Fig. 21.4 Hemoglobin electrophoresis. Sickle cell trait. Capillary electrophoresis

Q17. A 3-year-old child is being investigated for anemia. Results of CBC (Table 21.7), blood film (Fig. 21.5), and Hb electrophoresis (Fig. 21.6) are presented below. Interpret the results and comment on salient features of the disease.

Table 21.7 CBC

CBC parameter	Patient's result	Reference range
WBC	5.4	3.7–10 × 10^9/L
RBC	5.72	4.5–5.4 × 10^{12}/L
HB	11	110–140 g/L
Hct	0.33	0.33–0.43 L/L
MCV	60	83–101 fL
MCH	19	27–32 pg
MCHC	325	315–345 g/L
RDW	16	11.6–14.6%
PLT	183	130–430 × 10^9/L
MPV	9	7–11 fL
Poly#	2.0	1.7–6 × 10^9/L
Lymp#	2.9	1–3 × 10^9/L
Mono#	0.4	0.2–1.0 × 10^9/L
EO#	0.1	0.02–0.5 × 10^9/L
BASO#	00	0.02–0.1 × 10^9/L
RETIC%	2.8	0.5–1.5%
Absolute ret count	280	50–150 10^{12}/L
ESR	29	0–20 mm 1st h Westergren

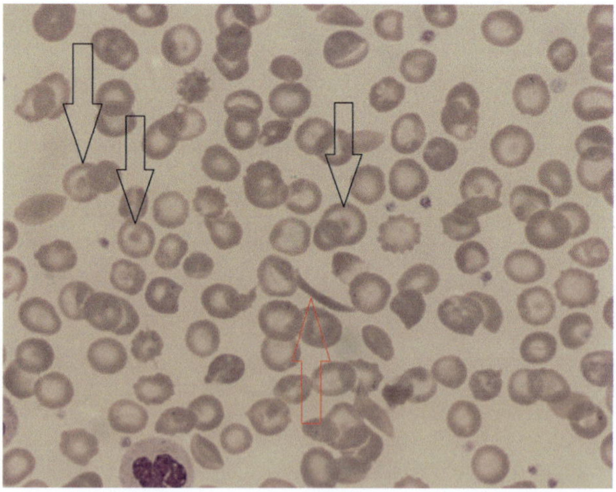

Fig. 21.5 PBF. SCA-thalassemia. Sickle cell, target cells with many microcytic hypochromic red cells

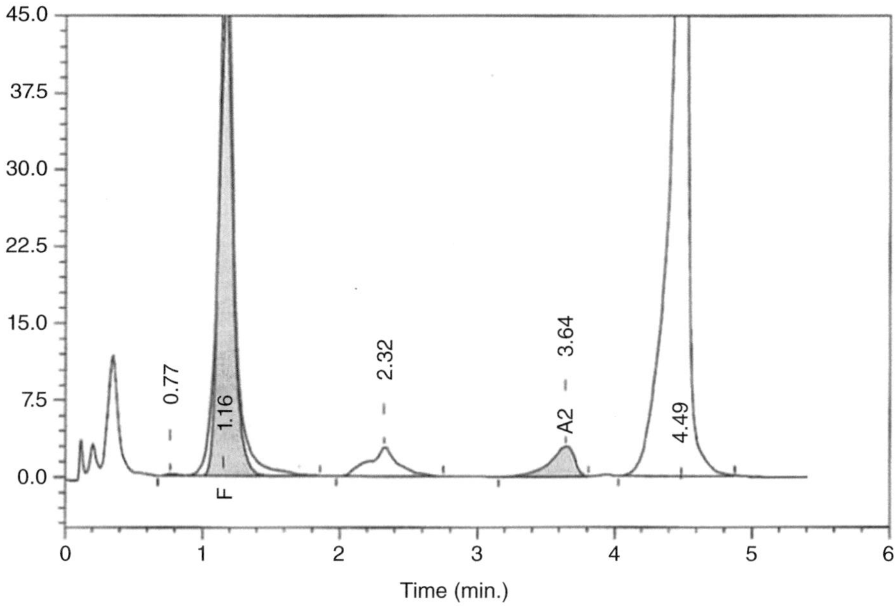

Fig. 21.6 Hemoglobin electrophoresis. Sickle cell/beta^0 thalassemia

Answer: The CBC shows microcytic hypochromic anemia with disproportionally increased red cell count (this combination is suggestive of thalassemia). There is mild reticulocytosis also. The blood film shows microcytic hypochromic red cells with few target cells (component of thalassemia) and few sickle cells. The Hb electrophoresis shows prominent bands at position of Hb F and HbS. There is no HbA. These findings correlate well with diagnosis of sickle cell- beta^0 thalassemia (Hb S/B^0 thalassemia).

Hb S/beta^0 thalassemia has phenotype similar to SCD but is slightly less severe. There is compound heterozygosity with one gene having structural defect (hemoglobin S) while the other has absent beta chain production (beta^0). The lower values for MCV and MCH differentiate this condition from homozygous SCD [2, 20, 22].

In some situations, the function of beta gene is not totally knocked out and some quantity of beta chain is still produced. So there will be some production of HbA. Such cases are labeled as HbS- beta$^+$ thalassemia. Further confirmation may be done through molecular genetic analysis. Given below (Fig. 21.7) is Hb electrophoresis done on patient with anemia, decreased MCV and MCH, and mild reticulocytosis.

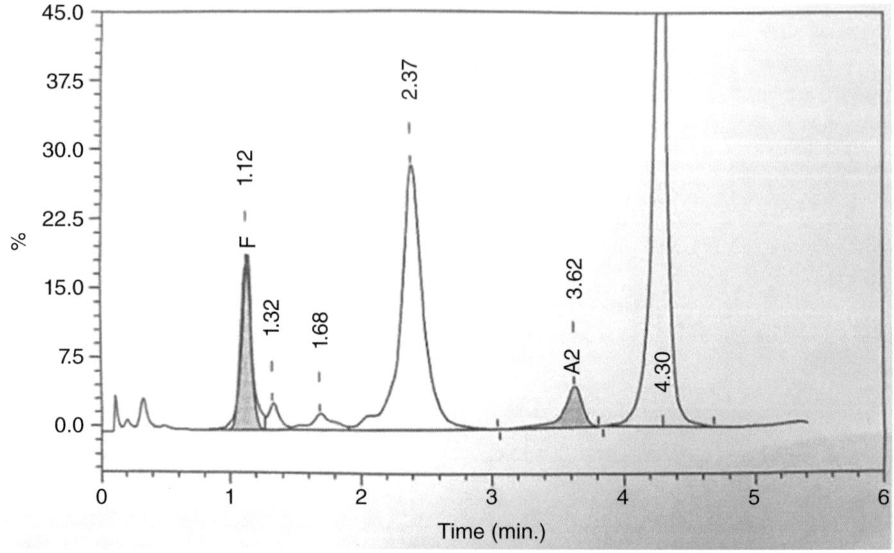

Fig. 21.7 Hemoglobin electrophoresis. Sickle cell/ beta + thalassemia

The electrophoresis shows prominent band at position of HbA, HbS, HbA2, and HbF. HbA is 38%, and HbS is 47.6%, in addition to slightly raised HbF (10%) and HbA2 (4.4%). Since this patient has low MCV and MCV, the diagnosis should be sickle cell / beta$^+$ thalassemia [20, 25–27].

Q18. A 14-year-old boy is being investigated for anemia with biochemical evidence of hemolysis (raised LDH and indirect bilirubin). Results of CBC (Table 21.8) and Hb electrophoresis (Fig. 21.8) are presented below. Interpret the results and comment on salient features of the disease.

Table 21.8 CBC

CBC parameter	Patient's result	Reference range
WBC	9.9	3.7–10 × 10^9/L
RBC	4.2	4.5–5.4 × 10^{12}/L
HB	99	110–140 g/L
Hct	0.29	0.33–0.43 L/L
MCV	88	83–101 fL
MCH	30	27–32 pg
MCHC	341	315–345 g/L
RDW	21	11.6–14.6%
PLT	295	130–430 × 10^9/L
MPV	10	7–11 fL
Poly#	4.0	1.7–6 × 10^9/L
Lymp#	4.7	1–3 × 10^9/L
Mono#	0.1	0.2–1.0 × 10^9/L
EO#	0.1	0.02–0.5 × 10^9/L
BASO#	00	0.02–0.1 × 10^9/L
RETIC%	3.6	0.5–1.5%
Absolute ret count	870	50–150 × 10^{12}/L

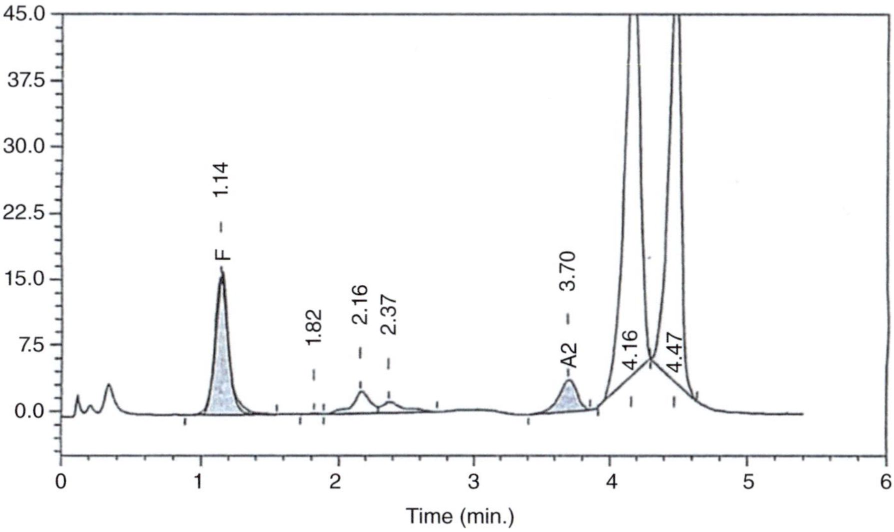

Fig. 21.8 Hemoglobin electrophoresis. Hemoglobin SD disease

Answer: The CBC shows normocytic normochromic anemia with reticulocytosis. The Hb- electrophoresis shows prominent bands at position of HbD (44%), HbS (39%), and Hb F (13.4%). There is no HbA. These findings correlate well with diagnosis of hemoglobin SD disease.

Hemoglobin SD disease is compound heterozygous state with both genes having structural abnormality-one gene with HbS (Beta^{6} Glu > Val) while the other has HbD (Beta^{121}Glu > Gln). Since both beta genes are defective, no normal HbA is produced. These compound heterozygotes are slightly less severe as compared to homozygous HbS, with clinical presentation of chronic hemolytic anemia and episodes of crises [28].

There are different variants of HbD and in double heterozygous state with HbS, the pattern of disease depicts much variability. HbD especially HbD Punjab (and Hb Los Angeles) is most important as it results in severe disease. HbS in combination with HbD-Ibadan is asymptomatic [29].

Other variants like HbD-Iran and Hb Korle-Bu are harmless. (Capillary electrophoresis is better way for their separation).

Q19. What are the common clinical presentations when HbS is seen in combination with HB-C, HB-E, HB-G, and HB-O Arab?

Answer: In Hb C, glutamic acid of the β-globin chain is replaced by lysine at sixth position. Hemoglobin C in combination with HbS (heterozygous SC disease) produces milder phenotype than pure SCD. The anemia is less severe, and Hb levels may be in normal range. Complications like avascular necrosis, hematuria, and proliferative retinopathy can occur. Blood film will show few sickle cells in addition to target cells, rod-like crystals, and boat-shaped cells. Hb electrophoresis will establish the diagnosis with bands at both HbS and HbC positions [26].

Combined heterozygosity for hemoglobin S and E (hemoglobin SE disease) is very rare benign clinical condition. There is HbS (beta ^{6} Glu to Val) and Hb E (Beta^{26} Glu > lys). Clinical manifestations include episodes of vaso-occlusion, hemolytic anemia, bone infarction, gallstones, and hematuria. Patients have mild anemia. HPLC will show bands in position of HBS (approximately 60–65%) and HBE (30–35%) [20, 26].

Hemoglobin S/O(Arab) disease is also a rare compound heterozygous disease in which there is HbS (beta^{6} Glu to Val) and Hb O- Arab (beta^{121} Glu to Lys). Patients have hemolytic anemia with episodes of recurrent vaso-occlusive events and can have complications like acute chest syndrome, dactylitis, gallstones, nephropathy, aplastic crises, avascular necrosis, and leg ulcers. The peripheral blood smear shows sickle cells, target cells, and polychromasia. Hb electrophoresis will show bands in position of Hb S and Hb O. Demonstration of ^{121}Glu to Lys on beta chain confirms the diagnosis [30].

The G-Philadelphia is a rare α-globin chain variant. Double heterozygous state HbG-Philadelphia/S trait is very rare. The clinical phenotype resembles HbS/ beta+ thalassemia or sickle cell trait. Hb electrophoresis will show bands in position of HbS and HbG. The demonstration of substitution of lysine for asparagine at position 68 of the α-globin chain is diagnostic for hemoglobin G-Philadelphia (alfa 68 Asn → Lys) [31].

21.3 Quick Information for Practicing Clinicians and Students

References [1–33]:

1. SCA (HbSS- homozygous form of SCD) is the most common form of structural hemoglobinopathy and shows phenotypic variation in clinical presentation.
2. The next most common form of SCD is the co-inheritance with HbS and HbC.
3. Co-inheritance of *HbS with beta^0 thalassemia* has a severe course of disease similar to homozygous HbSS patients.
4. SCA red cells are normocytic normochromic. Presence of microcytosis with or without hypochromia suggests presence of thalassemia or other structural hemoglobinopathy, if iron deficiency is excluded.
5. Alkaline gel does not distinguish between hemoglobin variants such as HbD and HbG, which co-migrate with HbS. Similarly, HbE and Hb 0-Arab have identical migration pattern to Hb C molecules.
6. HPLC and capillary electrophoresis are able to identify majority of clinically significant abnormal hemoglobins variants.
7. In presence of different Hb variants, capillary zone electrophoresis is even better than HPLC for quantifying HbA2.
8. In laboratories where advanced tests are not available, sickling test, HB electrophoresis on alkaline and acid gel, HPLC and HbA2 estimation by microcolumn chromatography are performed.
9. Genetic studies of patient and family screening are quite helpful for management.
10. Vaso-occlusive crisis: Painful crises are the most common clinical manifestation.
11. Pain is triggered by dehydration, fever, infections, or sudden change in weather.
12. Respiratory infections can trigger the sickle cell acute chest syndrome.
13. Splenic sequestration and acute chest syndromes are medical emergencies.
14. Indications of hemoglobin testing include:

    (a) Microcytic hypochromic anemia with reticulocytosis after iron deficiency has been ruled out.
    (b) Vascular obliteration crises of unknown cause in regions where HbS and/or HbC are widespread.
    (c) Testing of family members, diagnosis of partners for genetic counseling, prenatal diagnosis.
    (d) Investigate cause of hydrops fetalis.
    (e) Chronic non-spherocytic hemolytic anemia

To acquire further knowledge on the subject, following sources are advised:

1. BCSH guidelines
2. Br Jr. Hematology
3. ASH education book
4. Blood
5. NEJM
6. Int Jr. Lab Hematology

References

1. Shah A. Acquired hemolytic anemia. Indian J Med Sci. 2004;58:533–6.
2. Haley K. Congenital hemolytic anemia. Med Clin North Am. 2017;101:361–74.
3. Reddy MN, Franciosi RA. Rapid quantitation of hemoglobin S by isoelectric focusing. Ann Clin Lab Sci. 1994;24:401–6.
4. Clark BE, Thein SL. Molecular diagnosis of haemoglobin disorders. Clin Lab Haematol. 2004;26:159–76.
5. Kalita D, Singh S, Kudesia M, Mendiratta S, Mittal M, Mathur A. Detection of abnormal Hemoglobin variants by HPLC method: common problems with suggested solutions. Int Sch Res Not. 2014;2014:1–10.
6. Diggs LW, Naumann HN, Diggs BM. A solubility test for sickle cell-Hemoglobin. Lab Med. 1975;6:38–41.
7. Rentapalli B, Gade J, Dawood Sulemani D, Ganji SB, Kiranmai P, Revupalli S, Kavali S, Ramtenki A. Agar gel alkaline electrophoresis as A cost effective screening modality for abnormal Hemoglobins. IOSR J Dent Med Sci. 2017;16:39–43.
8. Hughes J. Comparison of electrophoresis on citrate agar, cellulose acetate, or starch for Hemoglobin identification system. Clin Chem. 1975;1076:1072–6.
9. Chen FTA, Liu CM, Hsieh YZ, Sternberg JC. Capillary electrophoresis—A new clinical tool. Clin Chem. 1991;37:14–9.
10. Steinberg MH. Genetic etiologies for phenotypic diversity in sickle cell anemia. Sci World J. 2009;9:46–67.
11. Manwani D, Frenette PS. Vaso-occlusion in sickle cell disease: pathophysiology and novel targeted therapies. Blood. 2013;122:3892–8.
12. Hebbel RP. Ischemia-reperfusion injury in sickle cell anemia: relationship to acute chest syndrome, endothelial dysfunction, arterial vasculopathy, and inflammatory pain. Hematol Oncol Clin North Am. 2014;28:181–98.
13. De Montalembert M. Management of children with sickle cell anemia: A collaborative work. Arch Pediatr. 2002;9:1195–201.
14. Brousse V, Buffet P, Rees D. The spleen and sickle cell disease: the sick (led) spleen. Br J Haematol. 2014;166:165–76.
15. Booth C, Inusa B, Obaro SK. Infection in sickle cell disease: A review. Int J Infect Dis. 2010;14:e2–e12. https://doi.org/10.1016/j.ijid.2009.03.010.
16. Morrissey BJ, Bycroft TP, Almossawi O, Wilkey OB, Daniels JG. Incidence and predictors of bacterial infection in febrile children with sickle cell disease. Hemoglobin. 2015;39:316–9.
17. Minhas PS, Virdi JK, Patel R. Double whammy-acute splenic sequestration crisis in patient with aplastic crisis due to acute parvovirus infection. J Commun Hosp Int Med Perspect. 2017;7:194–5.
18. Watson RJ, Burko H, Megas H, Robinson M. The hand-foot syndrome in sickle-cell disease in young children. Pediatrics. 1963;31:975–82.
19. Habara A, Steinberg MH. Minireview: genetic basis of heterogeneity and severity in sickle cell disease. Exp Biol Med. 2016;241:689–96.
20. Weatherall DJ, Clegg JB, Higgs DR, Wood WG. The hemoglobinopathies. In: Scriver CR, Beauder AL, Sly WS, Valle D, Mc G-H, editors. The metabolic basis of inherited disease. 8th ed. New York; 2000.
21. Steinberg MH. Sickle cell anemia, the first molecular disease: overview of molecular etiology, pathophysiology, and therapeutic approaches. Sci World J. 2008;8:1295–324.
22. Sichelzellkrankheit DR. Leitlinien Kinderheilkunde und Jugendmedizin. 2006;I:1–7.
23. Bender MA. Sickle cell disease. In: Adam MP, Ardinger HH, Pagon RA, et al., editors. GeneReviews® [internet]. Seattle, WA: University of Washington; 1993–2021.
24. Israr AS, Rabia Z, Imran AS et al. Hematological Parameters and Demographic Distribution of Hemoglobinopathies and Various Hemoglobin Variants. Cureus. 2022;14(12):e33115. Published online 2022. https://doi.org/10.7759/cureus.33115.

25. Kleihauer E, Kohne E, Kulozik AE. Anomale Hämoglobine und Thalassämie-Syndrome Grundlagen und Klinik. Landsberg: Ecomed Verlagsgesellschaft; 1996.
26. Steinberg MH, Forget BG, et al. Disorders of hemoglobin: genetics, pathophysiology and clinical management. Cambridge: Cambridge University Press; 2001. As above Weatherall DJ, Clegg JB, Higgs DR, Wood WG. The hemoglobinopathies. In: Scriver CR, Beauder AL, Sly WS, Valle
27. Olivieri NF. The ß-Thalassemias. N Engl J Med. 1999;341:99–109.
28. Jain RC. Hemoglobin D disease. Am J Clin Pathol. 1971;56:40–2. https://doi.org/10.1093/ajcp/56.1.40.
29. Desai DV, Dhanani H, Shah M, Dayal N, Kapoor A, Yeluri SV. Homozygous hemoglobin D disease: a case report. Internet J Pathol. 2004;3:1.
30. Ibrahim SA, Mustafa D. Sickle-cell haemoglobin O disease in a Sudanese family. Br Med J. 1967;3:715–7.
31. Schwartz HC, Spaet TH, Zuelzer WW, Neel JV, Robinson AR, Kaufman SF. Combinations of Hemoglobin G, Hemoglobin S and thalassemia occurring in one family. Blood. 1957;12:238–50.
32. Dickerhoff R, von Rücker A, Maschmeyer G, Heimpel H. Probleme erwachsener Sichelzellpatienten in Deutschland. Dtsch med Wschr. 2009;134:1179–84.
33. Thomas L. *Labor und diagnose*. 8th ed. Frankfurt: TH-Books Verlagsgesellschaftt; 2011. Hämoglobinopathien

Chapter 22
Non-Sickle Cell Structural Hemoglobinopathies

Case 1 A 9-year-old male child presented with complaints of repeated joint pains in arms and legs and vague abdominal pain for the last 1 week. The mother informed that the child was frequently complaining of these symptoms for the last 6 months for which local practitioner had given analgesics. He was also prone to upper respiratory infections since birth. He was looking pale and was feeling more tired after playing with peers. The family had good socio-economic status. None of the parents or siblings were ever investigated for anemia.

Examination revealed pallor and mild icterus. Mild tachycardia was also observed. Tip of spleen was palpable. A CBC done at presentation is given in Table 22.1.

Table 22.1 CBC

CBC parameter	Patient's result	Reference range
WBC	7.2	3.7–10 × 10^9/L
RBC	4.2	4.5–5.4 × 10^{12}/L
HB	106	130–160 g/L
Hct	0.315	0.33–0.43 L/L
MCV	74	83–101 fL
MCH	24	27–32 pg
MCHC	325	315–345 g/L
RDW	18	11.6–14.6%
PLT	210	130–430 × 10^9/L
MPV	10	7–11 fL
Poly#	3.8	1.7–6 × 10^9/L
Lymp#	2.2	1–3 × 10^9/L
Mono#	0.6	0.2–1.0 × 10^9/L
EO#	0.6	0.02–0.5 × 10^9/L
BASO#	00	0.02–0.1 × 10^9/L
RETIC%	3.5	0.5–1.5%
Absolute ret count	340	50–150 × 10^9/L
ESR	19	0–20 mm 1st h Westergren

A. Gupta, *Decision Making Through Problem Based Learning in Hematology*, https://doi.org/10.1007/978-981-99-8933-1_22

22.1 Questions

Q1. Interpret the CBC result given above and suggest investigations for further evaluation in such case.

Answer: The CBC result shows anemia (low values for red cells, hemoglobin, and hematocrit) and reticulocytosis. Values for MCV and MCH are low. RDW is slightly high.

So, there is mild microcytic hypochromic anemia with reticulocytosis. Causes of microcytic hypochromic anemia include; [1]

1. Iron deficiency, combined iron and B12/folic acid deficiency
2. Thalassemia
3. Sideroblastic anemia
4. Anemia of chronic disorders
5. Lead poisoning

To exclude these possibilities and reach at final diagnosis, further tests required include blood film examination, biochemical tests for liver, kidney, pancreatic functions including tests to establish hemolysis (total and indirect bilirubin, LDH, haptoglobin), serum iron profile, estimation of serum levels of vitamin B12 and folic acid (to exclude dual deficiency), CRP (to exclude anemia due to chronic disorders), hemoglobin electrophoresis (to exclude hemoglobinopathies), and estimation of serum levels of lead will be required. A bone marrow examination will be necessary to evaluate possibility of sideroblastic anemia.

Q2. Given are image from blood film (Fig. 22.1) and results from biochemical tests with hemolytic profile (Table 22.2), urine and stool examination (Table 22.3), serum iron profile and B12/folic acid levels, CRP (Table 22.4), and hemoglobin electrophoresis (Fig. 22.2). Interpret the results and suggest possible diagnosis

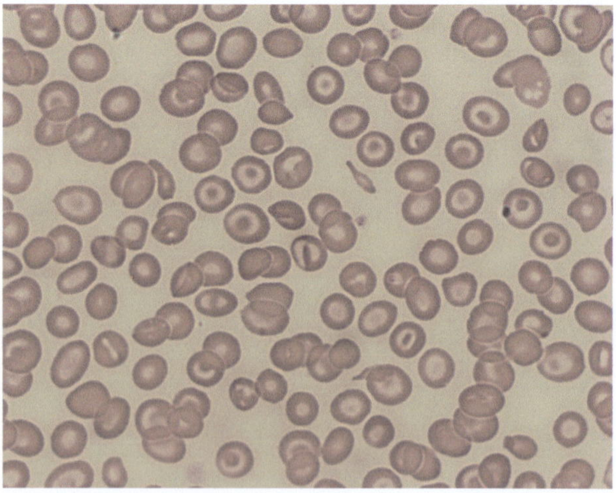

Fig. 22.1 PBF. Peripheral blood film. Microcytic hypochromic cells and many target cells Leishman stain ×100

Table 22.2 Biochemical tests

Test	Patient's result	Ref range
Glu	4.5	3.9–6.1 mmol/L
Urea	2.9	2.5–6.6 mmol/L
Creat	90	60–120 μmol/L
Na^+	139	136–146 mmol/L
K^+	4.5	3.7–5.0 mmol/L
Ca^+	2.3	2.2–2.6 mmol/L
Mg^+	1.0	0.08–1.1 mmol/L
T. Prot	68	63–80 mmol/L
Alb	25	35–47 mmol/L
Choles	2.5	1.5–5.2 mmol/L
TG	0.9	0.4–1.7 mmol/L
Urates	370	150–400 mmol/L
T Bil	37	3–20 μmol/L
D. Bil	6	0–5 μmol/L
I Bil	31	5–15 μmol/L
Alk Ph	41	26–88 IU/L
ALT	54	10–60 IU/L
AST	32	10–42 IU/L
GGT	20	7–64 IU/L
LDH	232	90–180 IU/L
Hapto	0.1	0.2–2.0 g/L
T4	10.6	7.8–16 pmol/L
TSH	3.99	0.27–4.2 μIU/mL

Table 22.3 Urine and stool examination

Urine examination	Patient's result	Reference range
SG	1.020	1.005–1.030
Ph	6	5–7
Leu	Neg	Neg
Nit	Neg	Neg
Pro	Neg	Neg
Glu	Neg	Neg
Ket	Neg	Neg
Uro	Negative	Neg
Bil	Neg	Neg
Hemosiderin	Negative	Neg
Stool examination		
Occult blood	Neg	Neg
Ova/cysts	Neg	Neg

Table 22.4 Serum iron profile, B12, folic acid, and CRP

Test	Patient's result	Ref range
S. Iron	35	11–31 µmol/L
Transferrin	2.9	2.1–3.6 g/L
Trans. sat %	40	20–40%
Ferritin	450	11–307 ng/mL
S. B12	665	150–700 pmol/L
S. folate	31.7	10–42 nmol/L
RBC folate	2554	1187–2854 nmol/L
CRP	9	0–10 mg/L

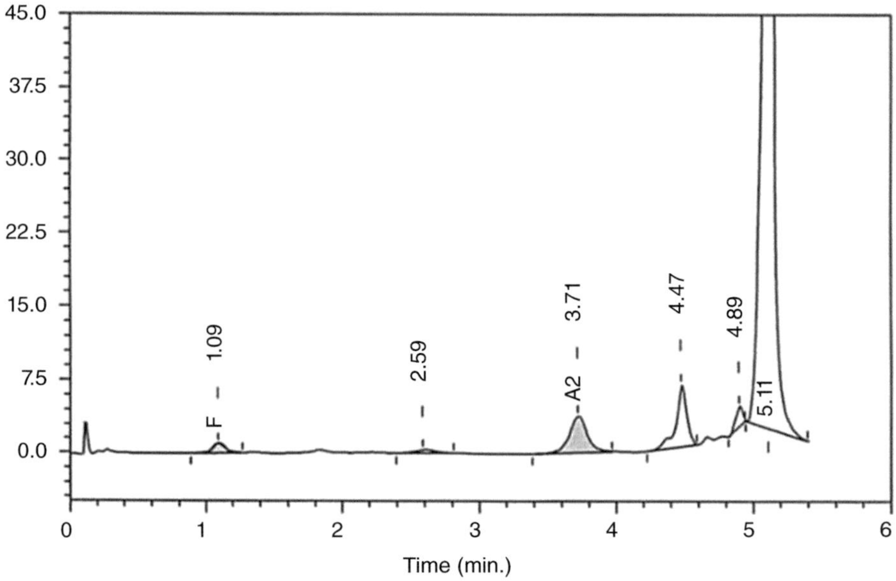

Fig. 22.2 HPLC. Biorad variant V-II: Hb A: 0%, Hb F: 4.5%, Hb A2: 3.5%, Hb C: 92%

Answer: The peripheral blood smears show low density of red cells. There are microcytic hypochromic red cells and large number of target cells. The biochemical tests show indirect hyper- bilirubinemia, high LDH, and reduced haptoglobin. The urine and stool examinations are normal. Serum iron profile, B12 and folic acid, and CRP levels are also normal. The hemoglobin electrophoresis shows a prominent band at position of Hb C- quantified at 92%. Also small quantities of Hb F and HbA2 are present. There is no HbA.

All these findings confirm a diagnosis of homozygous HbC (HbCC) disease.

Q3. Which further tests are indicated in such patients?

Answer: Once diagnosis of HbC is confirmed, a family screening is important to identify the presence of hemoglobinopathy in parents and siblings. In this patient, both parents had Hb C trait. Given below are image of blood film (Fig. 22.3) and HPLC (Fig. 22.4) of one of the parents with HB C trait.

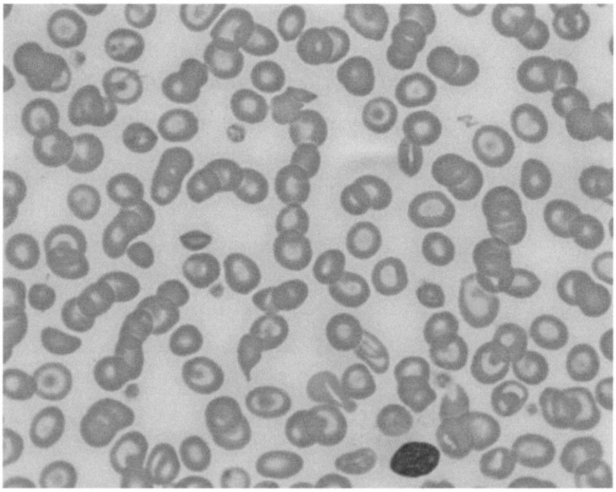

Fig. 22.3 PBF. Microcytic hypochromic cells and few target cells (as compared to patient). Leishman stain ×100

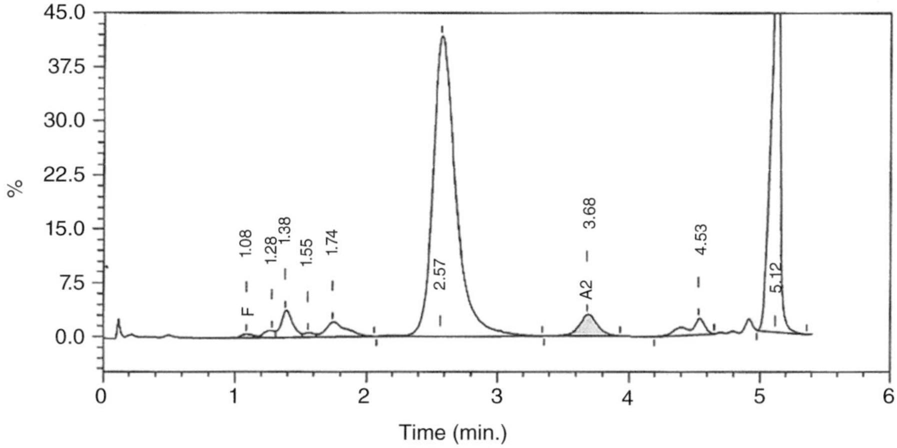

Fig. 22.4 HPLC: Hb A: 62%, Hb F: 0.7%, Hb A2: 3.2%, Hb C: 34.5%

The blood film shows mildly microcytic hypochromic red cells and target cells. The HPLC shows Hb A 62% and HbC 34.5%. These values are diagnostic of HbC trait. So both parents are suffering from HbC trait and inheritance from both resulted in HbC disease in this patient.

DNA-based diagnosis of Hb C is optional for confirmation and is usually requested before genetic counseling. However, HPLC is sufficient for diagnosis.

Q4. What are the clinical and pathophysiologic characteristics of HbE disease? What other conditions can be co-inherited with it?

Answer: Hb C results from change of lysine to glutamic acid at $beta^6$ position of globin chain. It is less soluble than HbA and can form crystals within red cells resulting in increased viscosity of blood [2–4].

Hb C disease has a mild phenotype with few symptoms of anemia and no effect on growth and development as such. Mild hemolytic anemia may occur. Patents may have mild jaundice, splenomegaly, and increased frequency of gall stones. The hemolytic markers are mildly elevated, and blood film shows microcytosis with target cells and occasional crystals.

Patients with Hb C trait are phenotypically normal. The condition becomes more significant when there is co-inheritance with other hemoglobinopathies such as HbS (sickle cell) and beta-thalassemia. When in combination with HbS, i.e., HbSC disease, clinical condition is mildly less severe than homozygous (HbSS) sickle cell disease. HPLC will show both Hb S and HB C which will clinch diagnosis. There is more frequency of proliferative retinopathy and avascular necrosis.

Co-inheritance of Hb C with beta-thalassemia, i.e., HbC/beta-thalassemia results in mild to moderate chronic hemolytic anemia. In HbC/$beta^0$-thalassemia, HPLC will show presence of HbC and mildly raised HbA2 and HbF with no Hb A. In HbC / $beta^+$ -thalassemia, Hb A is also present [5, 6].

Case 2 A 5-year-old male child was referred to pediatric clinic. The mother complained that the child was looking pale and was feeling more tired after playing with peers. These symptoms were gradually progressing. Also the child was getting repeated upper respiratory infections. The family had good socio-economic status. None of the parents or siblings were ever investigated for anemia.

Examination revealed pallor and mild icterus. Mild tachycardia was also observed. There was no organomegaly. Investigations revealed anemia and mildly raised hemolytic parameters on biochemical tests. All other relevant tests for anemia were non-contributory.

Q5. Given are result of CBC (Table 22.5) blood film (Fig. 22.5) and hemoglobin analysis by HPLC and capillary electrophoresis (Figs. 22.6, and 22.7). Interpret the results and suggest final diagnosis.

Table 22.5 CBC

CBC parameter	Patient's result	Reference range
WBC	6.2	3.7–10 × 10^9/L
RBC	4.2	4.5–5.4 × 10^{12}/L
HB	111	120–150 g/L
Hct	0.340	0.33–0.43 L/L
MCV	71	83–101 fL
MCH	27	27–32 pg
MCHC	320	315–345 g/L
RDW	19	11.6–14.6%
PLT	308	130–430 × 10^9/L
MPV	10	7–11 fL
Poly#	2.8	1.7–6 × 10^9/L
Lymp#	2.2	1–3 x10^9/L
Mono#	0.8	0.2–1.0 × 10^9/L
EO#	0.4	0.02–0.5 × 10^9/L
BASO#	00	0.02–0.1 × 10^9/L
RETIC%	3.2	0.5–1.5%
Absolute ret count	410	50–150 × 10^9/L
ESR	20	0–20 mm 1st h Westergren

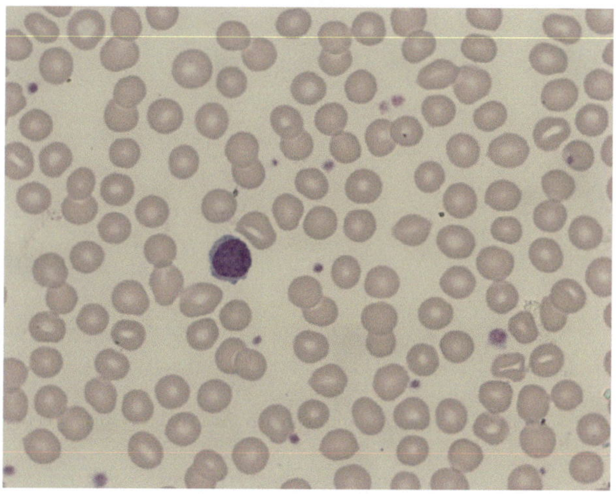

Fig. 22.5 PBF. Mild microcytosis. Hb E disease. Leishman ×100

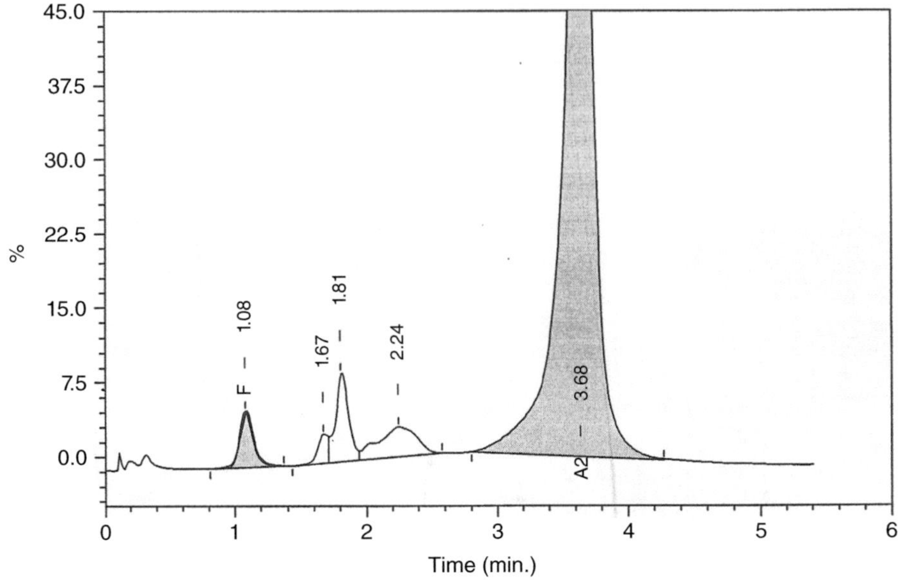

Fig. 22.6 HPLC(Biorad V-II) HbE disease: Hb E: 94%, Hb F: 2%, Hb A2: 4%. In HPLC, HbE band is seen in position of HbA2. For definite evaluation, capillary electrophoresis is helpful

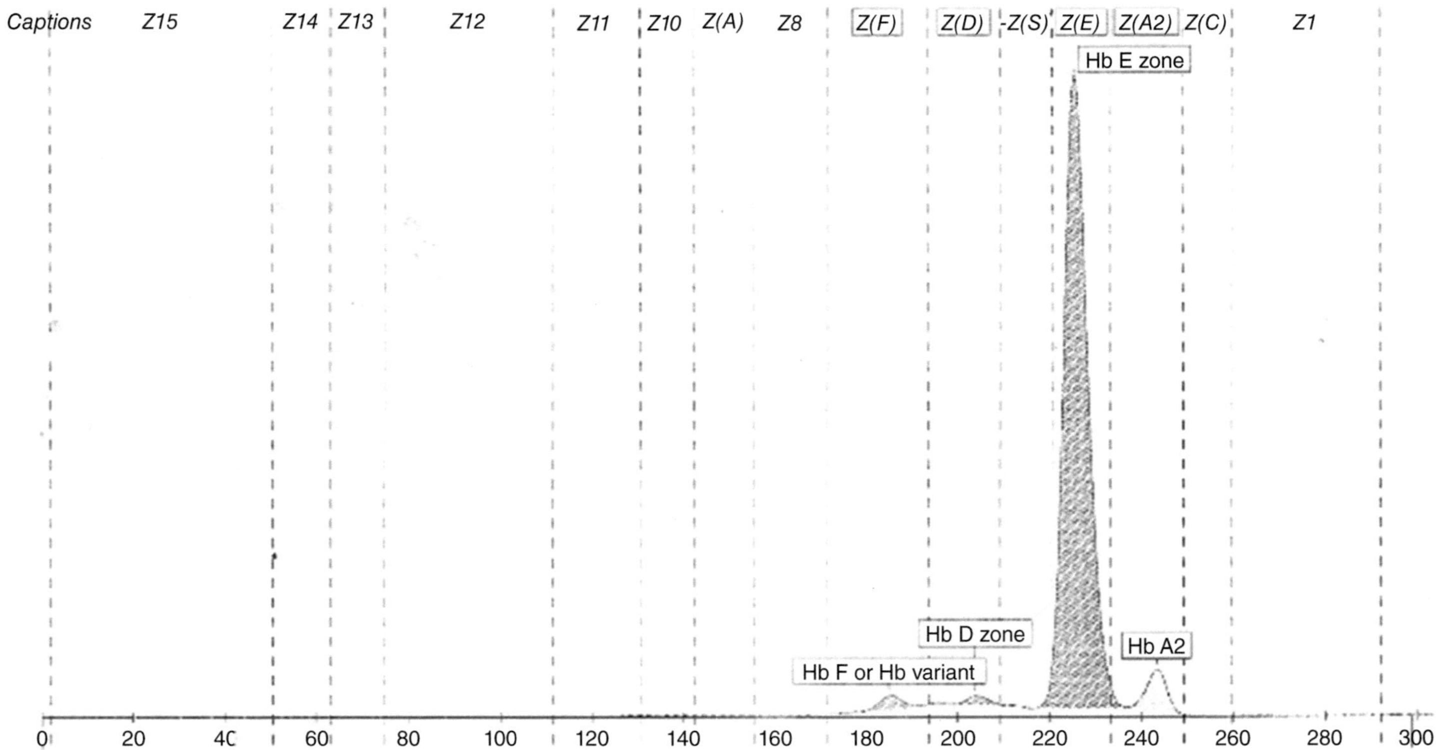

Fig. 22.7 Capillary electrophoresis: Hb EE disease: 95.4%, Hb A: 0%, Hb A2: 4.6%

Answer: The CBC result shows mild anemia. The MCV is low but MCH and MCHC are within normal limits. There is mild reticulocytosis. RDW is slightly high. So, there is mild microcytosis without hypochromia. Causes of microcytic anemia include iron deficiency, combined iron and B12/ folic acid deficiency, anemia of chronic disorders, and hemoglobinopathies.

The initial investigations for iron, B12/folic acid, and other relevant investigations for anemia of chronic disease were non-contributory. The blood film shows microcytic cells with few target cells. Hemoglobin analysis done by HPLC(Biorad V-II), and capillary electrophoresis shows a prominent band in the region of Hb E (92.4%). There is no Hb A. This confirms a diagnosis of homozygous HBE disease (HbEE).

Q6. Which further tests are indicated in such patient?

Answer: Once diagnosis of HB EE is confirmed, a family screening is important to identify the presence of hemoglobinopathy in parents and siblings. In this patient, both parents had Hb E trait with normal CBC except for mild microcytosis. Given below are images of blood film (Fig. 22.8) and hemoglobin electrophoresis (Fig. 22.9) from one of the parents.

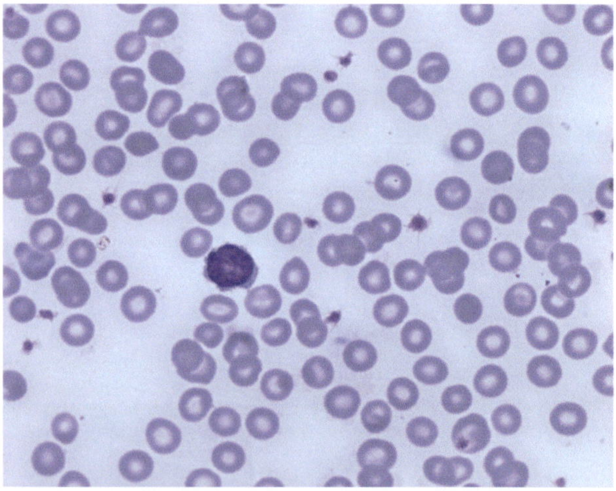

Fig. 22.8 PBF microcytic red cells. Leishman stain ×100

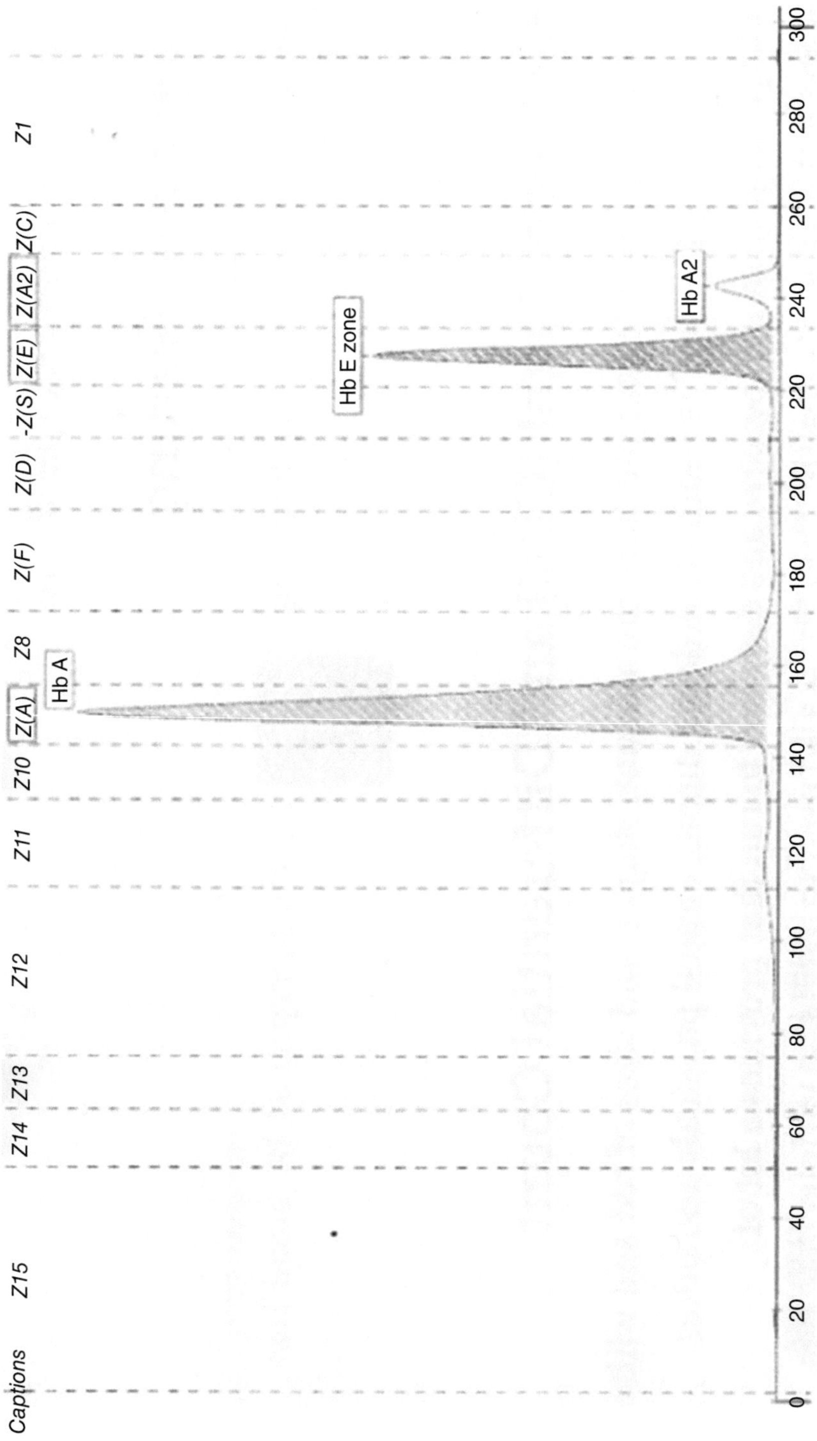

Fig. 22.9 Capillary electrophoresis: HbE trait .Hb A: 70%, Hb A2: 3.5%, Hb E: 26.5%

The blood film shows mildly microcytic red cells. The Hb electrophoresis shows Hb A 70% and HbE 26.5%. These values are diagnostic of HbE trait.

Since this child had homozygous HbEE disease, he has acquired one gene from each parent, which indicates that both parents of this child are heterozygous for HbE, i.e., they have HbE trait.

Further confirmation by DNA-based diagnosis of Hb E is optional and is considered only before genetic counseling. However, Hb electrophoresis is sufficient for diagnosis.

Q7. What are the clinical and pathophysiologic characteristics of hbE hemoglobinopathy?

Answer: Hb E is caused by a substitution of glutamic acid by lysine at position 26 of the β-globin gene ($Beta^6$ Glu to Lys). Homozygous state, HbEE, produces mild anemia and microcytosis, while heterozygous state (HbAE) is asymptomatic. Typical red cell morphology shows microcytosis and target cells.

Compound heterozygous state can occur with Hb E and alfa- or beta-thalassemia. The concomitant inheritance of α-thalassemia lowers the percentage of Hb E. Iron deficiency also lowers the Hb E percentage.

In Hb E β^0-thalassemia, Hb E ranges from 40% to 60%, with markedly increased HbF. No HbA is present. Phenotype is more like thalassemia major.

Hb E β^+-thalassemia patients usually have a mild anemia and show microcytic hypochromic red cells and a raised HbE and HbF. Hb A is also present. Phenotype is more like mild to intermediate thalassemia.

Compound heterozygous states with Hb E / Lepore and Hb E/ delta -beta-thalassemia present with mild phenotypes.

Compound heterozygous state of Hb E with HbS produces mild anemia with microcytic red cells. Electrophoresis will show both HbS (approx. 60%) and HbE (appox. 30%). The clinical presentation mimics sickle/ β^+-thalassemia with episodes of painful crises, sequestration, and avascular necrosis [7–10].

Case 3 A 25-year-old male was being investigated for hemoglobinopathies as a part of premarital screening policy. He was a completely healthy looking male with no history of any specific complaints. Physical examination was unremarkable. His parents were never screened for any inheritable disease.

Q8. Given are the result of CBC (Table 22.6) and hemoglobin analysis (Fig. 22.10) by capillary electrophoresis. Interpret the results and comment on further evaluation.

Table 22.6 CBC

CBC parameter	Patient's result	Reference range
WBC	8.5	3.7–10 × 10^9/L
RBC	4.8	4.5–5.4 × 10^{12}/L
HB	135	130–160 g/L
Hct	0.41	0.33–0.43 L/L
MCV	89	83–101 fL
MCH	29	27–32 pg
MCHC	329	315–345 g/L
RDW	14	11.6–14.6%
PLT	300	130–430 × 10^9/L
MPV	11	7–11 fL
Poly#	5.5	1.7–6 × 10^9/L
Lymp#	2.0	1–3 × 10^9/L
Mono#	0.5	0.2–1.0 × 10^9/L
EO#	0.5	0.02–0.5 × 10^9/L
BASO#	00	0.02–0.1 × 10^9/L
RETIC%	1.5	0.5–1.5%
Absolute ret count	160	50–150 × 10^9/L
ESR	10	0–20 mm 1st h Westergren

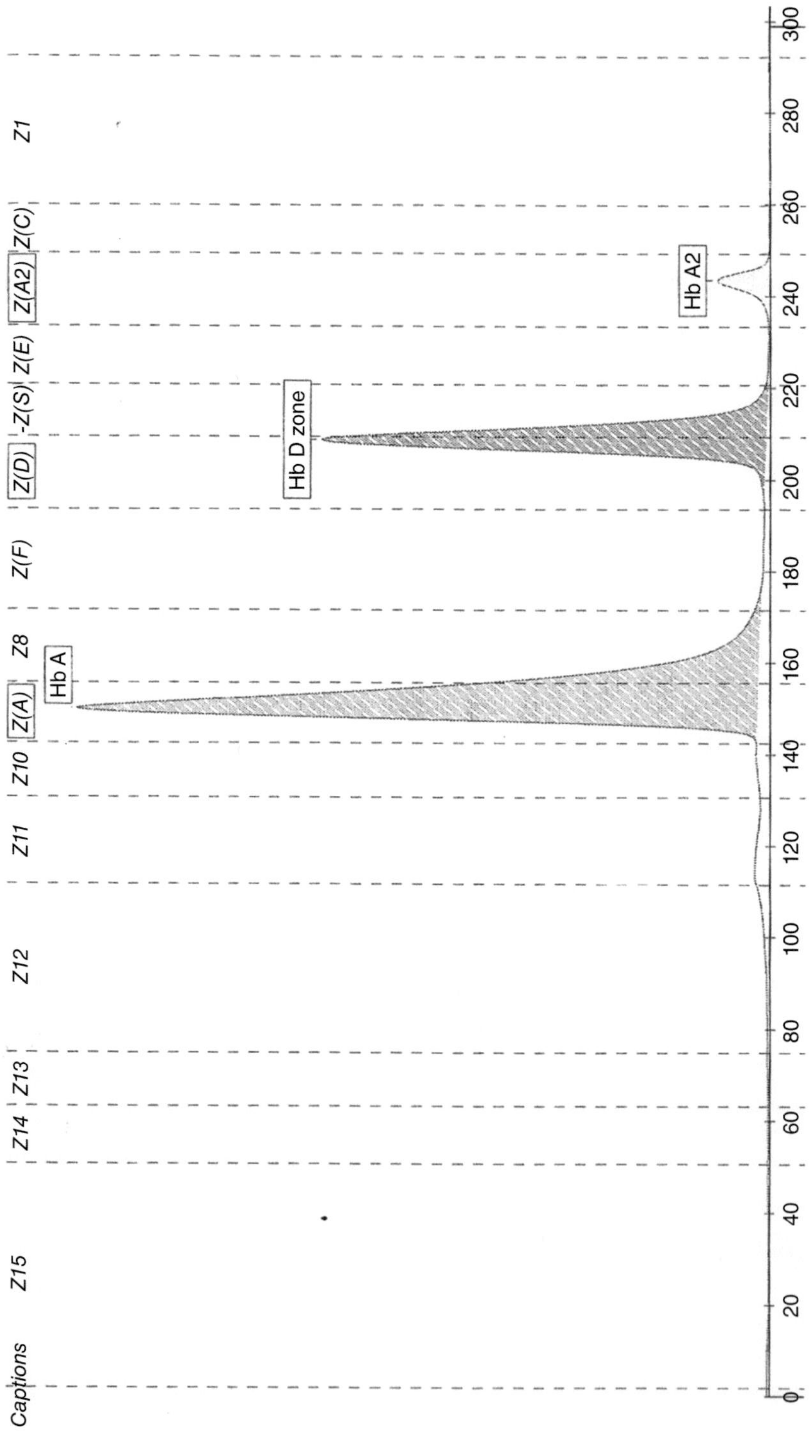

Fig. 22.10 Capillary electrophoresis: Hb A: 73%, Hb A2: 2%, Hb D: 25%

Answer: The CBC result is within normal limits. There is no anemia. However, the capillary electrophoresis shows reduced HbA (73%) and presence of HbD (25%). These findings are consistent with HbD trait. Further confirmation by DNA analysis is optional. The parents and siblings should also be screened. Since this is premarital investigation in this case, the spouse should also be investigated for hemoglobinopathies.

Q9. What are the clinical and pathophysiologic characteristics of hemoglobin D hemoglobinopathy?

Answer: Hemoglobin D is formed due to substitution of glutamine for glutamic acid at 121st position of beta chain (beta^{121} Glu to Gln).

Hemoglobin D hemoglobinopathy can occur in four different combinations:

1. Hb D trait (heterozygous state, Hb^A Hb^D) is a harmless clinical condition with normal hemogram. HbD is approximately 30–40%.
2. Hb D disease (homozygous HbD state, Hb^DHb^D) is also clinical silent condition. HbD is over 50–60%. They have normal Hb, red cell indices and no evidence of hemolysis.
3. Hb SD disease is a combination of Hb D and HbS (Hb^S $Hb^{D)}$. Episodes of sickling and hemolysis can be observed (please refer to section on sickle cell hemoglobinopathies).
4. Hb D in combination with beta-thalassemia- HbD/beta-thalassemia presents clinically with hemolytic anemia with or without splenomegaly depending on degree of thalassemic defect (Beta^0 or beta$^+$) [11–13].

22.2 Quick Information for Practicing Clinicians and Students

Hb C

1. (Hb CC) may present with mild chronic hemolysis, splenomegaly, and jaundice.
2. Peripheral blood shows mild microcytic hypochromic red cells and target cells.
3. It is less soluble than HbA and can form crystals within red cells resulting in increased viscosity of blood.
4. Hb C disease has a mild phenotype with few symptoms of anemia.
5. Patents may have mild jaundice, splenomegaly, and increased frequency of gall stones.
6. The condition becomes more significant when there is co-inheritance with other hemoglobinopathies such as HbS and beta-thalassemia.
7. There is more frequency of proliferative retinopathy and avascular necrosis in HbSC.

Hb E

8. Homozygous HbE disease produces mild anemia and microcytosis while heterozygous state (HbA/E) is asymptomatic. Typical red cell morphology shows microcytosis and target cells.

9. Concomitant α-thalassemia or iron deficiency lowers the Hb E percentage.
10. In Hb E β^0-thalassemia phenotype is more like thalassemia major.
11. Hb E β^+-thalassemia phenotype is more like mild to intermediate thalassemia.
12. Compound heterozygous state of Hb E with HbS produces mild anemia. The clinical presentation mimics sickle/ β^+-thalassemia with episodes of painful crises, sequestration, and avascular necrosis.

Hb D

13. HbD disease and traits are clinically silent conditions.
14. Compound heterozygous state of Hb D and HbS (Hb^S $Hb^{D)}$ presents with episodes of sickling and hemolysis.
15. Hb D in combination with beta-thalassemia- HbD/beta-thalassemia presents clinically with hemolytic anemia with or without splenomegaly depending on degree of thalassemic defect ($Beta^0$ or $beta^+$).

To acquire further knowledge on the subject, following sources are advised:

1. BCSH guidelines
2. Br Jr. Hematology
3. ASH education book
4. Blood
5. NEJM
6. Int Jr. Lab Hematology

References

1. Matos JF, Dusse LMS, Borges KBG, et al. A new index to discriminate between iron deficiency anemia and thalassemia trait. Rev Bras Hematol Hemoter. 2016;38(3):214–9. https://doi.org/10.1016/j.bjhh.2016.05.011.
2. Powars DR, Hiti A, Ramicone E, Johnson C, Chan L. Outcome in hemoglobin SC disease: a four-decade observational study of clinical, hematologic, and genetic factors. Am J Hematol. 2002;70(3):206–15.
3. Olson JF, Ware RE, Schultz WH, Kinney TR. Hemoglobin C disease in infancy and childhood. J Pediatr. 1994 Nov;125(5 Pt 1):745–7.
4. Rezende PV, Santos MV, Campos GF, Vieira LLM, Souza MB, Belisário AR, Silva CM, Viana MB. Clinical and hematological profile in a newborn cohort with hemoglobin SC. J Pediatr. 2018;94(6):666–72.
5. Chmel H, Bertles JF. Hemoglobin S/C disease in a pregnant woman with crisis and fat embolization syndrome. Am J Med. 1975;58(4):563–6.
6. Prindle KH Jr, McCurdy PR. Red cell lifespan in hemoglobin C disorders (with special reference to hemoglobin C trait). Blood. 1970;36(1):14–9.
7. Rees DC, Styles L, Vichinsky EP, Clegg JB, Weatherall DJ. The hemoglobin E syndromes. Ann N Y Acad Sci. 1998;850:334–43.
8. Fucharoen S, Winichagoon P. Clinical and hematologic aspects of hemoglobin E beta-thalassemia. Curr Opin Hematol. 2000;7:106–12.
9. Fucharoen S, Ketvichit P, Pootrakul P, Siritanaratkul N, Piankijagum A, Wasi P. Clinical manifestation of beta-thalassemia/hemoglobin E disease. J Pediatr Hematol Oncol. 2000;22:552–7.

10. Rees DC. Hemoglobin F and hemoglobin E/beta-thalassemia. J Pediatr Hematol Oncol. 2000;22:567–72.
11. Jain RC. Hemoglobin D disease. Am J Clin Pathol. 1971;56:40–2.
12. Adekile A, Mullah-Ali A, Akar NA. Does elevated hemoglobin F modulate the phenotype in Hb SD-Los Angeles? Acta Haematol. 2010;123:135–9. https://doi.org/10.1159/000276998.
13. Serjeant BE, Myerscough E, Serjeant GR, et al. Sickle cell-hemoglobin D Iran: a benign sickle cell syndrome. Hemoglobin. 1982;6:57–9.

Chapter 23
Copper Deficiency Anemia

A 45-year-old female patient was referred to hematology OPD with main complaints of gradually progressive weakness, lethargy, and feeling dyspneic on brisk walking for the past 3 months. She also gave a history of giddiness and palpitations while climbing stairs. One year back, she had been diagnosed to have type-2 diabetes mellitus and was started on anti-diabetic medications. Six months ago, she had COVID infection. During that period, she started developing signs of neuropathy and gradually increasing weakness, for which she was prescribed zinc supplements along with other multivitamins. Her social and economic status was satisfactory. There was no history of any other chronic illness, medication, or exposure to chemical/radiations. The examination showed anemia without jaundice. There was no lymphadenopathy or hepato-splenomegaly. Nothing abnormal was detected on chest, cardiovascular, or abdominal examination. Result of CBC done at presentation is given in Table 23.1.

A. Gupta, *Decision Making Through Problem Based Learning in Hematology*,
https://doi.org/10.1007/978-981-99-8933-1_23

Table 23.1 CBC

CBC parameter	Patient's result	Reference range
WBC	3.5	3.7–10 × 10^9/L
RBC	2.10	4.5–5.4 × 10^{12}/L
HB	8.5	130–160 g/L
Hct	0.25	0.33–0.43 L/L
MCV	90	83–101 fL
MCH	29	27–32 pg
MCHC	333	315–345 g/L
RDW	12	11.6–14.6%
PLT	170	130–430 × 10^9/L
MPV	12	7–11 fL
Poly#	1.6	1.7–6 × 10^9/L
Lymp#	1.2	1–3 × 10^9/L
Mono#	0.6	0.2–1.0 × 10^9/L
EO#	0.1	0.02–0.5 × 10^9/L
BASO#	00	0.02–0.1 × 10^9/L
RETIC%	0.8	0.5–1.5%
Absolute ret count	45	50–150 × 10^9/L
ESR	52	0–20 mm 1st h Westergren

23.1 Questions

Q1. Interpret the CBC result given above and suggest investigations for further evaluation in such case.

Answer: The CBC result shows decreased WBC count with decreased neutrophils. RBC count is low with decreased hemoglobin level and hematocrit. Platelet count is normal. ESR value is high. Reticulocyte percentage and absolute values are mildly reduced. So, there is bicytopenia. Anemia is normocytic normochromic. The possible causes of bicytopenia are as follows [1]:

1. Ineffective erythropoiesis as it happens in nutritional causes such as megaloblastic anemia, dual deficiency anemia, and myelodysplastic syndrome.
2. Bone marrow infiltration/ replacement as in leukemia, lymphomas, myeloma, or metastasis.
3. Bone marrow suppression by autoimmune disorders, CRF, hemophagocytic syndromes, PNH, aplastic anemia, myelofibrosis, and following chemotherapy for malignancies.

4. Fungal, tubercular, and viral infections like HIV, hepatitis, and Epstein–Barr virus.
5. Consumption as it happens in DIC or sequestration into spleen due to splenomegaly (portal HT with cirrhosis, myelofibrosis, storage diseases, etc.).

So all these diseases need to be excluded through history, physical examination, and appropriate investigations.

Next best investigation will be examination of blood film. Tests for renal, hepatic, pancreatic, and thyroid functions are recommended. Direct antiglobulin test (DAT) and immunology screen should also be done. As she is already on multivitamins, levels of serum B12 and folic acid will not reflect any genuine information. At this time, she does not have any evidence of infection. There is no organomegaly also.

Based on the result of these investigations, further tests of bone marrow examination as well as assessment with flowcytometric analysis of CD55 and CD59 on peripheral blood can be considered.

Q2. Given is image from blood film (Fig. 23.1) and results of kidney, liver, pancreas, and thyroid function tests (Table 23.2), DAT and immunology (Table 23.3) are provided. Interpret the results. What are the possible differential diagnoses? What further investigations will be required to exclude various possibilities?

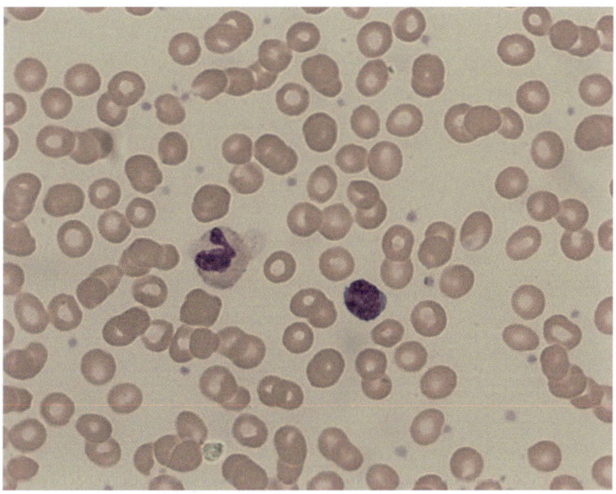

Fig. 23.1 PBF. Normocytic normochromic anemia and few hyposegmented neutrophils. Leishman stain ×40

Table 23.2 Biochemical tests

Test	Patient's result	Ref range
Glu (F)	7.1	3.9–6.1 mmol/L
Urea	2.9	2.5–6.6 mmol/L
Creat	101	60–120 μmol/L
Na^+	141	136–146 mmol/L
K^+	4.6	3.7–5.0 mmol/L
Ca^+	2.3	2.2–2.6 mmol/L
Mg^+	1.0	0.08–1.1 mmol/L
T. Prot	67	63–80 mmol/L
Alb	41	35–47 mmol/L
Choles	2.9	1.5–5.2 mmol/L
TG	0.9	0.4–1.7 mmol/L
Urates	300	150–400 mmol/L
T Bil	41	3–20 μmol/L
Indirect Bil	32	5–20 μmol/L
D. Bil	9	0–5 μmol/L
Alk Ph	80	26–88 IU/L
ALT	56	10–60 IU/L
AST	34	10–42 IU/L
GGT	30	7–64 IU/L
LDH	300	90–180 IU/L
Hapto	0.4	0.2–2.0 g/L
T4	10.2	7.8–16 pmol/L
TSH	3.90	0.27–4.2 μIU/mL
Amylase	20	28–100 IU/L
Lipase	33	0–160 U/L

Table 23.3 DAT and immunological tests

Test	Patient's result	Ref range
Direct Antiglobulin Test	Negative	Negative
Anti-ds-DNA Antibody	Negative	0–20 Iu/mL
ANA screen	Negative	Negative
AnA pattern	Negative	Negative
ANA titer	Negative	Negative
Sm B	Negative	Negative
RNP A and C	Negative	Negative
SS-A	Negative	Negative
SS-B	Negative	Negative
Scl-70	Negative	Negative
Jo-1	Negative	Negative
Ribosomal P	Negative	Negative
Histone	Negative	Negative
MPO Ab	Negative	Negative
Proteinase Ab	Negative	Negative

Answer: The blood film shows reduced red cell density, reduced leukocytes with occasional hyposegmented neutrophils. Platelets were normal. There was no immature cells. The biochemical tests showed mildly raised fasting blood glucose level (diabetic status), mildly raised total and indirect bilirubin and elevated LDH levels. The results of DAT and immunology profiles were within normal limits.

So possibilities of hematological malignancies, systemic conditions, and immunological diseases are excluded.

Next best test will be to do a bone marrow examination to rule out covert bone marrow infiltration/ aleukemic leukemia, lymphomas, impending aplastic anemia, myeloma, or myelodysplastic syndrome.

Q3. Given are images from bone marrow biopsy and aspiration (Figs. 23.2, 23.3, 23.4, and 23.5). Interpret the findings and suggest diagnosis.

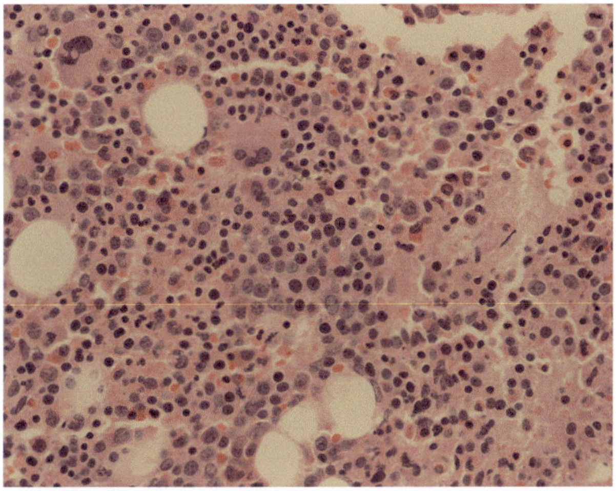

Fig. 23.2 BM trephine biopsy. Mildly hypercellular marrow showing erythroid hyperplasia. H/E stain ×40

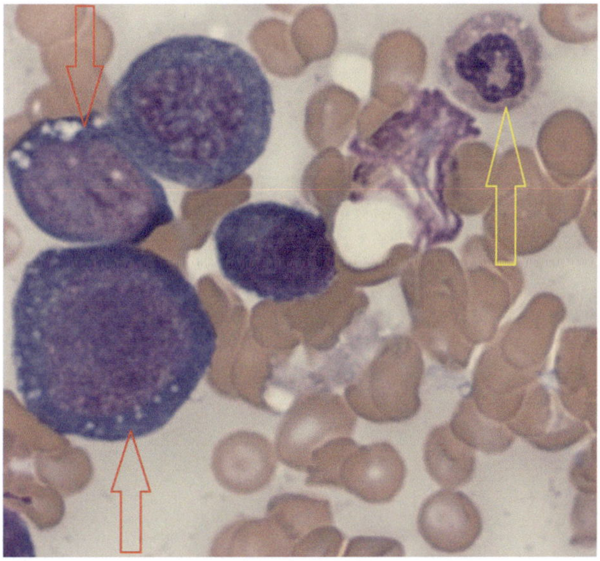

Fig. 23.3 BM aspiration. Erythroblasts with cytoplasmic vacuolations (red arrows) and a ring neutrophil(yellow arrow) Leishman stain ×100

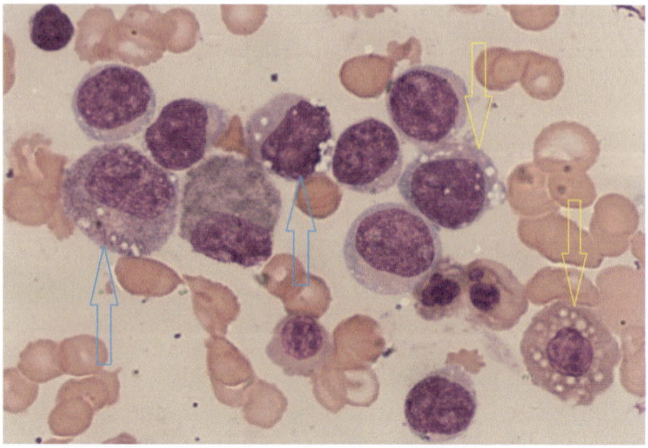

Fig. 23.4 Bone marrow aspiration. Vacuolations in Intermediate and late erythroblasts (yellow arrows) and myelocytes and metamyelocytes (blue arrows). Leishman stain ×40

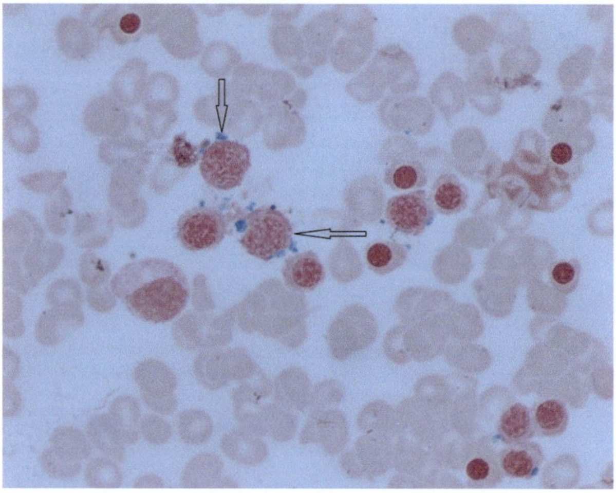

Fig. 23.5 Bone marrow aspiration. few sideroblasts are seen. Prussian blue stain ×40

Answer: The bone marrow biopsy shows mildly hypercellular marrow. The aspirate shows a mild erythroid hyperplasia. Many early and intermediate erythroid precursors show cytoplasmic vacuolation. Mild maturation arrest was noted in granulocytic precursors, many of which also showed cytoplasmic vacuolation.

The Prussian blue stain shows increased iron in reticuloendothelial cells and slightly increased number of sideroblasts (count was less than 5%). Megakaryocytes were normal.

So. there are findings of erythroid hyperplasia with vacuolation of erythroblasts and granulocytic precursors with presence of slightly increased number of sideroblasts. Mild maturation arrest is seen in granulocytic precursors. No cytogenetic abnormality was seen. Review of history reveals that she had been consuming zinc in addition to multivitamins. These characteristic findings in bone marrow along with peripheral blood anemia and neutropenia are strongly indicative of copper deficiency. However, it needs to be confirmed. So, the next investigation should be estimation of serum level of zinc and copper. All other differential diagnoses are excluded as there is no evidence of marrow infiltration, leukemia, lymphoma, and aplastic anemia. MDS is also ruled out as there is no significant dysplastic changes or chromosomal abnormality to support this diagnosis.

Q4. Given are results of serum zinc and copper levels (Table 23.4). Interpret the result and suggest final diagnosis.

Table 23.4 Serum zinc and copper level

Serum Zinc level	160 μg/L	N: 60–130
Serum copper level	300 μg/L	N: 810–1990

Answer: The results show high level of zinc and low copper. This confirms diagnosis of copper deficiency in this patient.

Q5. what are the causes of copper deficiency?

Answer: Copper is a trace element which is involved in the normal functioning of many cellular enzymes. It is coenzyme in which has many functions in superoxide dismutase, cytochrome-c oxidase, and ceruloplasmin.

Cooper is found in high quantity in seafood, mushrooms, tofu, sweet potatoes, sesame seeds, cashews, chickpeas, salmon, dark chocolate, and avocados.

Risk factors for deficiency include gastrointestinal tract surgery, prolonged malabsorption, total parenteral nutrition, and zinc excess. Inadequate dietary intake is very rare. Copper deficiency is also seen in renal failure and rare disease like Wilson's disease [2, 3].

Q6. What is the cause and pathogenesis of copper deficiency in this patient?:

Answer: This patient was consuming zinc for previous few months in addition to multivitamins, which also contained zinc. So daily intake of excess of zinc is cause of anemia in this patient. She did not have any other risk factors for development of copper deficiency. Prolonged and excessive zinc intake results in reduced copper absorption from intestines.

Normally, metallothionein acts as guard in intestines to reduce zinc toxicity by providing zinc binding sites. But these proteins have greater affinity for copper than zinc. Excessive presence of zinc in the body stimulates the production of metallothionein proteins. When metallothionein is in excess, it binds preferentially to copper. So the copper stays bound to enterocytes along with metallothionein and is excreted through feces when intestinal cells undergo sloughing. Thus copper is not absorbed into blood and subsequently, decreased levels of copper occur resulting in its deficiency [2, 4, 5].

Q7. What are the pathological effects of copper deficiency on iron metabolism?

Answer: Copper deficiency can cause decreased absorption of iron from the intestines and reduced release of iron from the reticuloendothelial system. It also produces ineffective erythropoiesis due to diminished activity of copper-containing enzymes and increased destructions of erythrocytes [6].

Q8. What is the cause of neutropenia in copper deficiency?

Answer: The granulocytic cell lines are also effected in copper deficiency. There is ineffective myelopoiesis, decreased number of progenitor cells, and excessive destruction of copper-deficient neutrophils. Also, there is increased clearance of such neutrophils and development of anti-neutrophilic antibodies [7, 8].

Q9. What are the indicators of ineffective erythropoiesis in this patient?

Answer: Elevated indirect bilirubin and high LDH indicate ineffective erythropoiesis.

23.2 Correlation of Results of Preliminary Investigations with Symptoms and Signs in Copper Deficiency Anemia

Q10. What are the classical hematological and clinical features of copper deficiency and how do they correlate with symptoms and sign in this patient?

Answer: Most common features observed are anemia and leukopenia. Sometimes, thrombocytopenia is also seen resulting in pancytopenia. Very rarely isolated neutropenia is seen. Sideroblastic anemia with neutropenia is mentioned in literature as common dual findings in copper deficiency [6, 9].

Clinical presentation also includes myelopathy and peripheral neuropathy.

Our patient also had symptoms of anemia in form of gradually progressive weakness, lethargy, and feeling dyspneic and had episodes of giddiness and palpitations. No signs or symptoms related to neutropenia were present. She also had history suggestive of peripheral neuropathy. Investigations confirmed anemia, neutropenia, vacuolated erythroblasts, and myeloid precursors. So both clinical findings and investigations correlate with diagnosis of copper deficiency. This was confirmed by changes in bone marrow and serum levels of copper.

Q11. What are the typical changes in bone marrow morphology in copper deficiency?

Answer: The bone marrow is hypercellular with erythroid hyperplasia. Cytoplasmic vacuolization of immature erythroid and granulocytic precursors has been described as very prominent features of copper deficiency [5, 10].

Q12. What is suggested triad of copper deficiency?

Answer: Anemia, leukopenia, and myeloneuropathy are being considered as triad of copper deficiency [11].

23.3 Quick Information for Practicing Clinicians and Students

References [1–11]:

1. Copper deficiency is an under-recognized cause of anemia and leukopenia.
2. Deficiency occurs after gastric resection, prolonged total parenteral nutrition, prolonged high levels of zinc intake, and general malnutrition.
3. An early clinical sign of copper deficiency is a reduction in the number of circulating neutrophils.
4. Anemia, leukopenia, and myeloneuropathy are being considered as triad of copper deficiency.
5. Patients presenting with anemia and neutropenia with or without associated neuropathy should suspected to have copper deficiency and investigated accordingly.

6. The bone marrow is hypercellular with erythroid hyperplasia. Cytoplasmic vacuolation of immature erythroid and granulocytic precursors has been described as prominent features of copper deficiency.
7. Myelodysplastic syndrome is a close differential diagnosis. Vacuolations in myeloid precursors are extremely rare in MDS.
8. If serum copper levels remain normal despite symptoms that suggest copper deficiency, measurement of ceruloplasmin levels can prove useful.
9. According to the World Health Organization expert consultation on vitamins and minerals requirements in humans, the upper limit of zinc intake in an adult is 45 mg/d; zinc intake higher than 50 mg/d starts disturbing copper homeostasis.

To acquire further knowledge on the subject, following sources are advised:

1. BCSH guidelines
2. Br Jr. Hematology
3. ASH education book
4. Blood
5. NEJM
6. Int Jr. Lab Hematology

References

1. Elizabeth PW, Daniel AA. The differential diagnosis and bone marrow evaluation of new-onset pancytopenia. Am J Clin Pathol. 2013;139:9–29.
2. Lazarchick J. Update on anemia and neutropenia in copper deficiency. Curr Opin Hematol. 2012;19(1):58–60. https://doi.org/10.1097/MOH.0b013e32834da9d2.
3. Dembinski K, Gargasz AE, Dabrow S, et al. Three distinct cases of copper deficiency in hospitalized pediatric patients. Clin Pediatr (Phila). 2012;51:759–62. https://doi.org/10.1177/0009922812446743.
4. Uauy R, Olivares M, Gonzalez M. Essentiality of copper in humans. Am J Clin Nutr. 1998;67(5):952S–S959.
5. Porea TJ, Belmont JW, Mahoney DH Jr. Zinc-induced anemia and neutropenia in an adolescent. J Pediatr. 2000;136(5):688–90.
6. Fischer PW, Giroux A, L'Abbe MR. Effects of zinc on mucosal copper binding and on the kinetics of copper absorption. J Nutr. 1983;113(2):462–9.
7. Deur CJ, Stone MJ, Frenkel EP. Trace metals in hematopoiesis. Am J Hematol. 1981;11(3):309–31.
8. Percival SS. Neutropenia caused by copper deficiency: possible mechanisms of action. Nutr Rev. 1995;53(3):59–66.
9. Merza H, Sood N, Sood R. Idiopathic hyperzincemia with associated copper deficiency anemia: a diagnostic dilemma. Clin Case Rep. 2015;3(10):819.
10. Wazir SM, Ghobrial I. Copper deficiency, a new triad: anemia, leucopenia, and myeloneuropathy. J Commun Hosp Intern Med Perspect. 2017;7(4):265–8.
11. World Health Organization. Vitamin and mineral requirements in human nutrition. 2nd ed. Geneva: World Health Organization; 2004. p. 1–362. https://apps.who.int/iris/bitstream/handle/10665/42716/9241546123.pdf?ua=1

Chapter 24
Inherited Bone Marrow Failure Syndrome–Fanconi Anemia

A 7-year-old male child presented to hematology clinic for evaluation of petechial spots on arms and abdomen. The mother had noticed that the child was having easy bruising tendency for the past 6 months. He was getting pale in appearance and had been getting repeated upper respiratory infections during the previous few months.

The socio-economic status of family was good. Mother informed that the child was diagnosed with congenital dislocation of hip which was successfully managed. There was no exposure to drugs, chemicals, or radiation. He was the first child with no siblings. Examination revealed slightly delayed developmental milestones. Physical examination showed moderate pallor. There was no jaundice. General physical examination revealed Café au lait spots and hypopigmented area over chest and back. There was hypoplasia of thumb and thenar eminence. Mild frontal bossing was also observed. Given is result of CBC done at presentation (Table 24.1).

A. Gupta, *Decision Making Through Problem Based Learning in Hematology*, https://doi.org/10.1007/978-981-99-8933-1_24

Table 24.1 CBC

CBC parameter	Patient's result	Reference range
WBC	2.6	3.7–10 × 10^9/L
RBC	2.5	4.5–5.4 × 10^{12}/L
HB	6.5	130–160 g/L
Hct	0.19	0.33–0.43 L/L
MCV	99	83–101 fL
MCH	27	27–32 pg
MCHC	320	315–345 g/L
RDW	23	11.6–14.6%
PLT	40	130–430 × 10^9/L
MPV	15	7–11 fL
Poly#	0.8	1.7–6 × 10^9/L
Lymp#	1.5	1–3 × 10^9/L
Mono#	0.2	0.2–1.0 × 10^9/L
EO#	0.1	0.02–0.5 × 10^9/L
BASO#	00	0.02–0.1 × 10^9/L
RETIC%	0.2	0.5–1.5%
Absolute ret count	20	50–150 × 10^9/L
ESR	50	0–20 mm 1st h Westergren

24.1 Questions

Q1. Interpret the CBC result given above and suggest investigations for further evaluation in such case

Answer: The CBC result shows decreased WBC count with markedly decreased neutrophils. RBC count is low with decreased hemoglobin level and hematocrit and high value for RDW. The MCV, MCH, and MCHC are within normal limits. Platelet count is markedly reduced. ESR value is high. Reticulocyte percentage and absolute values are markedly decreased.

So, there is pancytopenia with reticulocytopenia. The anemia is normocytic normochromic. The possible causes of pancytopenia with low reticulocyte count include [1–3]:

1. Pathologies involving bone marrow such as aplastic anemia, myelodysplastic syndrome, leukemia, and metastasis.
2. Infections (especially hepatitis A/B/C, HIV, EBV, parvovirus, and CMV infections).

3. Nutritional deficiencies (Vitamin B12, folate, copper, zinc, and ferritin).
4. Immunological diseases.
5. Rare possibilities like chronic renal, endocrine disorders, myelofibrosis, and PNH.

Next best investigation will be examination of blood film. Tests for renal, hepatic, pancreatic, and thyroid functions are recommended. In addition to viral screening, direct antiglobulin test (DAT) and immunology screen should also be done. Levels of serum b12, folic acid ferritin, copper, and zinc should be estimated. A bone marrow examination for evaluation of aplastic anemia, leukemia, MDS, and metastasis is must along with flowcytometric analysis of CD55 and CD59 and cytogenetic analysis for chromosomal status.

As the child has skeletal abnormalities, inherited bone marrow failure syndrome is important etiology to considered. Idiopathic aplastic anemia is a diagnosis by exclusion.

Q2. Given are the image of blood film (Fig. 24.1), results of renal, hepatic, pancreatic, and thyroid functions (Table 24.2); serum B12/, folic acid, copper, zinc, and ferritin levels (Table 24.3); virology screen (Table 24.4); DAT and immunology screening (Table 24.5); and screening for PNH (Table 24.6). Interpret these results and suggest provisional diagnosis. What further tests should be done to confirm this diagnosis?

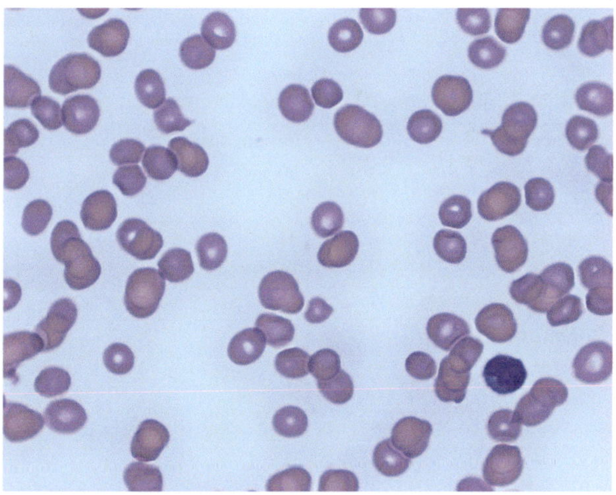

Fig. 24.1 PBF. Low density of red cells, reduced granuocytes, and platelets

Table 24.2 Biochemical tests

Test	Patient's result	Ref range
Glu	5.2	3.9–6.1 mmol/L
Urea	5.1	2.5–6.6 mmol/L
Creat	90	60–120 μmol/L
Na^+	141	136–146 mmol/L
K^+	4.4	3.7–5.0 mmol/L
Ca^+	2.4	2.2–2.6 mmol/L
Mg^+	1.0	0.08–1.1 mmol/L
T. Prot	70	63–80 mmol/L
Alb	42	35–47 mmol/L
Choles	3.5	1.5–5.2 mmol/L
TG	0.9	0.4–1.7 mmol/L
Urates	395	150–400 mmol/L
T Bil	15	3–20 μmol/L
D. Bil	2	0–5 μmol/L
Alk Ph	60	26–88 IU/L
ALT	66	10–60 IU/L
AST	40	10–42 IU/L
GGT	55	7–64 IU/L
LDH	140	90–180 IU/L
Hapto	1.6	0.2–2.0 g/L
T4	10.6	7.8–16 pmol/L
TSH	3.99	0.27–4.2 μlU/mL
Amylase	20	28–100 IU/L

Table 24.3 Serum iron, B12, folic acid, copper, and zinc levels

Lab test	Patient's result	Reference range
Ferritin	89	24–336
Serum B12	350	50–700 pmol/L
Serum folic acid	31	10–42 nmol/L
Red cell folate	1550	1187–2854 nmol/L
Serum copper	85	60–140 mcg/dL
Serum zinc	112	70–180 μg/100 mL

Table 24.4 Viral serology

Test name	Result	Ref range
CMV-DNA	Not detected by real-time PCR	Non-reactive
CMV-IgG	Reactive	Non-reactive
CMV-IgM	Non-reactive	Non-reactive
EBV-DNA	Not detected by real-time PCR	Non-reactive
EBV-IgG	Reactive	Non-reactive
EBV-IgM	Non-reactive	Non-reactive
HBs Ag	Non-reactive	Non-reactive
HCV-Ab	Non-reactive	Non-reactive
HCV-Ag	Not detected	Non-reactive
HIV Ag/Ab	Non-reactive	Non-reactive
Parvovirus B19 IgG	Non-reactive	Non-reactive
Parvovirus B19 IgM	Non-reactive	Non-reactive

Table 24.5 DAT and immunology profile

Test	Patient's result	Ref range
Direct Antiglobulin Test	Negative	Negative
Anti-ds-DNA Antibody	Negative	Negative
ANA	Negative	Negative
ANCA	Negative	Negative
Anti-LKM antibodies	Neg	Negative
Anti-mitochondrial antibodies	Neg	Negative
Anti-CCP antibodies	Neg	Negative
Rh-Factor	Negative	Negative
Rh titer	5	0–20 IU/mL
CRP	8	0–10 mg/L
C3	0.890 g/L	0.83–1.77 g/L
C4	0.45 g/L	0.20–0.8 g/L
IgG	14	6–16 g/L
IgM	1.3	0.5–2.0 g/L
IgA	3	0.8–4.0 g/L

Table 24.6 Screening for PNH. Flow cytometric analysis on peripheral blood for evaluation of red cell and granulocyte anchoring proteins

Cell type	Anchoring protein	Deficiency%
Red cells	CD55 and CD59	00% deficient
Neutrophils	CD24	00% deficient
Monocytes	CD 14	00% deficient

Answer: The blood film shows low density of red cells, reduced leukocytes, and decreased platelets. Leukocytes are morphologically normal. No immature cells are seen. The red cells are normocytic normochromic. No tear drop cells, nucleated cells, or any other abnormality of red cells are noted. There is no polychromasia.

The renal, hepatic, pancreatic, and thyroid functions are within normal limits. Serum B12, folic acid, copper and zinc levels are also normal. DAT and immunology profiles are negative. Virology screen does not show any evidence of active viral infection. There is no evidence of hemolysis. These investigations exclude systemic diseases, immunological, viral, and nutritional causes of pancytopenia. Also PNH is excluded as the anchor proteins are not deficient, and there is no evidence of hemolysis.

So, most likely cause of pancytopenia in this case is bone marrow pathology for which bone marrow biopsy is important. As the child has skeletal abnormalities, Inherited bone marrow failure syndromes are important diagnosis to consider, and chromosomal breakage test should be done. Bone marrow biopsy is required to exclude aplastic anemia, leukemia, MDS, and metastasis. Cytogenetic analysis for chromosomal studies should be included in investigations.

Q3. Given are the images from bone marrow aspirate and biopsy (Figs. 24.2, 24.3, and 24.4) and the results of chromosomal breakage from peripheral blood (Table 24.7). Interpret and suggest final diagnosis in this case.

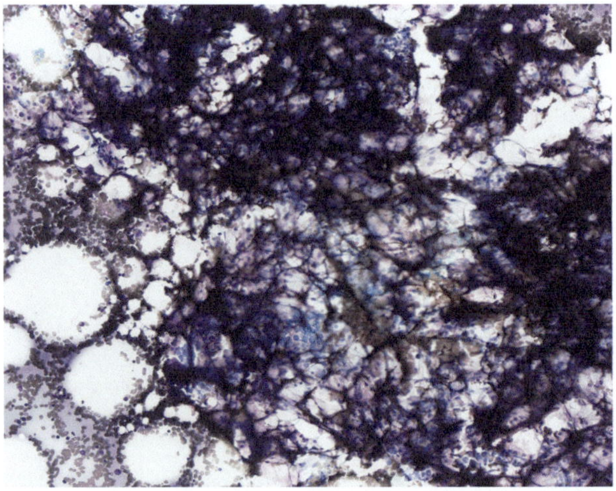

Fig. 24.2 Bone marrow aspirate. Hypocellular marrow particle. Leishman stain ×100

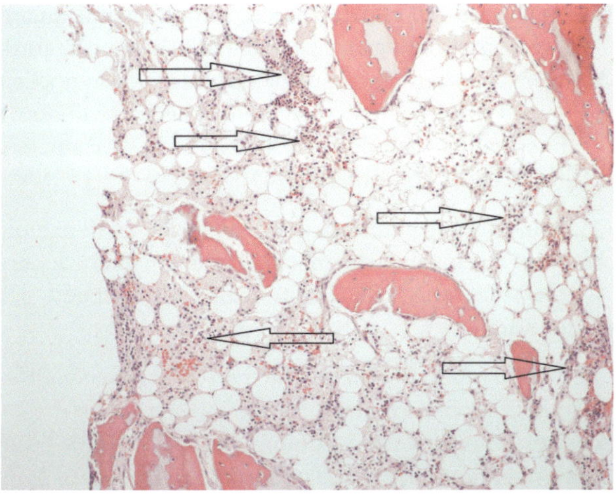

Fig. 24.3 Bone marrow trephine biopsy. Hypocellular marrow. Few remaining aggregates of hemopoietic cells are seen (arrows). H/E ×100

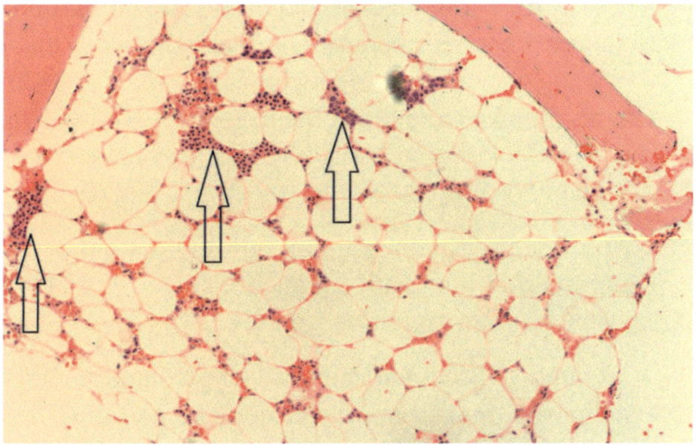

Fig. 24.4 Bone marrow trephine biopsy. Hypocellular marrow. Another area with few aggregates of hemopoietic cells are seen (arrows). H/E ×45

Table 24.7 Chromosomal breakage test

Chromosomal stress test using diepoxybutane (DEB)	Total metaphases analyzed: 20 Karyotype: 46XY. 20% structural aberrations (breaks)

Answer: The bone marrow aspirate is markedly hypocellular for age with particles composed mainly of fat cells. The trephine biopsy confirms hypocellularity. More than 90% of the spaces are replaced by fat. The normal hemopoietic cells are markedly reduced. Few granulocytic, erythroid precursors, and lymphocytes are noted. There is no evidence of hemopoietic or non-hemopoietic malignancy, evidence of infectious, or storage disorder.

Evaluation for chromosomal stability by stress test using DEB shows structural aberrations (breaks).

These findings confirm a diagnosis of chromosomal instability syndrome in this child most likely Fanconi's anemia.

Q4. What are the clinical pointers for Fanconi anemia. In which situations, this diagnosis should be suspected and subjected to further investigations?

Answer: Children who have cytopenias with hypoplastic or aplastic anemia, unexplained macrocytosis, myelodysplastic features, and characteristic physical abnormalities should be suspected to have Fanconi anemia and subjected to further tests for confirmation [4].

Q5. What are the confirmatory tests for Fanconi anemia?

Answer: To establish diagnosis of Fanconi anemia, chromosomal breakage is a reliable screening test. Identification of mutated gene remains optional but is confirmatory.

Q6. Which other inherited bone marrow failure syndromes present with hypoplastic or aplastic bone marrow?

Answer: Bone marrow failure syndromes are a group of bone marrow diseases presenting with reduced or absent production of single or multiple cell lines (erythroid, myeloid, or megakaryocytic) due to defect in hematopoietic stem cell. These can be inherited or acquired. The common examples of inherited conditions are Fanconi anemia, Diamond-Blackfan anemia, dyskeratosis congenita, amegakaryocytic thrombocytopenia, and Shwachman-Bodian-Diamond syndrome. Aplastic anemia is the most commonly acquired form. Similarly, myelodysplastic syndrome and PNH can also have clinical presentation like marrow failure syndromes.

Q7. What are the salient points to differentiate inherited bone marrow failure syndromes, other than Fanconi anemia?

Answer: Common conditions are [5–10]:

1. Diamond-Blackfan anemia—Short stature, congenital anomalies (like thumb abnormalities craniofacial defects, and cleft lip/palate), macrocytic anemia with reticulocytopenia, elevated levels of erythrocyte adenosine deaminase.
2. Dyskeratosis congenita:- Triad of abnormal skin pigmentation, nail dystrophy, and oral leukoplakia, in addition to aplastic anemia. Majority of patients (approximately 90%) of patients develop cytopenias. Telomere length less than the first percentile.
3. Amegakaryocytic thrombocytopenia: Thrombocytopenia which progresses to pancytopenia, severe to absent reduction in megakaryocyte number in bone marrow. Genetic abnormality is mutations in *MPL*, which encodes for the thrombopoietin receptor.
4. Shwachman-Diamond syndrome is a disorder of exocrine pancreatic dysfunction and bone marrow failure. Main hematological abnormality is neutropenia. Anemia, thrombocytopenia, or pancytopenia can occur. Skeletal abnormalities and poor growth are common. The diagnosis is based on clinical findings and exocrine pancreatic function tests. Genetic testing can be helpful to confirm the diagnosis. This is autosomal recessive disorder due to mutations in the Shwachman-Bodian-Diamond syndrome (*SBDS*) gene.

Q8. Based on above-mentioned possibilities, What additional investigations may be considered to evaluate differential diagnosis of bone marrow failure syndromes?

Answer:

1. Erythrocyte adenosine deaminase levels.
2. Studies for telomere length.
3. Mutational analysis for MPL gene.
4. Analysis for SBDS gene.
5. Erythropoietin levels.
6. Fetal hemoglobin level.

Q9. What are the important points to be considered in evaluating a case of suspected inherited bone marrow failure syndrome.

Answer: Most important is history, including family history (especially history of IBMFs or cancers), thorough physical examination for skeletal abnormalities, extensive lab investigations, fetal hemoglobin, ADA enzyme level, serum Epo level, radiological investigations like skeletal survey, U/S and MRI, bone marrow examination, chromosomal analysis, and genetic mutational assessment.

Q10. What is etiopathogenesis of Fanconi anemia?

Answer: Fanconi anemia is an autosomal recessive disorder resulting from mutations in approximately 23 types of genes. Mutations are homozygous or double heterozygous and result in defective DNA repair through defects in proteins as well as other enzymes involved in the repair of damaged DNA. Rare mutation of FANCB is X-linked, and FANCR is autosomal dominant. Normally FA genes encode for some proteins (e.g., ligase, helicase, BRCA2, etc.) which are responsible for DNA repair and resistance against DNA damage. When these genes are mutated, there is defective repair of DNA which results in genomic instability following exposure to cytotoxic agents.

Fanconi cells are hypersensitive to crosslinking agents like mitomycin C and diepoxybutane. The inability of the affected cells to withstand normal oxidative stress and oxygen free radicals causes oxidative damage [11–13].

Q11. What are the salient features of Fanconi anemia?

Answer [2, 4, 10, 14–16]:

1. Pancytopenia, history suggestive of anemia, bleeding tendency, and recurrent infections.
2. Low birth weight history, family history, and marriage history are important, particularly where the prevalence of consanguineous marriage system is high.
3. Approximately 75% of Fanconi anemia is associated with birth defects. On physical examination, the stature of the child may be short, and there are light-brown skin pigmentation ("cafe-au-lait") lesions in more than 50% of cases. Structural abnormalities of extremities (upper limb abnormalities) are more common.
4. Diagnosis may be delayed until the bone marrow failure develops.

5. Macrocytic anemia, high fetal hemoglobin levels, increased serum erythropoietin, and hypocellular bone marrow.
6. The chromosomal breakage test is most reliable for diagnosis. It has been suggested that such test should be done in all cases with ANC less than 1.0×10^9/L, Hb less than 100 g/L, reticulocyte count less than 40×10^9/L, platelet count less than 50×10^9/L, and bone marrow cellularity less than 25% [17]. Cell cycle analysis by flow cytometry is an alternative to the chromosomal breakage test.
7. Patients are prone to develop myelodysplasia/ acute myeloid leukemia. They are more prone to cancer at a young age. Such patients are very sensitive to chemotherapy and radiation. That makes it mandatory to exclude this diagnosis especially for those who are expected to go for bone marrow transplantation.

24.2 Correlation of Results of Preliminary Investigations with Symptoms and Signs in Fanconi Anemia

Q12. How do symptoms and signs in this patients corelate with diagnosis?

Answer: This child had symptoms of pancytopenia- anemia(pallor), leukopenia (history of repeated infections), and thrombocytopenia (history of bleeding). Physical examination showed evidence of skeletal abnormalities. Pancytopenia with skeletal abnormalities suggests possibility of inherited BM failure syndromes in a child, and these findings correlate well with diagnosis.

Q13. What were the laboratory tests which correlated with diagnosis of Fanconi anemia?

Answer: Pancytopenia and normocytic normochromic anemia with reticulocytopenia indicated bone marrow pathology as most likely cause. However, other possibilities were excluded by many laboratory tests. The findings in bone marrow biopsy and result of chromosomal stress test correlate well with diagnosis of Fanconi anemia.

24.3 Quick Information for Practicing Clinicians and Students

References [1–16]:

1. Bone marrow failure syndromes are a group of bone marrow diseases presenting with reduced or absent production of single or multiple cell lines.
2. Fanconi anemia, Diamond-Blackfan anemia, Dyskeratosis congenita, amegakaryocytic thrombocytopenia and Shwachman-Bodian-Diamond syndrome are most common.

3. Most important for diagnosis is family history particularly where the prevalence of consanguinity of marriage system is high. Thorough physical examination for skeletal abnormalities is recommended.
4. Approximately 75% of Fanconi anemia is associated with birth defects. On physical examination, the stature of the child may be short, and there are light-brown skin pigmentation ("cafe-au-lait") lesions in more than 50% of cases. Structural abnormalities of extremities (upper limb abnormalities) are more common.
5. Children who have cytopenia with hypoplastic or aplastic anemia, unexplained macrocytosis, myelodysplastic features, and characteristic physical abnormalities should be suspected to have Fanconi anemia and subjected to further tests for confirmation. Pancytopenia, history suggestive of anemia, bleeding tendency, and recurrent infections are common presentations.
6. Diagnosis may be delayed until the bone marrow failure develops. Early recognition is important.
7. The chromosomal breakage test is most reliable for diagnosis. Cell cycle analysis flow cytometry is an alternative to the chromosomal breakage test.
8. The assessment of telomere length (telomere length less than the first percentile for age) is highly sensitive but not specific to the diagnosis.
9. Patients are prone to develop myelodysplasia/ acute myeloid leukemia. They are more prone to cancer at a young age.
10. These patients are highly sensitive to chemotherapy and radiation. It is critical to rule out this diagnosis prior to transplant for any patient with unexplained pancytopenia.
11. Prenatal Fanconi anemia diagnosis can be accomplished by demonstration of chromosome breaks in cells obtained in utero from chorionic villus biopsy, amniocentesis, or cord blood (by cordocentesis) or by identification of Fanconi anemia gene mutations in DNA extracted from fetal cells.

To acquire further knowledge on the subject, following sources are advised:

1. BCSH guidelines
2. Br Jr. Hematology
3. ASH education book
4. Blood
5. NEJM
6. Int Jr. Lab Hematology

References

1. Bennett JM, Orazi A. Diagnostic criteria to distinguish hypocellular acute myeloid leukemia from hypocellular myelodysplastic syndromes and aplastic anemia: recommendations for a standardized approach. Haematologica. 2009;94:264–8.
2. Elizabeth PW, Daniel AA. The differential diagnosis and bone marrow evaluation of new-onset pancytopenia. Am J Clin Pathol. 2013;139:9–29.

3. Killick SB, Bown N, Jamie CJ. Guidelines for the diagnosis and management of adult aplastic anaemia. Br J Haematol. 2016;172:187–207.
4. Bagby GC, Alter BP. Fanconi anemia. Semin Hematol. 2006;43(3):147–56.
5. Taniguchi T, D'Andrea AD. Molecular pathogenesis of Fanconi anemia: recent progress. Blood. 2006;107(11):4223–33.
6. D'Andrea AD, Grompe M. The Fanconi anaemia/BRCA pathway. Nat Rev Cancer. 2003;3(1):23–34.
7. Diamond LK, Blackfan KD. Hypoplastic anemia. Am J Dis Child. 1938;15:307.
8. Zinsser F. Atrophia cutis reticularis cum pigmentations, dystrophia unguium at leukoplakis oris (poikioodermia atrophicans vascularis Jacobi) Ikonographia. Dermatologica. 1910;5:219–33.
9. Myers KC, Davies SM, Shimamura A. Clinical and molecular pathophysiology of Shwachman-Diamond syndrome: an update. Hematol Oncol Clin North Am. 2013;27(1):117–28., ix. https://doi.org/10.1016/j.hoc.2012.10.003.
10. Narla A. When to worry about inherited bone marrow failure and myeloid malignancy predisposition syndromes in the setting of a hypocellular marrow. Hematology Am Soc Hematol Educ Program. 2021;2021(1):153–6.
11. Meetei AR, Levitus M, Xue Y, Medhurst AL, Zwaan M, Ling C, Rooimans MA, Bier P, Hoatlin M, Pals G, de Winter JP, Wang W, Joenje H. X-linked inheritance of Fanconi anemia complementation group B. Nat Genet. 2004;36(11):1219–24.
12. Longerich S, Li J, Xiong Y, Sung P, Kupfer GM. Stress and DNA repair biology of the Fanconi anemia pathway. Blood. 2014;124(18):2812–9.
13. Wegman-Ostrosky T, Savage SA. The genomics of inherited bone marrow failure: from mechanism to the clinic. Br J Haematol. 2017;177(4):526–42. https://doi.org/10.1111/bjh.14535.
14. Giampietro PF, Adler-Brecher B, Verlander PC, Pavlakis SG, Davis JG, Auerbach AD. The need for more accurate and timely diagnosis in Fanconi anemia: a report from the International Fanconi Anemia Registry. Pediatrics. 1993;91:1116–20.
15. Dufour C. How I manage patients with Fanconi anaemia. Br J Haematol. 2017;178(1):32–47. https://doi.org/10.1111/bjh.14615.
16. Ogilvie P, Hofmann UB, Bröcker EB, Hamm H. Skin manifestations of Fanconi anemia. Hautarzt. 2002;53(4):253–7.
17. Arleen DA. Fanconi anemia and its diagnosis. Mutat Res. 2009;668(1–2):4–10. https://doi.org/10.1016/j.mrfmmm.2009.01.013.

Chapter 25
Cancer-Associated Anemia

A 62-year-old female is referred to hematology clinic with complaints of progressive weakness and difficulty in carrying out routine daily self-care. She was diagnosed to have carcinoma of the breast-right side, 6 months back, for which she was subjected to mastectomy followed by hormonal therapy. Currently she is complaining of loss of appetite, lethargy, and palpitations even with routine household chores. In addition, she admits to taking analgesics for frequent bony pains in the last 2 months. Examination showed pallor without jaundice. No hepatosplenomegaly or lymphadenopathy was observed. Local examination of breast showed a tiny nodule, less than 1 cm in right breast. CBC done at presentation is presented in Table 25.1.

A. Gupta, *Decision Making Through Problem Based Learning in Hematology*, https://doi.org/10.1007/978-981-99-8933-1_25

Table 25.1 CBC

CBC parameter	Patient's result	Reference range
WBC	2.2	3.7–10 × 10^9/L
RBC	2.9	4.5–5.4 × 10^{12}/L
HB	65	130–160 g/L
Hct	0.190	0.33–0.43 L/L
MCV	83	83–101 fL
MCH	27	27–32 pg
MCHC	325	315–345 g/L
RDW	16	11.6–14.6%
PLT	30	130–430 × 10^9/L
MPV	10	7–11 fL
Poly#	0.8	1.7–6 × 10^9/L
Lymp#	207	1–3 × 10^9/L
Mono#	0.3	0.2–1.0 × 10^9/L
EO#	0.4	0.02–0.5 × 10^9/L
BASO#	00	0.02–0.1 × 10^9/L
RETIC%	0.1	0.5–1.5%
Absolute ret count	15	50–150 × 10^9/L
ESR	19	0–20 mm 1st h Westergren

25.1 Questions

Q1. Interpret the result of CBC given above and suggest investigations for further evaluation in such case.

Answer: The CBC result shows pancytopenia-anemia, leukopenia, and thrombocytopenia. Anemia is normocytic normochromic with slightly high RDW. The reticulocyte count is markedly reduced.

Causes of pancytopenia in general include the following:

1. Aplastic anemia
2. Nutritional deficiency states like B12/folic acid deficiency with or without iron deficiency and copper deficiency
3. Myelodysplasia, leukemia, other hematopoietic neoplasms like lymphomas involving bone marrow
4. Bone marrow metastasis, storage disorders, granulomatous diseases
5. Post-chemo-/radiotherapy
6. Autoimmune disease with or without myelofibrosis, idiopathic myelofibrosis
7. Hypersplenism
8. Bone marrow suppression due to infections

Next best investigation will be to examine a blood film and to do baseline investigations for liver, kidney, thyroid, and bone profiles. Also serum iron profile and levels of B12/ folic acid and copper should be assessed.

Q2. Given are the images form blood film (Figs. 25.1 and 25.2) and results of baseline tests for liver, kidney, thyroid, and bone (Table 25.2) and serum levels of vitamin B12,folic acid, iron profile, and copper (Table 25.3) are provided. Interpret the results. What further investigations are required to reach at final diagnosis?

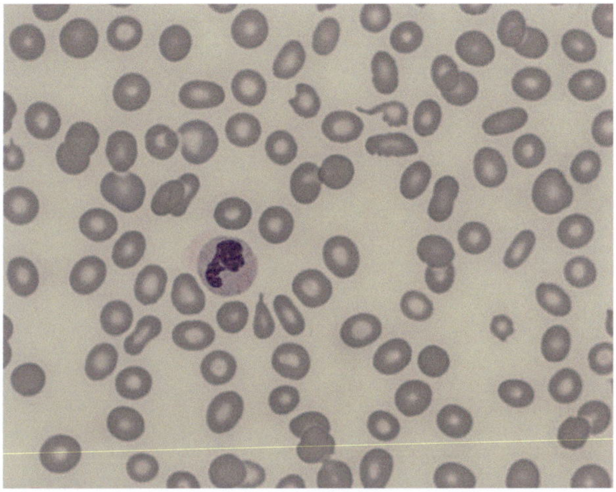

Fig. 25.1 Peripheral blood film. Reduced leukocytes, red cells, and platelets. Leishman stain ×100

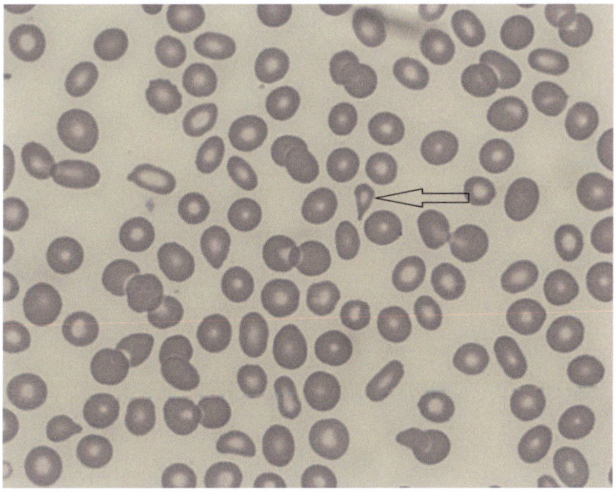

Fig. 25.2 Peripheral blood film. Normocytic normochromic red cells and occasional tear drop cells. Leishman stain ×100

Table 25.2 Biochemical tests

Test	Patient's result	Ref range
Glu (F)	6.0	3.9–6.1 mmol/L
Urea	2.9	2.5–6.6 mmol/L
Creat	90	60–120 μmol/L
Na^+	139	136–146 mmol/L
K^+	4.5	3.7–5.0 mmol/L
Ca^+	2.3	2.2–2.6 mmol/L
Mg^+	1.0	0.08–1.1 mmol/L
T. Prot	68	63–80 mmol/L
Alb	39	35–47 mmol/L
Choles	2.5	1.5–5.2 mmol/L
TG	0.9	0.4–1.7 mmol/L
Urates	300	150–400 mmol/L
T Bil	18	3–20 μmol/L
Indirect bil	16	5–20 μmol/L
D. Bil	2	0–5 μmol/L
Alk Ph	80	26–88 IU/L
ALT	55	10–60 IU/L
AST	32	10–42 IU/L
GGT	20	7–64 IU/L
LDH	170	90–180 IU/L
Hapto	0.9	0.2–2.0 g/L
T4	10.6	7.8–16 pmol/L
TSH	3.99	0.27–4.2 μlU/mL
Amylase	20	28–100 IU/L
Lipase	30	0–160 U/L

Table 25.3 Serum B12, folic acid, iron profile, zinc and copper levels

Test	Patient's result	Ref range
S. B12	650	150–700 pmol/L
S. Folate	31.7	10–42 nmol/L
RBC folate	2554	1187–2854 nmol/L
Ferritin	320	20–340 mcg/L
s. Iron	29	11–31 μmol/L
Transferrin	3.2	2.1–3.6 g/L
Tran sat%	30%	20–40%
Zinc	0.84	0.66–1.10 mcg/mL
Copper	100	65–140 mcg/dL

Answer: The blood films show reduced density of red cells and occasional white cell (reduced in number) and confirms thrombocytopenia. Red cells are predominantly normocytic normochromic. Few ovalocytes and rare tear drop poikilocytes are noted. No immature cells were seen.

The tests for functions of liver, kidney, thyroid, pancreas, and bone profiles are within normal limits. The hemolytic parameters (indirect bilirubin, LDH, haptoglobin) are also within normal range.

For further evaluation, next best step will be a bone marrow examination as in the present case, the patient has been recently diagnosed with carcinoma breast. It will also help in evaluating differential diagnosis of many conditions (mentioned above) which can result in pancytopenia. Radiological investigations for local recurrence and fine needle biopsy should also be planned.

Q3. Given are the images from bone marrow biopsy (Figs. 25.3, 25.4, and 25.5). What is the interpretation and final diagnosis?

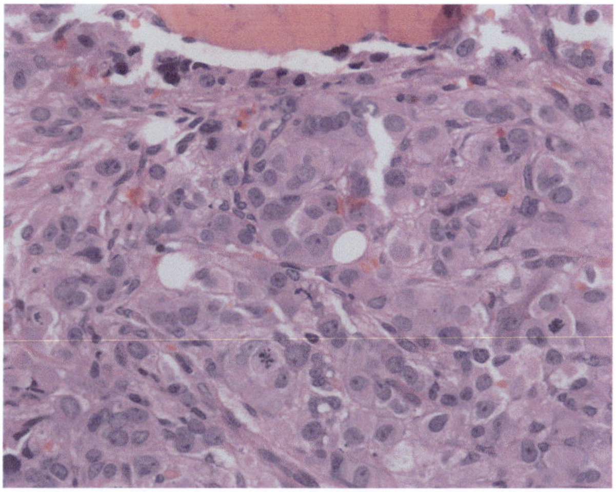

Fig. 25.3 Bone marrow biopsy. Metastatic deposits. H/E stain ×40

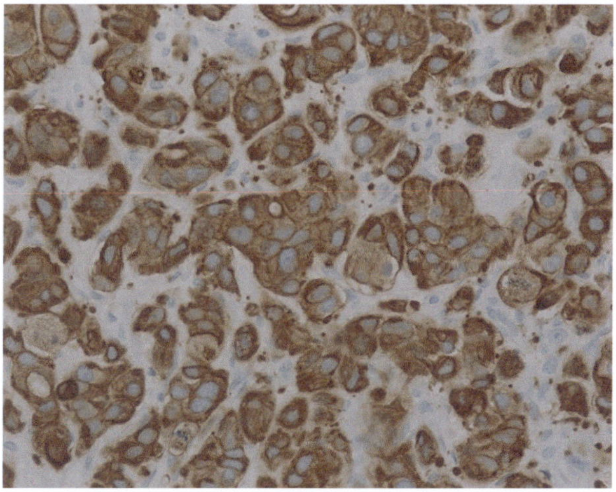

Fig. 25.4 Bone marrow biopsy. Immunostain cytokeratin (CK7) ×40

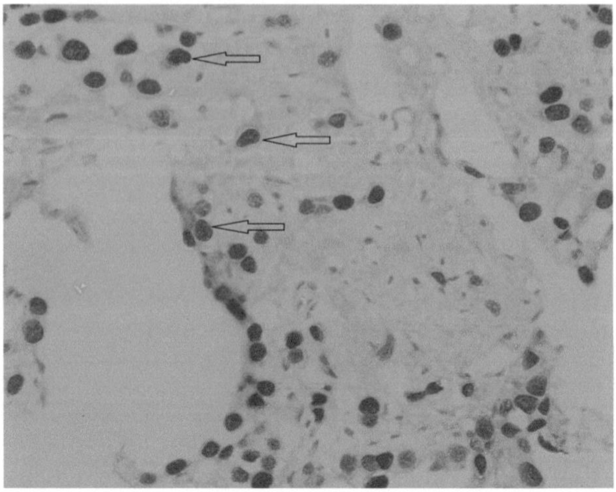

Fig. 25.5 Bone marrow biopsy. Estrogen receptors (ER) immunostain ×40

Answer: The trephibne biospy shows clusters and dispersed malignant cells. These cells are large with abundant cytoplasm. Many cells have vacuolated cytoplasm. Immunohistochemical stains show these cells to be positive for cytokeratin (CK7) and ER. The normal hematopoietic cells are markedly reduced in number. There is no evidence of fibrosis. These findings confirm a diagnosis of metastatic invasion of bone marrow by adenocarcinoma cells from breast. The pancytopenia in peripheral blood is due to replacement of normal hematopoietic cells by metastatic carcinoma cells.

Q4. Which are the most common cancers which metastasize to bone marrow and what pathogenetic mechanism is involved in settlement of tumor cells in bone marrow?

Answer: Carcinomas of breast, pancreas, lung, kidney, prostate, ovary, thyroid, and melanoma have greater tendency to spread to bones.

Some cancers cells especially breast and prostate express cytokine receptors which have high affinity for stromal cell-derived factor found in bone marrow stroma. IL-6, IL-8, IL-11, and vascular endothelial growth factor (VEGF) are secreted by breast cancer cells which promote osteolytic bone metastasis. Factors released by prostate cancer cells and some types of breast cancer stimulate osteoblasts. Endothelin-1 produced by tumor and vascular endothelial growth factor have a role in pathogenesis of osteoblastic bone metastasis [1].

Q5. What is definition of cancer-associated anemia and what is its pathophysiology?

Answer: Cancer-associated anemia is defined as Hb ≤11.9 g/dL for women and Hb ≤12.9 g/dL for men with cancer. It is caused by ineffective erythropoiesis, hemolysis, or blood loss. These mechanisms may be related primarily to main cancer or to drugs/ radiations, infectious associated diseases, etc. [2].

Q6. What is cancer-related anemia and what is pathophysiology?

Answer: Cancer-related anemia (CRA) refers to a condition occurring without bleeding, hemolysis, neoplastic bone marrow infiltration, kidney, and/or hepatic failure. It principally results from the synthesis of proinflammatory cytokines by both immune and cancer cells.

Proinflammatory cytokine, mainly IL-6, released by both tumor and immune cells suppresses erythropoiesis by affecting erythroid progenitor proliferation, erythropoietin production, red cell survival, and iron metabolism [3].

Q7. Sometimes, bone marrow is seen metastasized by cells of non-hemopoietic origin without evidence of overt primary malignancy. What is usual protocol for evaluation of primary cancer in case of bone metastasis of unknown origin?

Answer: Approximately 3% of malignancies diagnosed in bone marrow neoplastic conditions have unknown primary site, in spite of adequate clinical information and preliminary investigations. Such cases need extended workup on bone marrow biopsies [4, 5].

Within carcinoma, the most common subtypes of unknown primary are adenocarcinoma (60%), squamous carcinoma (5%), neuroendocrine carcinoma (5%), and poorly differentiated carcinoma (30%). For adenocarcinoma, the most common primary sites are lung and pancreas (both ~25%), then colon, stomach, and esophagus, breast, ovary, and prostate [6, 7].

Initially, CK7 and CK20 are advised. Based on results of this combination, further testing should be done. Suspicion of a primary site based on radiological and biochemical test results helps to tailor request for further immunostaining.

(a) CK7+ CK20-: Suggested panel - GATA3, ER, CK19,CDX2, PAX8, WT1, PAX2, P63. This panel will help confirm cancers of breast, upper GIT including pancreaticobiliary, ovarian, renal, and bladder origin.
(b) Both Ck7+ and CK20+: Suggested panel GATA3, P63, CK19, CDX2. This panel will help to confirm cancers of bladder, upper GIT including hepatobiliary and rectum
(c) CK7- CK20+: Suggested panel CDX2 for colorectal and upper GIT cancers.
(d) CK7-CK20-: TTF1, CK 5/6,P63, PAX8, PSA, Hepar1, CDX2, synaptophysin. This panel will help in confirmation of lung—small cell and squamous cell, renal, prostate, hepatic, gastric, and neuroendocrine carcinomas.

The NICE guidelines from UK suggest a minimum of CK7, CK20, PSA or estrogen receptor (ER), placental alkaline phosphatase (PLaP), and TTF-1. Another guideline suggests to include CKAE1-AE3 (Carcinoma), CLA (Lymphoma), S100, HMB-45, Melan-A (Melanoma) S100, Vimentin (Sarcoma) in initial panel [8–10].

25.2 Correlation of Results of Preliminary Investigations with Symptoms and Signs in Cancer-Associated Anemia

Q8. How do the symptoms and signs in this patient correlate with diagnosis of metastatic carcinoma?

Answer: She had complains of loss of appetite, lethargy, and palpitations even with routine household chores. She also complained of progressive weakness. These are symptoms of anemia. She also had frequent bony pains, indirectly suggesting involvement of bones by some pathological process. Examination showed anemia without jaundice or any organomegaly. These symptoms and signs correlate well with reduced production of hemopoietic cells especially red cells due to bone marrow invasion by carcinoma cells.

Q9. How do the investigations guide in correlating diagnosis with symptoms and signs in this patient?

Answer: There is pancytopenia with reticulocytopenia which indicates reduced production of hemopoietic cells. Blood film did not show any abnormal cells. The biochemical and other tests excluded the possibility of peripheral destruction of cells. There was no splenomegaly. Thus, after all causes of peripheral consumption/ destruction for pancytopenia were ruled out, the bone marrow biopsy confirmed the diagnosis by providing evidence of replacement of normal hemopoietic cells by metastatic carcinoma cells. Thus the investigations helped in correlating the symptoms and signs with diagnosis in this patient.

25.3 Quick Information for Practicing Clinicians and Students

References [1–15]:

1. The most common initial clinical symptom of bone metastasis is pain. This is because tumor cells produce substances like bradykinin and substance P that irritate unmyelinated C-fiber neurons. In addition, irritation of the periosteum due to small microfractures of the trabecular bone also produces pain.
2. In addition to pain, common complications include pathological fractures, spinal cord, and nerve compression syndromes and hypercalcemia, which can lead to kidney dysfunction, cardiac arrhythmias, and death.
3. Bone pain, hypercalcemia, raised levels of ALP and /or LDH, unexplained cytopenias, and lytic or sclerotic bony lesions on radiology suggest bone marrow metastasis.
4. The most sensitive method for assessing bone metastases in the bone marrow is MRI capturing details of 80–90% of bone marrow areas in a single scan.
5. BM metastasis has been reported in 65–90% in prostate cancer, 65–75% in breast cancer, 17–64% in lung cancer, and 10% in colorectal cancer.

6. An initial screening panel should be CK7 and CK20. Next panel should include the immunostains based on their result. A large panel of immunostains at initial screening should be avoided.

To acquire further knowledge on the subject, following sources are advised:

1. BCSH guidelines
2. Br Jr. Hematology
3. ASH education book
4. Blood
5. NEJM
6. Int Jr. Lab Hematology

References

1. Guise TA, Mohammad KS, Clines G, Stebbins EG, Wong DH, Higgins LS, Vessella R, Corey E, Padalecki S, Suva L, et al. Basic mechanisms responsible for osteolytic and osteoblastic bone metastases. Clin Cancer Res. 2006;12:6213s–6s. https://doi.org/10.1158/1078-0432.CCR-06-1007.
2. Macciò A, Madeddu C, Gramignano G, et al. The role of inflammation, iron, and nutritional status in cancer-related anemia: results of a large, prospective, observational study. Haematologica. 2015;100(1):124–32.
3. Gilreath JA, Stenehjem DD, Rodgers GM. Diagnosis and treatment of cancer-related anemia. Am J Hematol. 2014;89(2):203–12.
4. Pavlidis N, Briasoulis E, Hainsworth J, Greco FA. Diagnostic and therapeutic management of cancer of an unknown primary. Eur J Cancer. 2003;39:1990–2005.
5. Pavlidis N, Briasoulis E, Pentheroudakis G. Cancers of unknown primary site: ESMO Clinical Practice Guidelines for diagnosis, treatment and follow-up. Ann Oncol. 2010;21(Suppl 5):v228–31.
6. Pavlidis N, Pentheroudakis G. Cancer of unknown primary site. Lancet. 2012;379:1428–35.
7. Massard C, Loriot Y, K. Fizazi carcinomas of an unknown primary origin—diagnosis and treatment. Nat Rev Clin Oncol. 2011;8:701–10.
8. Clinical guideline. Metastatic malignant disease of unknown primary origin in adults: diagnosis and management. National Institute for Health and Clinical Excellence(NICE) guidelines Published: 26 July 2010 Last updated: 26 April 2023 www.nice.org.uk/guidance/cg104
9. Losa F, Soler G, Casado A, Estival A, Fernández I, Giménez S, et al. SEOM clinical guideline on unknown primary cancer (2017). Clin Transl Oncol. 2018;20(1):89–96.
10. Ariza A, Balañá C, Concha Á, Hitt R, Homet B, Matilla A, et al. Update on the diagnosis of cancer of unknown primary (CUP) origin. Clin Transl Oncol. 2011;13(7):434–41.
11. Coleman RE. Clinical features of metastatic bone disease and risk of skeletal morbidity. Clin Cancer Res. 2006;12:6243s–9s. https://doi.org/10.1158/1078-0432.CCR-06-0931.
12. Schmidt GP, Schoenberg SO, Reiser MF, Baur-Melnyk A. Whole-body MR imaging of bone marrow. Eur J Radiol. 2005;55:33–40. https://doi.org/10.1016/j.ejrad.2005.01.019.
13. D'Oronzo S, Coleman R, Brown J, Silvestris F. Metastatic bone disease: pathogenesis and therapeutic options: up-date on bone metastasis management. J Bone Oncol. 2019;15:10025. https://doi.org/10.1016/j.jbo.2018.10.004.
14. Chauhan K, Jain M, Grover S, Shukla P, Rusia U, Grover RK. Bone marrow metastasis in nonhematologic malignancies: data from a cancer hospital. Clin Cancer Invest J. 2016;5:103–9.
15. Shimozuma K, Sonoo H, Fukunaga M, Ichihara K, Aoyama T, Tanaka K. Biochemical markers of bone turnover in breast cancer patients with bone metastases: a preliminary report. Jpn J Clin Oncol. 1999;29:16–22.

MIX
Papier aus verantwortungsvollen Quellen
Paper from responsible sources
FSC® C105338

If you have any concerns about our products,
you can contact us on
ProductSafety@springernature.com

In case Publisher is established outside the EU,
the EU authorized representative is:
Springer Nature Customer Service Center GmbH
Europaplatz 3, 69115 Heidelberg, Germany

Printed by Libri Plureos GmbH
in Hamburg, Germany